Technological Advances in Exotic Pet Practice

Editor

MINH HUYNH

VETERINARY CLINICS OF NORTH AMERICA: EXOTIC ANIMAL PRACTICE

www.vetexotic.theclinics.com

Consulting Editor
JÖRG MAYER

September 2019 • Volume 22 • Number 3

ELSEVIER

1600 John F. Kennedy Boulevard • Suite 1800 • Philadelphia, Pennsylvania, 19103-2899
http://www.vetexotic.theclinics.com

**VETERINARY CLINICS OF NORTH AMERICA: EXOTIC ANIMAL PRACTICE Volume 22, Number 3
September 2019 ISSN 1094-9194, ISBN-13: 978-0-323-68218-3**

Editor: Colleen Dietzler
Developmental Editor: Laura Kavanaugh

Veterinary Clinics of North America: Exotic Animal Practice (ISSN 1094-9194) is published in January, May, and September by Elsevier, Inc., 360 Park Avenue South, New York, NY 10010-1710. Subscription prices are $284.00 per year for US individuals, $519.00 per year for US institutions, $100.00 per year for US students and residents, $338.00 per year for Canadian individuals, $626.00 per year for Canadian institutions, $352.00 per year for international individuals, $626.00 per year for international institutions and $165.00 per year for Canadian and foreign students/residents. To receive student/resident rate, orders must be accompanied by name of affiliated institution, date of term, and the *signature* of program/residency coordinator on institution letterhead. Orders will be billed at individual rate until proof of status is received. Foreign air speed delivery is included in all *Clinics* subscription prices. All prices are subject to change without notice. **POSTMASTER:** Send address changes to *Veterinary Clinics of North America: Exotic Animal Practice*, Elsevier Health Sciences Division, Subscription Customer Service, 3251 Riverport Lane, Maryland Heights, MO 63043. **Customer Service: Telephone: 1-800-654-2452** (U.S. and Canada); **1-314-447-8871** (outside U.S. and Canada). **Fax: 1-314-447-8029. E-mail: journalscustomerservice-usa@elsevier.com (for print support); journalsonlinesupport-usa@elsevier.com (for online support).**

Reprints. For copies of 100 or more of articles in this publication, please contact the Commercial Reprints Department, Elsevier Inc., 360 Park Avenue South, New York, New York 10010-1710. Tel.: 212-633-3874; Fax: 212-633-3820; E-mail: reprints@elsevier.com.

Veterinary Clinics of North America: Exotic Animal Practice is covered in *MEDLINE/PubMed (Index Medicus).*

Contributors

CONSULTING EDITOR

JÖRG MAYER, Dr med vet, MSc
Diplomate, American Board of Veterinary Practitioners (Exotic Companion Mammals); Diplomate, European College of Zoological Medicine (Small Mammals); Diplomate, American College of Zoological Medicine; Associate Professor of Zoological Medicine, Department of Small Animal Medicine and Surgery, University of Georgia College of Veterinary Medicine, Athens, Georgia, USA

EDITOR

MINH HUYNH, DVM
Diplomate, European College of Zoological Medicine (Avian); Diplomate, American College of Zoological Medicine; Head of Exotic Department, Centre Hospitalier Vétérinaire Frégis, Arcueil, France

AUTHORS

TARIQ ABOU-ZAHR, BVSc, CertAVP(ZooMed), MRCVS
Valley Vets, Cardiff, United Kingdom

CHIARA ADAMI, DMV, MRCVS, PhD
Diplomate, European College of Veterinary Anaesthesia and Analgesia; Diplomate, American College of Veterinary Anesthesia and Analgesia; Department of Clinical Sciences and Services, Royal Veterinary College, Hatfield, United Kingdom

SARAH ALBERTON, DMV, IPSAV
Veterinarian, Bird and Exotic Animal Department, Laval Veterinary Center, Laval, Quebec, Canada

SCOTT BIRCH, BA
CEO, Pixelbeaker, Chattanooga, Tennessee, USA

CAMILLE BISMUTH, Dr med vet
Diplomate, European College of Veterinary Surgeons; Service de Chirurgie, CHV Fregis, Arcueil, France

CARA BLAKE, DVM
Diplomate, American College of Veterinary Surgeons (Small Animal); Assistant Professor, Small Animal Surgery, Department of Veterinary Clinical Sciences, Center for Veterinary Health Sciences, Oklahoma State University, Stillwater, Oklahoma, USA

JOÃO BRANDÃO, LMV, MS
Diplomate, European College of Zoological Medicine (Avian); Assistant Professor, Zoological Medicine, Department of Veterinary Clinical Sciences, Center for Veterinary Health Sciences, Oklahoma State University, Stillwater, Oklahoma, USA

DANIEL CALVO CARRASCO, LV, CertAVP(ZooMed), MRCVS
Diplomate, European College of Zoological Medicine (Avian); Great Western Exotic Vets, Swindon, United Kingdom; Wildfowl & Wetlands Trust, Slimbridge, United Kingdom

LUCILE CHASSANG, Dr med vet, IPSAV (Zoological Medicine)
Service NAC, CHV Fregis, Arcueil, France

JESSICA COMOLLI, DVM, LVT
Department of Small Animal Medicine and Surgery, Zoological Medicine Service, University of Georgia, Athens, Georgia, USA

THOMAS COUTANT, Dr med vet, IPSAV (Zoological Medicine)
Service NAC, CHV Fregis, Arcueil, France

DARIO D'OVIDIO, DMV, MSc, SPACS, PhD
Diplomate, European College of Zoological Medicine (Small Mammal); Private Practitioner, Arzano, Naples, Italy

NICOLA DI GIROLAMO, DVM, MS, PhD
Diplomate, European College of Zoological Medicine (Herpetology); Editor-in-Chief, *Journal of Exotic Pet Medicine*, Associate Professor, Zoological Medicine, Center for Veterinary Health Sciences, Oklahoma State University, Stillwater, Oklahoma, USA; Tai Wai Small Animal and Exotic Hospital, Sha Tin, New Territories, Hong Kong

STEPHEN J. DIVERS, BSc, BVetMed, FRCVS, DZooMed
Diplomate, European College of Zoological Medicine (Herpetology, Zoo Health Management); Diplomate, American College of Zoological Medicine; Professor of Zoological Medicine, Department of Small Animal Medicine and Surgery, College of Veterinary Medicine, University of Georgia, Athens, Georgia, USA

HARRIET HAHN, DMV
Diagnostic Imaging Department, Centre Hospitalier Vétérinaire Frégis, Arcueil, France

MINH HUYNH, DVM
Diplomate, European College of Zoological Medicine (Avian); Diplomate, American College of Zoological Medicine; Head of Exotic Department, Centre Hospitalier Vétérinaire Frégis, Arcueil, France

DELPHINE LANIESSE, Dr med vet, DVSc, IPSAV (Zoological Medicine)
Diplomate, European College of Zoological Medicine (Avian); Eläinsairaala Evidensia Tammisto Vantaa, Vantaa, Finland

JÖRG MAYER, Dr med vet, MSc
Diplomate, American Board of Veterinary Practitioners (Exotic Companion Mammals); Diplomate, European College of Zoological Medicine (Small Mammals); Diplomate, American College of Zoological Medicine; Associate Professor of Zoological Medicine, Department of Small Animal Medicine and Surgery, University of Georgia College of Veterinary Medicine, Athens, Georgia, USA

MIKEL SABATER GONZÁLEZ, LV, CertZooMed
Diplomate, European College of Zoological Medicine (Avian); Exoticsvet, Valencia, Spain

RODNEY SCHNELLBACHER, DVM
Diplomate, American College of Zoological Medicine; Dickerson Park Zoo, Animal Health, Springfield, Missouri, USA

IZIDORA SLADAKOVIC, BVSc (Hons I), MVS
Diplomate, American College of Zoological Medicine; Director of Avian and Exotics Service, Northside Veterinary Specialists, Terrey Hills, New South Wales, Australia

NOÉMIE SUMMA, DMV, IPSAV
Diplomate, American College of Zoological Medicine; Faculté de médecine vétérinaire, Clinical Instructor, Service de Médecine Zoologique, Université de Montréal, Saint-Hyacinthe, Québec, Canada

JOHN M. SYKES IV, DVM
Diplomate, American College of Zoological Medicine; Zoological Health Program, Wildlife Conservation Society, Bronx Zoo, Bronx, New York, USA

CLAIRE VERGNEAU-GROSSET, DMV, IPSAV, CES
Diplomate, American College of Zoological Medicine; Faculté de médecine vétérinaire, Assistant Professor, Service de Médecine Zoologique, Université de Montréal, Saint-Hyacinthe, Québec, Canada

GRAHAM ZOLLER, DMV, IPSAV (Zoological Medicine)
Exotic Pet Department, Centre Hospitalier Vétérinaire Frégis, Arcueil, France

Contents

Controlling the environment appropriately ensures the health and welfare of captive reptiles and amphibians. This article summarizes some of the technological advances and products currently available, including lighting, climate control, and recordkeeping.

medicine, recent technological advances allowed its application not only to small animals but also to exotic pets. This article reviews the literature available about some of these techniques (negative wound pressure therapy, photobiomodulation [laser therapy], electrical stimulation therapy, therapeutic ultrasonography, hyperbaric oxygen therapy), and other advances in wound management (skin expanders, xenografts, and bioengineered autologous skin substitutes) in exotic pet species.

Surgery can be challenging in exotic pets owing to their small size and blood volume, and their increased anesthetic risk compared with small animals. Various devices are available to facilitate suturing, cutting, and hemostasis in the human and veterinary fields. These surgical equipment improve the simplicity, rapidity, and effectiveness of surgery. Vessel-sealing devices, radiosurgery, lasers, and ultrasound devices are commonly used because of their ease of use and increase in surgical efficiency. Other surgical devices are available (eg, stapling devices) but are not discussed in this article.

The aim of this article is to review some of the technological advances in endoscopy and endosurgery. The article focuses on a few key areas relevant to exotic pets, including advances in urolith management, visualization, and laparoscopic surgery.

Reducing the frequency of drug administration in the treatment of exotic pets is advantageous because it may decrease handling frequency and thus potential stress and injury risk for the animal, increase owner compliance with the prescribed treatment, and decrease need for general anesthesia in patients that cannot be handled safely. Increasing efficient drug plasma concentration using sustained-released delivery systems is an appealing solution. Potential candidates that could provide a promising solution have been investigated in exotic pets. In this article, the technologies that are the closest to being integrated in exotic pet medicine are reviewed: osmotic pumps, nanoparticles, and hydrogels.

Medical devices are defined as implantable if they are intended to remain in the body after the procedure. In veterinary medicine, use of such devices is marginal but may find some indications. Use in exotic pet medicine is even more challenging due to size restriction and the limited data available. This review focuses on the esophageal and tracheal stent in the case of stricture, ureteral stent and subcutaneous ureteral bypass in the case of

VETERINARY CLINICS OF NORTH AMERICA: EXOTIC ANIMAL PRACTICE

SERIES OF RELATED INTEREST

Veterinary Clinics of North America: Small Animal Practice
Available at: https://www.vetsmall.theclinics.com/

THE CLINICS ARE NOW AVAILABLE ONLINE!
Access your subscription at:
www.theclinics.com

Preface

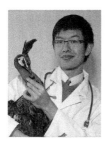

Minh Huynh, DVM, DECZM (Avian), DACZM
Editor

Over the past 20 years, technology has evolved to impact our daily life, inducing major societal changes. The health industry has also followed this trend, with technological devices being more accessible and globalized. It is expected that such revolution would have consequences on veterinary medicine, including exotic pet practice.

In my experience, exotic pet patient management usually involves innovation and creativity. Many aspects of exotic pet medicine and surgery are either unexplored or new, which implies that the clinician must extrapolate from small animal companion medicine or think outside of the box. One of the great examples in our field is the advent of endoscopic coelioscopy in the avian patient. This examination method was a perfect blend of anatomic specificity knowledge, use of a technological device (a rigid cystoscope) deviated from its original purpose, clinician technique, and imagination. This innovation is now considered a standard procedure in most avian practice.

This issue develops several aspects related to new technologies in exotic pet practice. "New" is always a relative term, and it is expected that techniques developed in each article will become more and more common until they become completely integrated in our practice. Some of those technologies described may fall into oblivion, probably because of their limited use, or because we would have found another way to treat disease. Some other major technologies not mentioned in this issue may arise in the next few years and become very important. Future is a difficult prediction.

The issue focuses on all aspects of veterinary medicine: diagnostics (diagnostic imaging, endoscopy, clinical pathology), surgical aspects such as development of bone plating, 3D medical printing, permanent implantable medical devices, soft tissue surgery, wound management, and other conventional aspects, such as anesthesia and therapeutics. A special article has been created for herpetology, which may benefit from the technological advances. More specifically, this issue also develops some aspects related to smartphones use in veterinary medicine and Internet.

Most of the data developed in this issue are not specific to the exotic patient. Evidence-based data and research still need to grow. I hope that reading this issue will encourage creativity, help to communicate with medical engineers, give

Vet Clin Exot Anim 22 (2019) xiii–xiv
https://doi.org/10.1016/j.cvex.2019.06.008
1094-9194/19/© 2019 Published by Elsevier Inc.

perspectives, and stimulate research projects for providing enhanced medical care in the exotic pet patient.

Ultimately, I will never stress enough that technology cannot replace veterinarian skills. The art of veterinary medicine is based on experience and clinical sense, not on technology. Care must be taken to treat clinical signs rather than data and to use the best technique rather than the newest technique.

Your brain is still the best technology to date.

I would like to thank all the colleagues and friends who have contributed to this issue for their hard work. I have no doubt that their skills and knowledge is and will be leading our discipline.

Minh Huynh, DVM, DECZM (Avian), DACZM
Centre Hospitalier Vétérinaire Frégis
43 Avenue Aristide Briand
94110 Arcueil, France

E-mail address:
nacologie@gmail.com

Medical Three-Dimensional Printing in Zoological Medicine

Cara Blake, DVM, DACVS-SA[a],*, Scott Birch, BA[b,1],
João Brandão, LMV, MS, DECZM (Avian)[c]

KEYWORDS

- Biomaterials • Fused deposition modeling (FDM) • Stereolithography (SLA)
- Selective laser sintering (SLS) • Exotic animals • Wildlife • Zoo animals

KEY POINTS

- Creating a 3-dimensional model of biological anatomy requires executing a sequence of steps by using a variety of computer-aided design software applications.
- Once the medical data is digitally prepared and the anatomic 3-dimensional model is created, it can be used by specialized 3-dimensional printers.
- Three-dimensional printing in human and veterinary medicine is gaining popularity and is used for the development of prosthetics, surgical implants and instrumentation, anatomic models, tissue engineering, drug delivery, and educational training.
- The application of 3-dimensional printing in zoological medicine species is in its infancy, resulting in a limited number of peer-reviewed publications in which it has been described.
- This modality will likely gain popularity and may aid veterinarians working with zoological medicine species to improve the quality of care provided to their patients.

INTRODUCTION

Technological advancements have shaped the current reality and serve as the stepping stone for the future. Many of the processes developed and used in mechanical and chemical engineering are commonly translated into use for medical applications. Medical 3-dimensional (3D) printing is a prime example of a 21st century computer-based application that has been adapted for use in human medicine, and to a certain extent, veterinary medicine.

Disclosure Statement: The authors have nothing to disclose.
[a] Small Animal Surgery, Department of Veterinary Clinical Sciences, Center for Veterinary Health Sciences, Oklahoma State University, 2065 West Farm Road, Stillwater, OK 74078, USA; [b] Pixelbeaker, 4834 Hillsdale Circle, Chattanooga, TN 37416, USA; [c] Zoological Medicine, Department of Veterinary Clinical Sciences, Center for Veterinary Health Sciences, Oklahoma State University, 2065 West Farm Road, Stillwater, OK 74078, USA
[1] Present address: 2065 West Farm Road, Stillwater, OK 74078.
* Corresponding author.
E-mail address: cara.blake@okstate.edu

Vet Clin Exot Anim 22 (2019) 331–348
https://doi.org/10.1016/j.cvex.2019.05.004
1094-9194/19/© 2019 Elsevier Inc. All rights reserved.

In 1984, Charles W. "Chuck" Hull registered the first 3D printer.[1,2] Unlike the traditional ink-based printers that create a 2-dimensional object, Hull described "a system for generating 3D objects by creating a cross-sectional pattern of the object to be formed at a selected surface of a fluid medium capable of altering its physical state in response to appropriate synergistic stimulation."[1,3] Three-dimensional printing was rapidly accepted and used in the automotive and aeronautic industries owing to the ability to produce rapid prototypes. The US military and health care professionals recognized the potential use of this technology in medical applications. Although initial use was limited to anatomic models and prosthetic implants, the current applications of its use are widespread, touching virtually every aspect of human medical specialties. The use of 3D printing in veterinary medicine is growing and its application in various indications across multiple species will most likely expand with increased clinical experience and availability of the technology.

FROM DIAGNOSTIC IMAGING TO 3-DIMENSIONAL MODEL: DIGITAL IMAGING AND COMMUNICATIONS IN MEDICINE TO STEREOLITHOGRAPHY FORMAT FILE PROCESS OR IMAGE SEGMENTATION

Creating and distributing a 3D model of biological anatomy requires executing a sequence of steps by using a variety of computer-aided design software applications

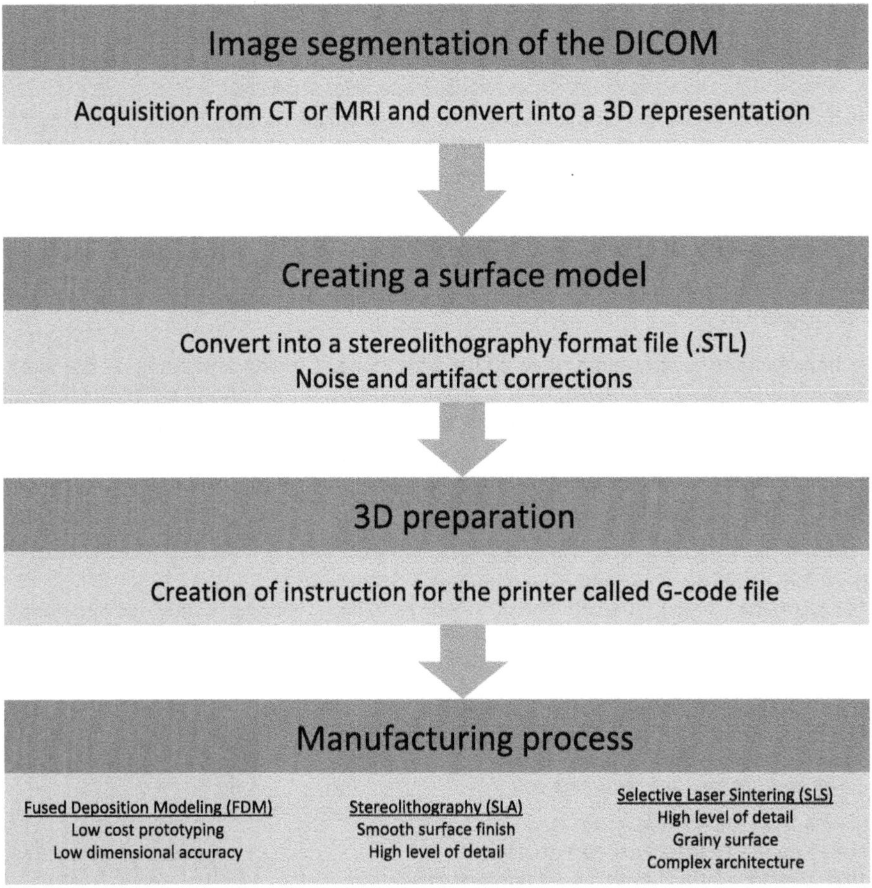

Image segmentation of the DICOM

Acquisition from CT or MRI and convert into a 3D representation

Creating a surface model

Convert into a stereolithography format file (.STL)
Noise and artifact corrections

3D preparation

Creation of instruction for the printer called G-code file

Manufacturing process

Fused Deposition Modeling (FDM)	Stereolithography (SLA)	Selective Laser Sintering (SLS)
Low cost prototyping	Smooth surface finish	High level of detail
Low dimensional accuracy	High level of detail	Grainy surface
		Complex architecture

Fig. 1. Step-by-step process of creating a 3D printed model.

(**Fig. 1**). It can be challenging and time consuming, but worth the effort to create a high-quality reconstruction. The visually transformed data can be shared digitally—in augmented reality/virtual reality or online environments—or physically, where tactile or ocular examination in real life takes priority.

If the decision is made to 3D print patient anatomy, the process starts with image segmentation of the digital imaging and communications in medicine (DICOM) dataset. In veterinary medicine, this commonly exists as a 2-dimensional image sequence acquired from computed tomography (CT) scans or an MRI. Entire bodies can be imaged, depending on their size, or particular regions of interest such as tumors or fractures can be prioritized.

Image segmentation is the process of converting the information contained in the DICOM files into realistic 3D representations or visualizations. In the case of CT scans, segmentation is accomplished through the automatic or manual detection of boundaries based on tissue classes or the variations of tissue density, measured in Hounsfield units, with an application such as Materialise Mimics (Materialise, Leuven, Belgium) or the open-source 3D Slicer (https://www.slicer.org). Because of these density differences, the anatomic structures or systems such as bone, soft tissue, blood volume, and air around the subject can be isolated.

These isolated structures or regions of interest become virtual 3D layers, perfectly nested around each other in the surrounding internal environment. These layers can then be volumetrically visualized on a computer screen in real time, with a variety of color and transparency settings allowing a customized viewing experience. This visualization method alone is often enough for the practitioner or clinician to corroborate a diagnosis or understand the disease present in the patient. A few more steps are necessary if a 3D print is needed.

Once the boundaries for the anatomic structures that are to be 3D printed are identified, the next step in the process is to create a surface model. Unlike a volumetric 3D visualization, a surface model is a group of connecting polygons that define the border of the tissue density range of interest. These connecting polygons are called a mesh, and they form the skin or thin outside shell of the 3D model, with the inside of the mesh being hollow, much like a balloon. This mesh is exported from the segmentation application as the initial stereolithography (SLA) format file (.STL) and is ready for mesh refinement, the last step before printing.

DICOM files are generated from a wide variety of imaging workstations, and each dataset can contain errors, discontinuities, low contrast, artifacts, and other anomalies or have an individual slice thickness greater than 4 mm, which can create stair-stepping in bones or tissue. The initial .STL model often needs to be repaired, smoothed, cropped, or appended. The model will need to be watertight, with no holes or overlapping polygons in the mesh. To avoid print failure, the model needs a minimum wall layer thickness that matches the tolerance range of the printer. Artifacts created from scan noise need to be removed, unnecessary structures cropped out, and holes in the mesh repaired. If the model initially contains an excessively large number of polygons, a decimation process can reduce this polycount, making the model less taxing to a workstation and easier to archive or upload. Global smoothing filters in applications such as Autodesk Meshmixer (Autodesk Inc., San Rafael, CA) or Pixologic zBrush (http://pixologic.com) can improve model topology, and a variety of sculpting tools or brushes can further refine the mesh, adjust mesh density, and isolate various structures.

Once the repair and optimization process is complete, the model will need to be prepared for the 3D printing process with a software slicing application such as Ultimaker Cura (Ultimaker, Geldermalsen, the Netherlands) or Simplify3D (https://www.

simplify3d.com). These applications work with a wide assortment of printers and have a powerful toolset to optimize the chances for print success. These printers translate the 3D models into instructions that the printer can understand, also called a G-Code file. These instructions include model placement and setup in the build chamber, slicing and infill percentage settings, support structure placement, and machine control information for the sintering laser, UV curing light, or extruder nozzle. Once the printer settings are selected and final preparations have been made, the G-Code file is exported so that it can be loaded into the 3D printer via USB key or a network drive.

FROM STEREOLITHOGRAPHY FORMAT FILE TO 3-DIMENSIONAL PRINTING ANATOMIC MODELS

Once the medical dataset is segmented, cleaned, and repaired, the anatomic 3D model created and exported to a G-Code file, the .STL file can be manufactured. There are a wide variety of computer-controlled 3D printing processes, but each uses a material, such as plastic, nylon, or metal, that is added together, joined, or solidified into a 3D object. Each printer has unique specifications defining resolution, layer thickness, and X–Y resolution in dots per inch or micrometers, and it is crucial to match the correct .STL mesh resolution with the printer settings to optimize the print speed and quality.

Contemporary printing methods can construct a model in a few hours or over the course of several days, depending on the size and complexity of the anatomy. Each printer has a maximum build chamber size, which can limit the number of models produced simultaneously; this sizing varies widely among printer models and brands. Unless it is necessary to print a very large specimen, anatomic regions of interest will fit into a standard size build chamber, regardless of which printing process is used.

A large number of additive processes are available, each with its own advantages and disadvantages. The main considerations when 3D printing biological anatomy are the speed of the printer, the materials available, the cost of each print, and the way in which the printer manages the support structures needed during the model build process. Anatomy models, especially vascular systems, can be very complex and diminutive, and printers need to be capable of processing the irregular topographies while maintaining a high level of accuracy (**Fig. 2**). This review will focus on 3 types of additive manufacturing processes: fused deposition modeling (FDM), SLA, and selective laser sintering (SLS).

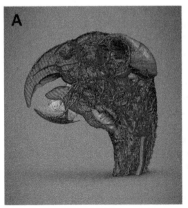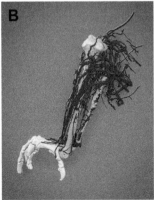

Fig. 2. (*A*) 3D rendered images highlighting the vasculature of the cranial-cervical region (*B*) and right distal limb of a Psittacine.

FDM is the most widely available technology and is mainly used for low-cost prototyping and design verification with fast turnaround times. FDM printers produce a model by extruding small beads or streams of material that harden immediately to form layers. The material is fed into a heated extrusion nozzle that traverses the build chamber, assembling the model layer by layer according to the instructions contained in the G-Code file. Material options include polylactic acid and acrylonitrile butadiene styrene plastics, nylon, wood fill, and even metal. Although quite affordable and relatively easy to use, FDM printing is limited in use by the size and complexity of the model, the need for support structures, extensive postprocessing of printed models, and the low dimensional accuracy and resolution compared with other printing processes.

SLA is a 3D printing technology that converts liquid materials or resins into solid, hardened parts, layer by layer, by selectively curing them with a light source such as a UV laser or projector. This process is also called vat photopolymerization. Models created with the SLA process have a smooth surface finish and a high level of detail. Support structures are required during the printing process; therefore, the model requires postprocessing to remove unwanted artifacts once the scaffold is removed. Printed models can be easily sanded, polished, and painted. A wide range of material and color choices are available for use, including clear, flexible, and castable resins.

SLS is a process that fuses together, or selectively sinters, particles of a thermoplastic polymer powder that builds a model layer by layer. This 3D printing process is used for both functional and mechanical prototyping, product development, and small production runs of parts requiring a very high degree of accuracy at a reasonable cost. Creating models with the SLS process does not require support structures, because the model is supported by unfused powder during the build. Because of this, biological anatomy with previously impossible geometries and models with complex interior structures such as hearts or kidneys can be created with a greater degree of accuracy. Although printed models will retain a high level of detail, parts tend to have a grainy surface finish that may require postprocessing and a sealant applied to reduce porosity if water tightness is required.

Of the 3 processes described, the SLS process, in these authors' opinion, has the best potential for creating high-quality anatomic models reconstructed from CT scans or MRI medical images. By eliminating the need for support structures during printing, complex organic arrangements and anatomic structures can be best represented, specifically, vascular systems and/or blood volume. On-demand online marketplaces, such as 3D Systems (Rock Hill, SC, USA) or 3D Hubs (Amsterdam, The Netherlands), provide SLS printing services, decreasing or eliminating the need to purchase and maintain a printer. The files of structures to be printed can be uploaded, customized, and models received back by the end user in just a few business days.

HUMAN MEDICINE

Three-dimensional printing was introduced into the human medical field in the mid-1990s. During this time, the technology was primarily used to create anatomic models and surface coating of prosthetic implants.[4,5] The US military recognized the usefulness of using CT scans to fabricate 3D medical models for craniofacial and orthopedic structures. Several groups worldwide, simultaneously and independently, worked to investigate and advance the potential uses of 3D printing in the human medical field.[2,5,6]

Initial reports of the use of 3D printing for clinical indications were published in the early 2000s. Some of the initial applications described for the use of 3D printing included the development of prostheses and implants for orthopedic and craniomaxillary procedures.[7–9] Since the introduction of 3D printing into the human medical field, its use has increased to include prosthetics, surgical implants and instrumentation, anatomic models, tissue engineering, drug delivery, and educational training.[5,10–12]

Three-dimensional printing has currently been reported in almost every human medical specialty, including but not limited to cardiology, interventional radiology, neurology, neurosurgery, orthopedic surgery, craniomaxillofacial surgery, and urology.[13–15] One of the primary applications is surgical planning. Before the advent of 3D model fabrication, surgeons relied on reviewing images obtained from advanced imaging such as CT scans and MRI on computer screens. In a recent study, surgery residents developed preoperative plans based on 3D rendered images or 3D printed models. There was a significant difference between the groups, with those developing a plan using the 3D printed models scoring higher.[16] These 3D printed models of complex fractures, large tumors, and anatomic anomalies provides the surgeon the opportunity to not only visualize, but manipulate the structure(s) of interest in advance of the procedure. The ability to rehearse surgical procedures has been reported to improve the surgeon's confidence and decrease surgical time and blood loss. In orthopedic procedures requiring implants, the 3D models are used to confirm the appropriate size of the implant(s), which may then be precontoured and sterilized before surgery. It should be noted however, that there may a trade off with respect to the amount of time saved during these procedures. The overall surgical and anesthesia time may be decreased, which suggests the preoperative preparation results in an improved intraoperative plan, benefiting both the patient and the surgical team. The time saved during the surgical procedure may be spent during the preoperative period with the design and fabrication of the models, in addition to the time spent practicing the procedure.[17–21]

Anatomic models can be printed using various materials such as thermoplastics, ceramics, epoxy resins, and plastics.[4,12] Therefore, models generated for surgical planning and rehearsal may be fabricated using a biomaterial that most closely resembles the tissue of primary interest. Three-dimensional models of craniofacial bones fabricated from salt were found to closely simulate the bone when cut, improving the tactile experience while practicing procedures using the models.[22]

A significant benefit of 3D printing is the ability to fabricate patient-specific surgical guides, instruments, and implants. Custom-made titanium implants have been created for patients undergoing surgery for conditions involving the cervical spine, thoracic wall, pelvis, and acetabulum.[23–25] Tracheobronchomalacia is a life-threatening disease in children owing to severe collapse of the airways. Three pediatric patients with tracheobronchomalacia were successfully treated with custom-made tracheobronchial splints. The 3D printed splints were constructed of a bioresorbable and biocompatible polymer (polycaprolactone), which allowed for growth of the bronchial tree and would resorb over several years, until resolution of disease.[26]

The use of 3D printed anatomic models goes beyond the surgeon and surgery team. Patients may benefit from a verbal explanation from the surgeon combined with tactile and visual information gained from the opportunity of handling the anatomic model. Models can also be used to demonstrate to patients the degenerative changes to organs subjected to progressive disease states, such as a brain affected by Alzheimer's disease.[27]

Three-dimensional models have also been reported to augment the education and training of medical students, residents, and less experienced surgeons. In addition, when repeatedly performing the same surgical procedure, procedure time for trainees and less experienced surgeons decreased. Three-dimensional models fabricated using a biomaterial similar to that of brain tissue provided neurosurgery residents the ability to learn how to atraumatically retract brain tissue.[28]

The 2 areas of 3D printing in which further research is required are drug delivery and tissue engineering. Medications formulated using 3D printing technology may provide individualized medications, specifically dosed for the individual. Depending on the underlying condition, drugs could be formulated as extended release and/or as combination therapy, with multiple drugs within the same tablet. Medicated devices such as vaginal rings or subcutaneous devices may also be fabricated with size and dosing specifications tailored to the patient.[12,29]

Tissue engineering and regenerative therapies use stem cells to generate cells lines and specific tissue types. A bioscaffold is typically required once cells have been grown in culture. Bioprinting is the process of using 3D printing technology to deposit small numbers of cells with high precision on a substrate or scaffold. Bioprinting can be used to generate a sheet of a specific tissue type in which drug safety may be evaluated. Another potential use of this technology is the ability to generate an entire organ from a patient either for transplantation or to assess drug efficacy. This process would eliminate the need for organ donors, immunosuppressive therapy, and potential organ rejection. Clinical trials investigating the safety and efficacy of a drug could be carried out without subjecting patient to a drug with unknown benefits.[12,29]

SMALL ANIMAL

Although use of 3D printing technology had been reported for use in human medical procedures since the 1990s, the first reported use in veterinary medicine was not until the early 2000s. Harrysson and colleagues[30] described using CT images to create polyurethane stereolithographic models via rapid prototyping for a dog with angular limb deformities. Three models were generated to allow for presurgical planning and intraoperative reference. The authors reported benefits of the rehearsal of the procedures included increased comfort with the surgical plan, and the generation and placement of the fixation construct, thus leading to fewer intraoperative decisions and decreased operative time. Since this initial report, there have been several case reports and case series documenting the use of SLA and 3D printing in dogs with antebrachial and femoral deformities. In these reports, rehearsal surgeries, patient-specific guides, and precontoured implants allowed for simplified intraoperative corrections and decreased surgical time.[31–33]

For dogs sustaining traumatic injuries resulting in bone loss or those with tumors affecting the bones of the appendicular skeleton, treatment options often include amputation. Although most canine patients do well after an amputation, it does result in gait and posture adaptations to accommodate for ambulation on 3 limbs. Limb-sparing surgery with endoprostheses may be considered a viable treatment option for these patients. There have been several reports of patient-specific endoprosthesis use in dogs with bone tumors of the mandible, tibia, and radius, in addition to 1 dog that sustained a gunshot wound to the stifle.[34,35] Three-dimensional printing was used to assess prosthetic fit in addition to the fabrication of metallic endoprostheses. There were implant-associated complications reported in several dogs in which endoprostheses were placed owing to bone tumors. These complications may be due to surgical technique, implant design and/or implant fabrication.[34] This is a consideration when using these novel, custom-designed implants, because they may not undergo the rigorous biomechanical testing of other surgical implants.

The stabilization of the vertebral column typically requires the placement of screws, pins, or wires into the pedicles or vertebral bodies. Preoperative CT 3D images can aid with preoperative planning of these surgical procedures. It does not however, provide intraoperative guidance during surgical procedure. Free-hand placement of implants, even with the use of fluoroscopic guidance can result in violation of the vertebral canal.[36,37] Patient-specific 3D printed drill guides have been used for the placement of cervical transpedicular screws in canine patients. The use of the drill guides resulted in decreased surgical times and accurate placement for the majority of screws.[38,39]

Caudal mandibular fractures in feline patients can be challenging to repair owing to limited bone stock and difficulty accessing the fracture site. A lack of anatomic reconstruction of these fractures can lead to malocclusion.[40] Caudal mandibular fractures in 2 cats were repaired with the assistance of 3D printed models. CT images were used to generate models of the skulls. Preoperative planning included evaluation of the fracture configurations, plate placement, and contouring. A stainless steel drill guide was also created to facilitate implant placement during surgery. Fracture reduction and normal occlusion were achieved.[41]

Owing to an enhanced understanding of bone biology and healing, there has been a paradigm shift toward biologic fracture repair. Fracture stabilization using minimally invasive osteosynthesis, in which the fracture site remains intact, preserving the fracture hematoma and vascular supply, is preferred, when appropriate. Preoperative imaging (radiographs, CT scans) are used to assess fracture configuration and contour implants. Intraoperatively, fracture reduction and implant placement are performed under fluoroscopic guidance. Although there is a biologic benefit with regard to fracture healing with this approach, it does expose both the patient and surgical team to ionizing radiation.[42–44] Therefore, processes that may mitigate or eliminate exposure to radiation during these minimally invasive fracture repairs should be considered. A comminuted midshaft diaphyseal humeral fracture in a cat was successfully repaired using minimally invasive osteosynthesis techniques with the aid of a 3D- printed patient-specific guide. The fracture reduction guides were created using computer-aided design software and subsequently printed and sterilized. A bone model of the contralateral humerus was used to contour the plate preoperatively. Intraoperative fluoroscopy was not used during the procedure as the patient specific guides were used for fracture reduction. Postoperative CT scans revealed appropriate implant placement with minimal varus and torsional malreduction.[45]

Several in vitro studies have been performed evaluating a freeform custom bone cutting jig and plates. In 1 study, freeform biodegradable plates were found to be biomechanically comparable with other stabilization methods (Kirschner wire, metal plate) for the repair of distal femoral fractures.[46] The biodegradable plates however, cost between 2.3 and 19.0 times the standard methods of repair. Although this amount may decrease with design and fabrication experience, it may be cost prohibitive in a clinical setting. Another point discussed by the authors was the use of a bioresorbable plate with unknown effects from the polymer on the periosteum, bone healing, and surrounding soft tissues. Further, in vivo testing would be required to assess for any untoward side effects. Another in vitro study evaluated a custom bone cutting jig and plates in tibia replicas created using SLA.[47] An osteotomy was created in the proximal tibia either freehand or using a custom jig. The use of the custom jig improved the accuracy of the osteotomy and the speed at which it was created. There was also an increase in stiffness in the constructs created with the custom jig. Although no mention of the cost to fabricate the plates or jig, the time to prepare the jig was approximately 9 hours. This study suggests that custom cutting jigs and plates may decrease surgical time and improve construct stability owing to the improved accuracy of osteotomy and implant placement. As has been reported in the human medical literature, the decrease in surgical time is a result of the preoperative planning, design, and fabrication of the 3D models, of which the time spent in preparation must be accounted.

The accuracy of the bone models generated by 3 different methods of 3D printing (SLA, FDM, and SLS) was evaluated in a recent study investigating various CT scan protocols and 3 freeform fabrication methods using a cadaveric canine femur. The results revealed the biomodels created using higher radiation settings were more accurate. The biomodels overestimated cortical thickness for all methods. Overall, there was no difference between the methodologies, but the reproducibility for model fabrication seems to have a greater effect on variability as compared with CT scan protocol or fabrication method.[48] Any variability in model or implant fabrication could negatively impact the success of the procedure performed. Therefore, the process by which the images are obtained in addition to the accuracy and quality of the 3D-generated objects should be evaluated to avoid a potential technical error owing to model inaccuracy.

THREE-DIMENSIONAL PRINTING IN ZOOLOGICAL MEDICINE

Three-dimensional printing is gaining popularity and its use is increasing in nontraditional species. However, the majority of the reports of its application in clinical cases and research projects are primarily found in non–peer-reviewed publications or advertised via social media. The following information reviews the information currently available in peer-reviewed publications.

Three-Dimensional Printing in Birds

A 21-year-old red-lored Amazon parrot (*Amazona autumnalis*) with a preexisting amputation of the distal left leg at the tibiotarsal–tarsometatarsal joint, was presented with new injuries to the right leg caused by another bird.[49] Pododermatitis type 2 was noted on the right foot.[49] To prevent further damage to the right foot, and improve the quality of life, a 3D-printed prosthetic limb was created[49] (**Fig. 3**). Several iterations and modifications of the prosthetic were required to fabricate an adequate device.[49] The parrot did not attempt to remove the prosthesis and there were no outward signs of discomfort during use. However, a small superficial scab was observed in the caudal posterior area of the distal stump indicating a pressure sore. This sore was managed by modifying the socket[49] (**Fig. 4**).

Beak deformities and beak trauma may necessitate the development of prosthetic devices. A limited number of published cases reports of custom-made beak prostheses for birds can be found in the literature,[50–52] but anecdotal reports of 3D-printed beak prostheses can be easily found in news articles from around the world. Recently, the construction of a 3D-printed beak prosthetic for a 10-year-old captive red-crowned crane (*Grus japonensis*) was been reported.[53] Necrosis of the distal cranial maxillary rhinotheca, secondary to a suspected infection resulted in the loss of the bird's ability to prehend food.[53] A customized titanium alloy beak was created using a combination of FDM and selective laser melting.[53] Thirty minutes after the placement of the prosthetic, the animal was able to eat.[53] Similar designs may be useful for other bird species; however, beak prosthetics will always pose some technical challenges associated with the normal growth and use of the beak. As the rhamphotheca grows and the bird applies forces with its gnathotheca, rhinothecal prostheses have a tendency to dislodge.[54] Alternatively, a 3D helmet can be printed to be used as an orthodontic device for beak correction and is currently under investigation (**Fig. 5**) (Minh Huynh, personal communication, 2019).

Three-Dimensional Printing in Reptiles

In these authors' opinion, chelonians may be the group of exotic animals that may benefit the most from the advances in 3D printing. The development of protective

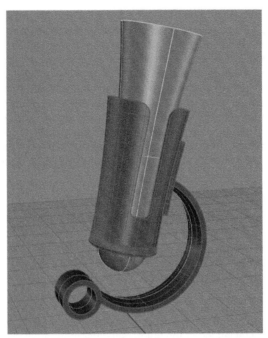

Fig. 3. 3D digital rendering of a prosthetic limb created for a red-lored Amazon parrot (*Amazona autumnalis*) that suffered a traumatic limb amputation (*Courtesy of* Drs. Cecilia Galicia, Vanessa Hernandez Urraca, Jaime Samour).

devices for shell wounds may be relatively straightforward. The authors have developed a protective shield for a breeding male adult African spurred tortoise (*Centrochelys sulcata*) to provide additional protection for a healing wound.[55] The animal developed a surgical plastrotomy site infection and the wound was improving and healing. To facilitate the transfer of the animal back to its outdoor enclosure and

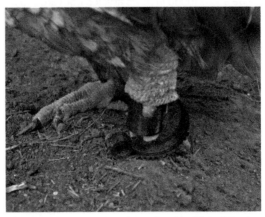

Fig. 4. Prosthetic limb created using a 3D printer for a red-lored Amazon parrot (*Amazona autumnalis*). (*Courtesy of* Drs. Cecilia Galicia, Vanessa Hernandez Urraca, Jaime Samour).

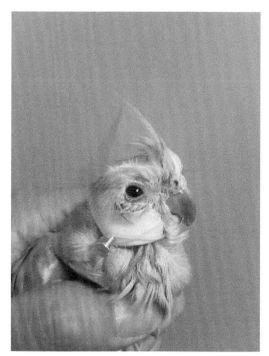

Fig. 5. 3D printed helmet created using a 3D printer, used as an orthodontic device for a cockatiel (*Nymphicus hollandicus*). (*Courtesy of* M. Huynh, DVM, Arcueil, France).

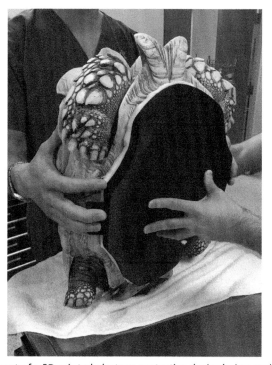

Fig. 6. The placement of a 3D printed plastron protective device being evaluated in an adult male African-spurred tortoise (*Centrochelys sulcata*). (*Courtesy of* I. Kanda).

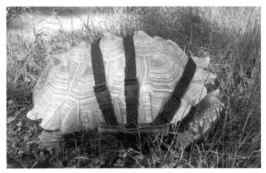

Fig. 7. An adult male African-spurred tortoise (*Centrochelys sulcata*) with a custom-made 3D printed protective device secured in place with fabric straps. This device was created to provide additional protection to a healing plastrotomy site while allowing the animal to live in its regular enclosure and breed. (*Courtesy of* I. Kanda).

engage in breeding activities, a protective shield was printed from images acquired from a whole body CT scan (**Figs. 6** and **7**). Chelonians that have lost the function of their limbs may benefit from the development of custom 3D-printed carts (**Fig. 8**). Similar to a recent report describing the management of pododermatitis using an orthotic boot in a southern Isabela giant tortoise (*Chelonoidis vicina*), 3D printing may be used to develop custom prosthetic limbs or protective limb devices.[56]

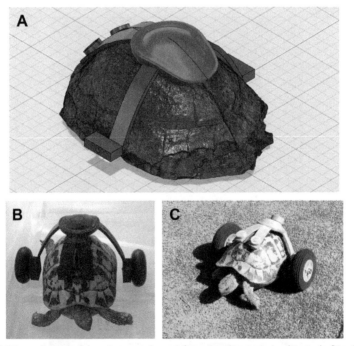

Fig. 8. (*A*) 3D rendering of a custom-made cart for a Russian tortoise (*Testudo [Agrionemys] horsfieldii*) with hindlimb dysfunction secondary to trauma. (*B, C*) The cart was 3D printed and fitted to the animal. (*Courtesy of* Massimo Mostosi and Nicola Di Girolamo).

Three-Dimensional Printing in Small Mammals

Although some reports of the use of 3D printing in exotic mammals (eg, wheelchair in a guinea pig) can be found on social media websites and in news reports, there is a lack of peer-reviewed publications about its application in clinical cases of exotic pet mammals. Nonetheless, exotic mammal species, such as rabbits, have been used as an animal model for the research of 3D printing, primarily investigating scaffolds for bone and cartilage regeneration.[57–60] Biphasic osteochondral composite scaffolds created with 3D printing using poly(ethylene glycol) hydrogel and β-tricalciumphosphate ceramic were implanted in critical sized defects in a rabbit trochlea model. Poly(ethylene glycol) hydrogels have been applied extensively for in vitro and in vivo cartilage tissue engineering and β-tricalciumphosphate ceramic is widely used for subchondral bone and autologous bone graft.[59] At 52 weeks, the treated tissue was normal in color with a smooth surface comparable with sham groups, whereas the untreated defects were insufficiently filled with red fibrous tissue, had rough surfaces, and entire defect margins were visible.[59] Studies involving testing of bone bioprinted material for bone defects have been performed in rabbit, rat, and mouse models.[61] These research projects may yield low clinical applicability at this time owing to limited availability and cost. Nevertheless, as technology becomes more available and affordable, it may be of use for exotic animal clinicians in the near future.

Endotracheal intubation is challenging in rodents because of the anatomy of the pharynx and, although the use of laryngoscopes have been reported in rats, many of these devices are not commercially available.[62] A design for a laryngoscope blade to be printed with a 3D printer using polylactide filament material has been published and the authors made it publicly available (https://www.thingiverse.com/thing:148315).[62] The authors of this publication were able to intubate 35 rats successfully.[62] Hypothetically, similar designs can be developed for other species.

Three-Dimensional Printing in Wildlife

The development of novel pharmaceutical forms is a constant practice in research, development, and innovation in laboratories, being of interest to researchers in both academia and industry.[63] Injection molding consists in the injection, under high-pressure conditions, of heat-induced softened materials into a mold cavity where they are shaped.[64] An ingenious use of 3D printing was the development of a 3D-printed, biodegradable projectile for the delivery of extended-release contraceptive for free-ranging animals.[65] Three concentrations of progesterone (2%, 5%, and 10% w/w) with polylactic acid was prepared as a 1.75-mm filament by hot melt extrusion, which was designed to create a projective shaped device.[65] The projectile was shown to provide sufficient kinetic energy to penetrate thin (sheep skin) and medium (horse skin) thickness skins.[65] The authors of this study suggest that a 3D-printed ballistic drug delivery system offers several potential advantages: (i) multiple pharmaceutical delivery, (ii) flexibility to create hollow reservoirs to accommodate solid, semisolid, or liquid formulations, (iii) customized dosages for each individual, (iv) target animal specificity, (v) the possibility of marking the animal with colors or electrical identification devices along with the administration of the therapeutics, (vi) low treatment costs, (vii) minimum direct contact with wild animals, and (viii) no anesthetization requirement.[65] The use of polylactic acid for extended-release drug delivery may be useful for other species.

Mating behavior and mate selection studies are useful for the biologist to monitor and understand wild animal biology. Three-dimensional printed northern map turtle

(*Graptemys geographica*) female decoys of multiple sizes were used to determine if male turtles would prefer larger females.[66] Males interacted and attempted to mate significantly more with the larger decoys.[66] The authors suggest that the use of 3D printed decoys and submersible action cameras involves minimal stress and disturbance and should be a valuable tool to document the mating and social behaviors of species that are prone to captivity stress or that are easily disturbed by observers in the field.[66] Similarly, under laboratory conditions, the possibility of using 3D printing technology to understand the role of body size on the social behavior of the zebrafish model organism has been reported.[67] Subjects exhibit an avoidance reaction for larger replicas, and they are attracted to and influenced by smaller replicas.[67]

Coevolutionary relationships between brood parasites and their hosts are often studied by examining the egg rejection behavior of host species using artificial eggs.[68] Three-dimensional printing may reduce human error, enable more precise manipulation of egg size and shape, and provide a more accurate and replicable protocol for generating artificial stimuli than traditional methods.[68] Three-dimensional printed artificial eggs that encompass the natural range of shapes and sizes of brown-headed cowbirds (*Molothrus ater*) eggs, painted to resemble either American robin (*Turdus migratorius*) or cowbird egg color, and artificially placed in nests of breeding wild robins were used.[68] Similar to previous studies, robins accept mimetically colored and reject nonmimetically colored artificial eggs.[68] Three-dimensional printing can provide time and cost savings to ecologists and, with recent advances in less toxic, biodegradable, and recyclable print materials, ecologists can choose to minimize social and environmental impacts associated with 3D printing.[69]

The impact of poaching in wildlife conservation is well-known. The production of synthetic rhinoceros horns as a substitute for that sourced from the wild (natural horn) to help relieve pressure on rhinoceros populations caused by trade demand has been suggested.[70] The use of 3D printing technology to produce solid synthetic horns that are physically indistinguishable from natural horns has been considered.[70] However, other investigators suggest that synthetic horn producers would benefit more by promoting their products as being superior to wild horns, but this could increase natural horn prices and lead to more rhino poaching.[71]

ANATOMY AND MUSEUM USE

Museums commonly exhibit skeletons of extant and extinct species. Only 7 skeletons of the extinct subspecies of plains zebra (*Equus quagga quagga*) are known to exist in museum collections worldwide; however, in the specimen from the Grant Museum of Zoology (London, UK), the left hind leg and right scapula have been missing for many years.[72] To remount the skeleton, the left scapula and articulated right hind limb were scanned using CT so that mirrored data could be used to 3D print the missing bones.[72] The 3D-printed models installed on the original specimen do more than provide an anatomically complete skeleton and improve the physical stability of the specimen; the black 3D printed bones contrast with the rest of the skeleton, which highlights the work undertaken and provides a more engaging exhibit.[72]

SUMMARY

Medical 3D printing in zoological medicine is still in its infancy, but is an area with great growth potential. The ability to train and plan for surgical procedures using a realistic model of the anatomic area of interest may be extremely useful for nontraditional species. This ability may also allow for the development of customized, patient-specific surgical instruments and implants, which may overcome certain size limitations that are frequently encountered with for small size patients.

Given the paucity of data available for the use of this technology in exotics animal species, one of the major challenges at this point, is the lack of experience in specific clinical cases for the application of 3D printing. Appropriate case selection, printing medium and printer type are all critical to the successful use of this technology in the treatment of patients. Thinking outside the box and considering previous applications of medical 3D printing in other species should provide some guidance to clinicians when considering its use to maximize the benefits of this invaluable medical modality.

REFERENCES

1. Hull CW. Apparatus for production of three-dimensional objects by stereolithography: US Patent 4,575,330, 1986.
2. Ventola CL. Medical applications for 3D printing: current and projected uses. P T 2014;39:704–11.
3. Schubert C, Van Langeveld MC, Donoso LA. Innovations in 3D printing: a 3D overview from optics to organs. Br J Ophthalmol 2014;98:159–61.
4. Hoang D, Perrault D, Stevanovic M, et al. Surgical applications of three-dimensional printing: a review of the current literature & how to get started. Ann Transl Med 2016;4:456.
5. Ballard DH, Trace AP, Ali S, et al. Clinical applications of 3D printing: primer for radiologists. Acad Radiol 2018;25:52–65.
6. Hespel AM, Wilhite R, Hudson J. Invited review–Applications for 3D printers in veterinary medicine. Vet Radiol Ultrasound 2014;55:347–58.
7. Melican MC, Zimmerman MC, Dhillon MS, et al. Three-dimensional printing and porous metallic surfaces: a new orthopedic application. J Biomed Mater Res 2001;55:194–202.
8. Curodeau A, Sachs E, Caldarise S. Design and fabrication of cast orthopedic implants with freeform surface textures from 3-D printed ceramic shell. J Biomed Mater Res 2000;53:525–35.
9. Hong SB, Eliaz N, Leisk GG, et al. A new Ti-5Ag alloy for customized prostheses by three-dimensional printing (3DP). J Dent Res 2001;80:860–3.
10. Malik HH, Darwood AR, Shaunak S, et al. Three-dimensional printing in surgery: a review of current surgical applications. J Surg Res 2015;199:512–22.
11. Rankin TM, Giovinco NA, Cucher DJ, et al. Three-dimensional printing surgical instruments: are we there yet? J Surg Res 2014;189:193–7.
12. Tappa K, Jammalamadaka U. Novel biomaterials used in medical 3d printing techniques. J Funct Biomater 2018;9 [pii:E17].
13. Pucci JU, Christophe BR, Sisti JA, et al. Three-dimensional printing: technologies, applications, and limitations in neurosurgery. Biotechnol Adv 2017;35:521–9.
14. Westerman ME, Matsumoto JM, Morris JM, et al. Three-dimensional printing for renal cancer and surgical planning. Eur Urol Focus 2016;2:574–6.
15. Mok SW, Nizak R, Fu SC, et al. From the printer: potential of three-dimensional printing for orthopaedic applications. J Orthop Translat 2016;6:42–9.
16. Zheng Y-x, Yu D-f, Zhao J-g, et al. 3D printout models vs. 3D-rendered images: which is better for preoperative planning? J Surg Educ 2016;73:518–23.
17. Maini L, Sharma A, Jha S, et al. Three-dimensional printing and patient-specific pre-contoured plate: future of acetabulum fracture fixation? Eur J Trauma Emerg Surg 2018;44:215–24.

18. Martelli N, Serrano C, van den Brink H, et al. Advantages and disadvantages of 3-dimensional printing in surgery: a systematic review. Surgery 2016;159:1485–500.

19. Lal H, Patralekh MK. 3D printing and its applications in orthopaedic trauma: a technological marvel. J Clin Orthop Trauma 2018;9:260–8.

20. Wang Y-T, Yang X-J, Yan B, et al. Clinical application of three-dimensional printing in the personalized treatment of complex spinal disorders. Chin J Traumatol 2016; 19:31–4.

21. Zeng C, Xiao J, Wu Z, et al. Evaluation of three-dimensional printing for internal fixation of unstable pelvic fracture from minimal invasive para-rectus abdominis approach: a preliminary report. Int J Clin Exp Med 2015;8:13039.

22. Okumoto T, Sakamoto Y, Kondo S, et al. Salt as a new colored solid model for simulation surgery. J Craniofac Surg 2015;26:680–1.

23. Xu N, Wei F, Liu X, et al. Reconstruction of the upper cervical spine using a personalized 3D-printed vertebral body in an adolescent with Ewing sarcoma. Spine (Phila Pa 1976) 2016;41:E50–4.

24. Wang L, Cao T, Li X, et al. Three-dimensional printing titanium ribs for complex reconstruction after extensive posterolateral chest wall resection in lung cancer. J Thorac Cardiovasc Surg 2016;152:e5–7.

25. Wong K, Kumta S, Geel N, et al. One-step reconstruction with a 3D-printed, biomechanically evaluated custom implant after complex pelvic tumor resection. Comput Aided Surg 2015;20:14–23.

26. Morrison RJ, Hollister SJ, Niedner MF, et al. Mitigation of tracheobronchomalacia with 3D-printed personalized medical devices in pediatric patients. Sci Transl Med 2015;7:285ra264.

27. Marks M, Alexander A, Matsumoto J, et al. Creating three dimensional models of Alzheimer's disease. 3D Print Med 2017;3:13.

28. Mashiko T, Konno T, Kaneko N, et al. Training in brain retraction using a self-made three-dimensional model. World Neurosurg 2015;84:585–90.

29. Awad A, Trenfield SJ, Gaisford S, et al. 3D printed medicines: a new branch of digital healthcare. Int J Pharm 2018;548:586–96.

30. Harrysson OL, Cormier DR, Marcellin-Little DJ, et al. Rapid prototyping for treatment of canine limb deformities. Vet Comp Orthop Traumatol 2003;9:37–42.

31. Dismukes DI, Fox DB, Tomlinson JL, et al. Use of radiographic measures and three-dimensional computed tomographic imaging in surgical correction of an antebrachial deformity in a dog. J Am Vet Med Assoc 2008;232:68–73.

32. Crosse KR, Worth AJ. Computer-assisted surgical correction of an antebrachial deformity in a dog. Vet Comp Orthop Traumatol 2010;23:354–61.

33. DeTora MD, Boudrieau RJ. Complex angular and torsional deformities (distal femoral malunions). Preoperative planning using stereolithography and surgical correction with locking plate fixation in four dogs. Vet Comp Orthop Traumatol 2016;29:416–25.

34. Bray JP, Kersley A, Downing W, et al. Clinical outcomes of patient-specific porous titanium endoprostheses in dogs with tumors of the mandible, radius, or tibia: 12 cases (2013–2016). J Am Vet Med Assoc 2017;251:566–79.

35. Liska WD, Marcellin-Little DJ, Eskelinen EV, et al. Custom total knee replacement in a dog with femoral condylar bone loss. Vet Surg 2007;36:293–301.

36. Hettlich BF, Fosgate GT, Levine JM, et al. Accuracy of conventional radiography and computed tomography in predicting implant position in relation to the vertebral canal in dogs. Vet Surg 2010;39:680–7.

37. Tran JH, Hall DA, Morton JM, et al. Accuracy and safety of pin placement during lateral versus dorsal stabilization of lumbar spinal fracture-luxation in dogs. Vet Surg 2017;46:1166–74.
38. Oxley B, Behr S. Stabilisation of a cranial cervical vertebral fracture using a 3D-printed patient-specific drill guide. J Small Anim Pract 2016;57:277.
39. Hamilton-Bennett SE, Oxley B, Behr S. Accuracy of a patient-specific 3D printed drill guide for placement of cervical transpedicular screws. Vet Surg 2018;47:236–42.
40. Milella L. Occlusion and malocclusion in the cat: what's normal, what's not and when's the best time to intervene? J Feline Med Surg 2015;17:5–20.
41. Southerden P, Barnes DM. Caudal mandibular fracture repair using three-dimensional printing, presurgical plate contouring and a preformed template to aid anatomical fracture reduction. JFMS Open Rep 2018;4. 2055116918798875.
42. Kim TW, Jung JH, Jeon HJ, et al. Radiation exposure to physicians during interventional pain procedures. Korean J Pain 2010;23:24–7.
43. Widmer WR, Shaw SM, Thrall DE, et al. Effects of low-level exposure to ionizing radiation: current concepts and concerns for veterinary workers. Vet Radiol Ultrasound 1996;37:227–39.
44. Rashid MS, Aziz S, Haydar S, et al. Intra-operative fluoroscopic radiation exposure in orthopaedic trauma theatre. Eur J Orthop Surg Traumatol 2018;28:9–14.
45. Oxley B. A 3-dimensional-printed patient-specific guide system for minimally invasive plate osteosynthesis of a comminuted mid-diaphyseal humeral fracture in a cat. Vet Surg 2018;47:445–53.
46. Marcellin-Little DJ, Sutherland BJ, Harrysson OL, et al. In vitro evaluation of free-form biodegradable bone plates for fixation of distal femoral physeal fractures in dogs. Am J Vet Res 2010;71:1508–15.
47. Marcellin-Little DJ, Harrysson OL, Cansizoglu O. In vitro evaluation of a custom cutting jig and custom plate for canine tibial plateau leveling. Am J Vet Res 2008;69:961–6.
48. Fitzwater KL, Marcellin-Little DJ, Harrysson OL, et al. Evaluation of the effect of computed tomography scan protocols and freeform fabrication methods on bone biomodel accuracy. Am J Vet Res 2011;72:1178–85.
49. Galicia C, Hernandez Urraca V, del Castillo L, et al. Design and use of a 3D prosthetic leg in a red-lored amazon parrot (Amazona autumnalis). J Avian Med Surg 2018;32:133–7.
50. Crosta L. Alloplastic and heteroplastic bill prostheses in 2 ramphastidae birds. J Avian Med Surg 2002;16:218–22.
51. Thengchaisri N, Soonthornphisaj C, Pusaksrikit S. Correction of upper beak fracture with chrome-cobalt-alloy model in a fighting cock. Symposon of the Asian Zoo and Wildlife Medicine, 2nd Workshop of the Asian Zoo and Wildlife Pathology. Faculty of Veterinary Science, Chulalongkorn University Bangkok, Thailand, 26-29 October, 2006.
52. Morris PJ, Weigel JP, Wolf L. Methacrylate beak prosthesis in a marabou stork (Leptoptilos crumeniferus). Journal of the Association of Avian Veterinarians 1990;4:103–7.
53. Song C, Wang A, Wu Z, et al. The design and manufacturing of a titanium alloy beak for Grus japonensis using additive manufacturing. Mater Des 2017;117:410–6.
54. Schnellbacher RW, Stevens AG, Mitchell MA, et al. Use of a dental composite to correct beak deviation in psittacine species. Journal of Exotic Pet Medicine 2010;19:290–7.

55. Faulkner E, Sypniewski L, Kanda I, et al. Use of an Airtight Plastic Food Storage Container as a Protective Wound Device in 2 Chelonians. Proceedings of the 3rd International Conference on Avian, Herpetological, and Exotic Mammal Medicine. 25th-29th March, 2017, Venice, Italy.

56. Waugh L, D'Agostino J, Cole GA, et al. management of pododermatitis with an orthotic boot in a Southern Isabela Giant Tortoise (Chelonoidis vicina). J Zoo Wildl Med 2017;48:594–7.

57. Ge Z, Tian X, Heng BC, et al. Histological evaluation of osteogenesis of 3D-printed poly-lactic-co-glycolic acid (PLGA) scaffolds in a rabbit model. Biomed Mater 2009;4:021001.

58. Do AV, Khorsand B, Geary SM, et al. 3D printing of scaffolds for tissue regeneration applications. Adv Healthc Mater 2015;4:1742–62.

59. Zhang W, Lian Q, Li D, et al. Cartilage repair and subchondral bone migration using 3D printing osteochondral composites: a one-year-period study in rabbit trochlea. Biomed Res Int 2014;2014:746138.

60. Wang X, Ao Q, Tian X, et al. 3D bioprinting technologies for hard tissue and organ engineering. Materials (Basel) 2016;9:802.

61. Chia HN, Wu BM. Recent advances in 3D printing of biomaterials. J Biol Eng 2015;9:4.

62. Vongerichten A, Aristovich K, Dos Santos GS, et al. Design for a three-dimensional printed laryngoscope blade for the intubation of rats. Lab Anim (NY) 2014;43:140.

63. Bilhalva AF, Finger IS, Pereira RA, et al. Utilization of biodegradable polymers in veterinary science and routes of administration: a literature review. J Appl Anim Res 2018;46:643–9.

64. Zema L, Loreti G, Melocchi A, et al. Injection molding and its application to drug delivery. J Control Release 2012;159:324–31.

65. Long J, Nand AV, Ray S, et al. Development of customised 3D printed biodegradable projectile for administrating extended-release contraceptive to wildlife. Int J Pharm 2018;548:349–56.

66. Bulté G, Chlebak RJ, Dawson JW, et al. Studying mate choice in the wild using 3D printed decoys and action cameras: a case of study of male choice in the northern map turtle. Anim Behav 2018;138:141–3.

67. Bartolini T, Mwaffo V, Showler A, et al. Zebrafish response to 3D printed shoals of conspecifics: the effect of body size. Bioinspir Biomim 2016;11:026003.

68. Igic B, Nunez V, Voss HU, et al. Using 3D printed eggs to examine the egg-rejection behaviour of wild birds. PeerJ 2015;3:e965.

69. Behm J, Waite BR, Hsieh ST, et al. Benefits and limitations of three-dimensional printing technology for ecological research. BMC Ecol 2018;18(1):32.

70. Broad S, Burgess G. Synthetic biology, product substitution and the battle against illegal wildlife trade. TRAFFIC Bulletin 2016;28:23. Available at: http://www.rhinoresourcecenter.com/.

71. Chen F. the economics of synthetic rhino horns. Ecol Econ 2017;141:180–9.

72. Larkin NR, Porro LB. Three legs good, four legs better: making a quagga whole again with 3D printing. Collection Forum 2016;30(1):73–84.

Smartphone-Based Device in Exotic Pet Medicine

Minh Huynh, DVM, DECZM (Avian), DACZM

KEYWORDS

- Smartphone • ECG • Fundoscope • Thermography • Endoscope
- Hand-carried ultrasound

KEY POINTS

- Heart rate can be measured with a smartphone, but studies are required to standardize the process, evaluate the accuracy, and assess the electrocardiograph.
- The smartphone can be used for fundoscopic evaluation, and some devices have been evaluated in rabbits.
- Smartphone-based thermal imaging can be performed, but further studies are needed for clinical interpretation.
- An endoscope adapter allows the connection of a smartphone to a regular endoscope.
- A reduced ultrasound device may be linked to a smartphone and may provide point-of-care evaluation.

INTRODUCTION

The introduction of smartphones has been a major social revolution in everyday life. Nowadays it is one of the most ubiquitous technological objects worldwide. Its original use in telecommunication has been overtaken by its processing capacity, turning it into a miniaturized mobile personal computer. Medical use of smartphones is an increasing trend in human medicine and also likely in veterinary medicine. Surveys have indicated that 80% of physicians and nurses use their smartphone.[1] Exotic pet medicine has several specificities that may be addressed by point-of-care technology. One of which is the difficulty of transporting some zoo or wild animals, which may require on-site examination. Another is the need of emergent care in the case of debilitated animals, where transportation may be a risk. Finally, the smartphone can help in everyday consultation as for any other veterinary discipline and can play a major role in telemedicine.

Disclosure Statement: The author possesses several devices used in this issue (AliveCor [(AliveCor Inc, San Francisco, CA, USA), Peek Retina (Peek Vision, London, UK), Clearscope, FLIR ONE (FLIR system Inc, Wilsonville, OR, USA), Lumify) but has no commercial link or interest with the company selling the products.
Centre Hospitalier Veterinaire Fregis, 43 Avenue Aristide Briand, Arcueil 94110, France
E-mail address: nacologie@gmail.com

Vet Clin Exot Anim 22 (2019) 349–366
https://doi.org/10.1016/j.cvex.2019.05.001
1094-9194/19/© 2019 Elsevier Inc. All rights reserved.

TECHNOLOGY

The smartphone is usually based on a cellular phone with an integrated camera, a global positioning system, Internet connection capacity, and an operating system able to execute various applications. The smartphone is generally equipped with a powerful light which can be used as a light source for oral examination, pupillary reflexe evaluation or even egg candling (**Fig. 1**). Most mobile phones use either an Android system or an iOS, each system being exclusive. Some smartphones possess a micro-USB or a USB-C port, allowing connection of additional devices.

APPLICATIONS

Mobile applications, commonly called "apps," are software applications designed to run on a mobile device. The software must take into account that mobile devices have less powerful processors than personal computers and have more features, such as camera and location detection. General apps using social media and instant communication may improve communication and information among clinician (see Nicola Di Girolamo's article "Advances in retrieval and dissemination of medical information", in this issue).

The veterinary app is a relatively narrow field among the variety of medical apps available. The use of apps is mainly limited to drug formulary, reference books, and calculators among physicians and students. Many review articles point out that medical apps can be developed without validation by a health care professional; therefore, information must be critically reviewed by users.[2–4] It is noteworthy that an app called Veterinary Care of Exotic Pets, developed by a veterinarian (M. Rowland), offers information about exotic animals, including a drug formulary, blood reference range, and visual content on various exotic species.

Some medical apps may have an interest for the exotic veterinary practitioner. A novel technique using augmented reality has been used to operate cerebral hematomas in humans.[5] Using a PACS (picture archiving and communication system) and an Android smartphone app, Sina neurosurgical assist, a computed tomographic (CT) scan image of the lesion was projected on the surgical site, facilitating endoscopic insertion.[5] Another app can help the clinician in planned needle insertion in CT-guided intervention. Needle insertions vastly rely on the assessment of the operator when fluoroscopy is not

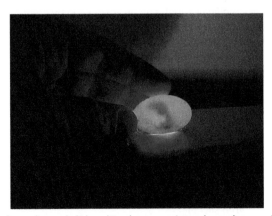

Fig. 1. Candling of a red eared sliders (*Trachemys scripta elegans*) egg with a smartphone. (*Courtesy of* Ian Kanda, Oklahoma State University).

available. The app Smart puncture calculates the angle and display needle insertion guidelines using the motion sensor inside the smartphone, which is placed adjacent to the patient.[6] Ultimately, there are several apps that can be useful, such as leukocyte count app (White blood cell counter) and various calculators (Vet Calculator Plus).

CARDIOLOGY

Heart rate can be measured efficiently with a smartphone in human medicine.[7–9] The phone's camera along with its light-emitting diode (LED) light source can measure heat rate accurately compared with a standard electrocardiogram (ECG).[7–9] Several apps have used this principle, called photoplethysmography (PPG). Blood absorbs more light than the surrounding tissue, and variation in blood volume (diastole and systole) affects the reflectance of light. There are contact and noncontact PPG. In contact PPG, the camera is placed directly on the skin of the human patient. In noncontact PPG, the camera is used in front of the patient's face. However, noncontact PPG has been found less accurate than contact PPG.[8] Contact PPG has been found to correlate well with standard ECGs.[7,8] The use of the earlobe as a surface contact was more accurate than with the finger in children using this application.[9]

Heart auscultation can be performed with the microphone of the smartphone. Several apps have been developed with this perspective.[10] The heartbeat could be interpreted with a specific stethoscope app in 65% of the patients.[10] The EkoCore stethoscope is a device that is added to a standard stethoscope for recording and transferring the sound wave in a smartphone.[11]

ECGs can be recorded on the smartphone using an external device. The AliveCor device is a bipolar electrode used for ECG recording in humans. The signal is transmitted with a high-pitched sound by the bipolar device and recorded by the smartphone microphone. Environmental noises as well as the electric field generated by the heating device or other smartphone may alter the signal.

The AliveCor system has been evaluated in small animal medicine.[12,13] There was minimal disagreement in the polarity of depolarization in dogs but frequent disagreement in cats.[12] Generally, heart rate and rhythm were accurately measured with the smartphone.[12,13] ECG is best obtained when the patient is placed in right lateral recumbency with alcohol or coupling gel applied on the electrode to enhance conduction.[12] The electrode is placed over the point of maximal intensity of the cardiac beat on the left side of the thorax with the positive electrode placed caudally, similar to a standard lead III.[12]

AliveCor was also evaluated in large animals, where it was validated in the horse and was found to provide a higher-quality ECG compared with a standard ECG in the goat.[14,15] The device was successfully used in bottlenose penguins.[16] It is noteworthy that dolphin vocalizations have created artifacts in the smartphone recording.[16]

D-Heart (D-Heart SRL, Genova, Italy) is another smartphone-based ECG device that streams the tracing via Bluetooth (**Fig. 2**). The ECG is acquired with 4-lead electrodes connected to a Bluetooth hand-sized transmitter. It was successfully evaluated in dogs.[17]

Both devices have demonstrated validities in various species. There are no specific reports in exotic pet medicine. The main advantage of the AliveCor system is the single-lead device, which is easier to place than a standard 4-lead ECG and provides major perspective in exotic animals when tolerance of 4-lead placement can be difficult. Furthermore, accurate measurement of heart rate by auscultation is difficult in some mammals and birds because of their very fast-paced heart rate. Standard validation of the graph and heart rate is still required (**Fig. 3**; **Table 1**).

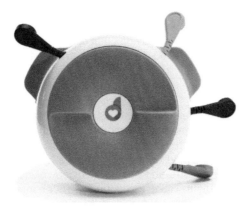

Fig. 2. D-Heart system.

OPHTHALMOLOGY

Use of the smartphone in fundoscopy by human ophthalmologists was first described in 2010.[18] Indirect and direct ophthalmoscopy have been described. The smartphone can be used simply with the camera and the flash mode on, illuminating the eye through an aspheric ophthalmic lens.[18–20] To facilitate the procedure, a 3-dimensional (3D) printed adapter can be placed on the smartphone, which holds the lens in a fixed position in front of the camera.[21]

Direct acquisition of images from the anterior chamber has been evaluated with an iPhone 5. Images have been found to be reliable but tend to produce oversaturation of the anterior segment under low-light settings.[22] It is also possible to attach a smartphone to an external optic fundus camera.[23]

Two devices have been developed specifically for direct ophthalmoscopy using a smartphone.

A specific device called D-eye (D-Eye SRL, Padova, Italy) adapted for iPhone and Samsung smartphones has also been evaluated in human medicine[24,25] (**Fig. 4**). The device is composed of lenses, polarizing filters, a beam splitter, a diaphragm, and a mirror attached to a smartphone. The device has been evaluated as an educational tool for the ophthalmologist, which make it easy to use by beginners because of its recording features and larger image display.[24,25]

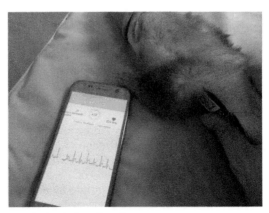

Fig. 3. Use of Alivecor electrode in a ferret.

Table 1			
Smartphone-based electrocardiographic recording device			
Device	Emitting System	Transmission	System
AliveCor, AliveCor Inc, San Francisco, CA, USA	Bipolar electrode	Microphone	iOS Android
D-Heart, D-Heart SRL, Genova, Italy	4-lead electrode	Bluetooth	iOS Android

It has been evaluated in dogs, cats, and rabbits.[26] Posterior segment structures could be identified in all animals.[26] Focal light artifacts were common when photographing the tapetum lucidum.[26]

A device called Peek Retina can be used by any type of smartphone (**Fig. 5**). The smartphone-based adapter consists of a plastic clip that covers the telephone camera and flash (white LED) with a prism assembly. The prism deflects light from the flash to match the illumination path with the field of view of the camera to acquire images of the retina. The phone camera and clip are held in front and close to the eye, which allows the camera to capture images of the fundus.[27] Preliminary work has been first investigated in a cohort of human patients.[28] Acquisition of optic disc imaging by nonclinically trained personnel was acceptable, making it very interesting in low-resource environments.[27]

Those devices bring perspective for fundic examination especially in avian wildlife casualties, whereby posterior chamber disorders are thought to be common in the case of trauma[29] (see **Fig. 5**). Mydriasis needs to be induced first using antimuscarinic drugs (tropicamide) in mammals or a neuromuscular blocker in birds (rocuronium) (**Fig. 6**).

INFRARED THERMOGRAPHY

Infrared thermography is a method that analyzes infrared energy emitted from object and converts it to temperature and display images of temperature distribution. This

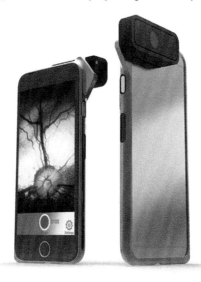

Fig. 4. D-eye fundoscope.

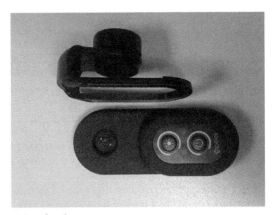

Fig. 5. Peek retina Vision fundoscope.

method has gained popularity in thermal screening and evaluation of breast cancer, diabetes neuropathy, and peripheral vascular disorder in humans.[30] It also helps in assessing efficacy of anti-inflammatory agents.[31] The principle is that any object above absolute zero emits electromagnetic radiation known as infrared or thermal radiation. The infrared emission from the skin can be recorded with an infrared camera. The warm areas are white, and the cooler areas are dark. The main advantage is that the process is completely noninvasive. The camera works like a digital video camera using a specific lens with semiconducting properties, allowing the transmission of heat waves.

There are several limitations and artifacts associated with the use of thermography. First, any feathers or hairs will impair propagation of the infrared.[32] Any alcohol, water, or mud creates artifacts.[32] The temperature of the environment should be controlled, especially with high ambient temperature.[32]

Inflammation (especially for pododermatitis) and pregnancy are good indications of infrared thermography in zoo animals.[32] The technology has been used successful in a flamingo with avascular necrosis of the wing and in turkeys with subclinical pododermatitis.[33,34] On the other hand, use in pododermatitis screening in penguins was unreliable, although feet with pododermatitis were warmer than feet with no lesion.[35] Infrared thermography has been evaluated in birds by Beaufrere[36] using a conventional FLIR EG portable thermal camera. It was mainly used as a monitoring tool rather

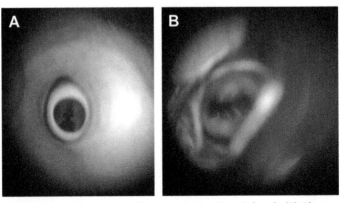

Fig. 6. (*A*) Observation of the fundus of an anesthetized Harris hawk. (*B*) Observation of the fundus of an anesthetized African gray parrot.

than a diagnostic tool. The camera allowed screening of inflammatory conditions from a distance, some having no hematologic or radiologic abnormalities.[36] Use of anti-inflammatory drugs allowed normalization of temperature signal from the inflammatory foot.[36] Other indications include assessment of the feather coverage in layer hens, stress evaluation in birds, or estrous detection in chinchillas.[37–39]

The American Academy of Thermology defines veterinary guidelines for infrared thermography.[40] Detector resolution of greater than 640×480 sensors or 320×240 sensors with lens and firmware innovations may approach 640×480 sensors. Repeatability and precision of $\leq \pm 0.5°C$ detection of temperature difference is recommended.[40]

FLIR ONE and Seek Thermal Compact XR (Seek Thermal, Santa Barbara, CA, USA) are thermographic devices connected to the smartphone (**Fig. 7**). The thermal resolution is 160×120 sensors. Although its precision for temperature assessment is not accurate compared with a conventional thermograph used in human medicine, its use has been investigated in a medical context. It is more affordable, more portable than a compact thermographic camera, and allows instant transmission through Internet or mobile phone. In a study about subclinical foot inflammation in diabetic patients, the absolute temperature could not be determined with the FLIR ONE, but the relative temperature difference was sufficient to assess inflammation.[31,41] Experimental assessment of limb perfusion in a swine model was adequately evaluated with the FLIR ONE as well as adequacy of tourniquet placement.[42] Lower-extremity ischemia in humans has been further evaluated with this same device.[43] Burn wounds have been assessed successfully with the FLIR ONE and showed the difference between the burn wounds and healthy skin, although it may overestimate unsalvageable tissue area.[44,45] Finally, there was a high concordance between thermographic images obtained by the FLIR ONE and CT angiography for detecting skin hotspots, which are cutaneous zones with higher temperature.[46]

Its use in exotic pet medicine needs to be further investigated, especially for avascular necrosis, such as pododermatitis, which is relatively common in birds and small mammals (see **Fig. 7**). Wound healing, inflammatory condition of the limb, frostbite, and atherosclerotic lesions are potential indications for use of this technology (**Fig. 8**).

ENDOSCOPY

Use of the smartphone for endoscopic or laryngoscopic procedures is relatively recent. It can be very simple, such as using the flashlight function of the phone to replace a laryngoscope for illumination.[47]

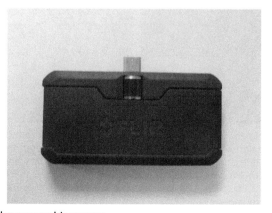

Fig. 7. FLIR ONE thermographic camera.

Otoscopy was one of the first fields to be explored. A prototype was adapted to a standard otorhinoendoscope.[48] This principle was further refined by using a plastic piece, which aligned a magnifying lens and a fiber-optic illumination system with the camera and the LED flash of a smartphone (Cellscope [Cellscope Inc, San Francisco, CA, USA]), increasing portability and accessibility.[49] This device has proven diagnostic abilities in clinical settings in humans. It could also be used easily by nonprofessional users (parents for their children).[50]

Airtraq (Prodol Meditec S.A., Vizcaya, Spain) and King Vision (King systems, Noblesville, IN, USA) are indirect laryngoscopes that allow visualization of the glottis

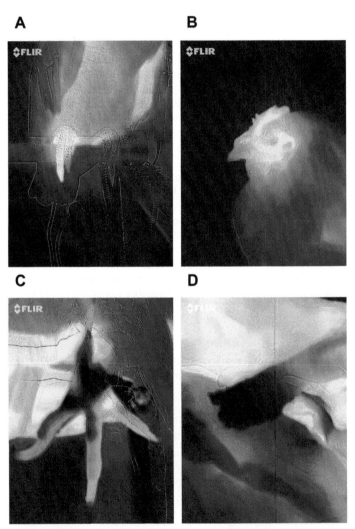

Fig. 8. (*A*) Thermal image of a parrot with lameness taken with an FLIR ONE. Note the higher temperature signal on the affected foot. (*B*) Thermal image of a chicken with an FLIR ONE. Only the skin and adnexal, which are not covered by feathers, are displaying a thermal signature. (*C*) Thermal image of pododermatitis in a red tail hawk with an FLIR ONE. Inflammation can be seen around the ulcerative lesion. (*D*) Thermal image of foot necrosis in a guinea pig with an FLIR ONE.

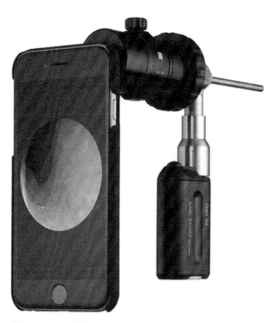

Fig. 9. Smartscope. (*Courtesy of* Karl Storz).

in human patients. Airtraq can be equipped with a smartphone adaptor for the iPhone coupled with an AirView app. It allowed quicker identification of epiglottis, quicker intubation, and easier tracheal tube insertion.[51,52] Coupling smartphone with a flexible fiber-optic endoscope allowed laryngoscopy as well as awake intubation.[53,54]

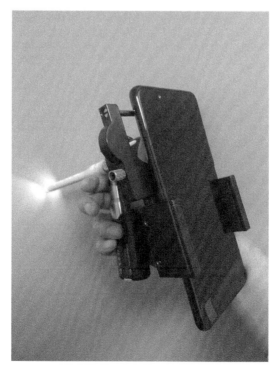

Fig. 10. Clearscope.

Several couplers have been developed to adapt the smartphone on the eyepiece of an endoscope, allowing direct visualization of the smartphone. The main principle is to align and secure the eyepiece of the endoscope, which is usually standard (32 mm), with the high-definition camera of the smartphone. The image is autofocused and reconstructed digitally with the smartphone to be viewed on the screen. There are devices that rely only on the digital zoom to display the image (Endoscope-i, VetOvation) and devices that add a lens that magnifies optically the image (Clearscope, Endokscope [Orange, CA, USA], Smartscope) (**Figs. 9** and **10**). The price is usually higher for the latter device, and because it adds a coupling element, and the whole apparatus is heavier and less handy. To fix the endoscope to the smartphone, a specific metallic or plastic case can be used (Endokscope, Smartscope, VetOvation, Mobile Optx) or a clamp system, which needs adjustment before use. When a case is used, it needs to be fitted with the smartphone, making it specific for each smartphone model.

The overall resolution of cystoscopic images acquired with an iPhone equipped with the Endokscope was comparable to an HD camera, although the latter was superior in quality images.[55] The accessibility was excellent, and training with this device encouraged more endoscopic procedures in urologists in developing countries.[56] Diagnostic accuracy in otorhinolaryngoscopy on human patients was comparable using a Clearscope device compared with an endoscopic traditional tower.[57] Laryngoscopic examinations performed with the Mobile Optx device were also successful[53] (**Table 2**).

Table 2
Smartphone adaptors for endoscope

Device	Technical Characteristics	Smartphone Adapted	Indication	Reference
Endoscope-i (Endoscope-i Ltd, Birmingham, UK)	Very small	iPhone series	Otorhinolaryngoscopy, anesthesia, urology	Mistry et al,[58] 2017
RVA Smart-Clamp (RVA Synergies, Gloucester, UK)		Universal		
VetOvation endoscope adaptor (VetOvation Inc, Raleigh, NC, USA)	Mechanical fixturing	iPhone series	Otoscopy Rhinoscopy	
Endoscope (Endoscope, Orange, CA, USA)	Builtin 8× magnification Mechanical fixturing	iPhone series	ENT, anesthesia, gynecology	Sohn et al,[55] 2013 & Yoon et al,[56] 2018
Clearscope (Clearwater Clinical Limited, Ottawa, Canada)	Built in 8× magnification	Universal	Otoscopy, urology, gynecology	Lee et al,[52] 2016
Smartscope (Karl Storz, Tuttlingen, Germany)	Builtin 8× magnification Mechanical fixturing	iPhone, Samsung Galaxy	Rigid endoscopy	
Mobile Optx (Mobile Optx, Philadelphia, PA, USA)	Built n 8× magnification Mechanical fixturing	iPhone series		Brant et al,[53] 2018

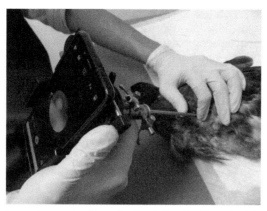

Fig. 11. On-site endoscopic examination of a Harris hawk affected with aspergillosis with a Clearscope.

Several pocket smartphone endoscopes or boroscopes can be found on the market. The camera is usually connected to the smartphone with the mini-USB or the USB-C port. The price is usually minimal, but the image quality is variable; orientation of the camera is difficult, and there are no possibilities to adjust the focus of the lens, which usually relies only on the autofocus of the phone.

The main advantage for using a smartphone over a conventional endoscopic unit is the increased portability, accessibility, transmission, and lower price. Recording of the procedure and teletransmission can be performed instantaneously, which in turn makes it a unique educational tool. Beyond the initial diagnostic purpose, smartphone adapters have improved cross-departmental communications and have been successfully used for teaching and learning. Staff physicians have reported that the frequency of repeat endoscopies to confirm diagnoses has decreased.[59] Discussion between physicians about the video recorded by the smartphone during procedure-improved learning in 81% to 88% of cases.[60]

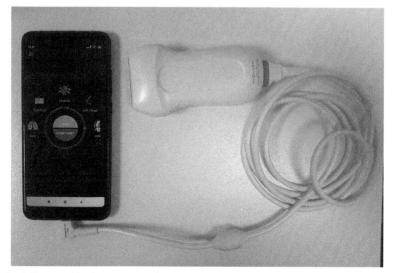

Fig. 12. Philips Lumify Linear L12-4 ultrasound probe.

Endoscopy in exotic pets has multiple applications, including sexing, health check, and surgery[61] (**Fig. 11**). Typically, those procedures could be performed in the field providing safe anesthetic support, avoiding stressful translocation of sensitive individuals. Increased portability of the endoscopic device may facilitate such an examination procedure.

ULTRASOUND

Point-of-care ultrasonography has been developed in emergency medicine as well as cardiology and obstetric medicine. Several ultrasound devices have been developed on the smartphone. The Philips Lumify is a probe that may connect to a smartphone or a tablet via mini-USB or USB-C port (**Fig. 12**). Three probes are developed, a convex 4- to 1-MHz probe, a convex probe 5 to 2 Mhz, and a linear probe 12 to 4 MHz. The device is used with the Android system. It has been successfully evaluated for education purposes, such as identification of wrist structures.[62] It has also been used in plastic surgery to deliver local anesthesia in the abdominal muscular layer and identify the largest perforators flap for reconstructive surgery.[63] Other types of ultrasonography smartphone-based devicea are wireless hand-carried ultrasound. The handheld probe generates a personal wifi connection to the apps, which is installed on an iOS or Android smart device. Three manufacturers have Food and Drug

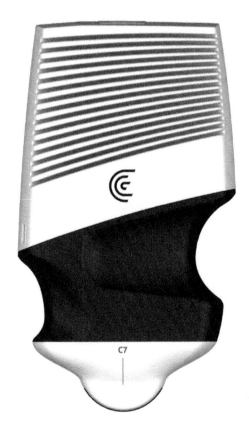

Fig. 13. Clarius wireless ultrasound probe.

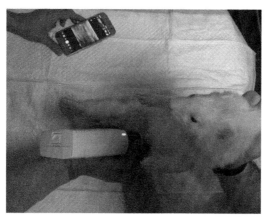

Fig. 14. Use of Clarius wireless ultrasound probe in a ferret presented for acute abdomen.

Adminstration–approved wireless ultrasound (Clarius, Healcerion, Sonostar) (**Fig. 13**). The transducers are relatively heavy because they carry a battery and a generator. The wireless mobile ultrasound device was used and was found useful for cervical assessment during labor in obstetric medicine.[64] Interventional puncture guidance in percutaneous nephrolithotomy has been successfully performed in human patients with such a device.[65]

An immediate application of smartphone-based ultrasound is the FAST (focused assessment with sonography for trauma) ultrasound technique. Although less common in exotic patients compared with dogs and cats, rapid evaluation of the thorax and abdomen can be performed to screen for effusion in emergent situations (**Fig. 14**). Other applications would include local anesthesia, interventional surgery, and field examination (**Fig. 15; Table 3**).

MICROSCOPE

Smartphones can be converted into high-performance microscopes with some additional external hardware. Those devices were initially developed for global health application. One of the most advanced devices, the Cellscope, has been evaluated for tuberculosis and blood-borne parasite screening.[66,67] The Cellscope is a platform consisting of a finite conjugate imaging pathway built into a 3D printed casing,

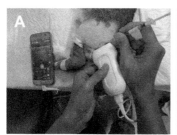
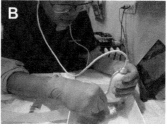

Fig. 15. (*A*) Use of a Philips Lumify to perform a sciatic nerve block in a rabbit undergoing an orthopedic procedure. (*B*) Use of a Philips Lumify to perform an abdominal ultrasound in a goldfish.

Table 3
Smartphone-based hand-carried ultrasound

Manufacturer	Series	Probe	Weight	Connection	Reference
Philips, Reedsville, PA, USA	Lumify S4-1 Lumify C5-2 Lumify L12–4	Microconvex 1–4 MHz Convex 2–5 MHz Linear 4–12 MHz	152 g 136 g 108 g	Cable mini-USB or USB-C Android only	Maetani et al,[62] 2018 & Miller et al,[63] 2018
Clarius Mobile Health Corp, Burnaby, Canada	C3 convex L7 linear C7 Microconvex EC7 endocavity	Convex 2-6 MHz Linear 3–10 MHz Microconvex 4–13 MHz Endo 3–10 MHz	540 g	Wifi iOS or Android	
Healcerion Inc, Seoul, North Korea	Sonon 300C Sonon 300L	Convex 3.5 MHz Linear 5–10 MHz	390 g 370 g	Wifi iOS or Android	Kim et al,[64] 2018
Sonostar Technologies Co Ltd, Guanzou, China	Uprobe-2/3 convex Uprobe-2/3 linear	Convex 3.5-5 MHz Linear 7–10 MHz	308 g	Wifi iOS only	Chen et al,[65] 2018

illuminated with a white LED flashlight. Those types of microscopes can be used in the field, and they open new possibilities regarding quantitative analysis. Quantitative microscopy with the Cellscope device could be performed with multiple smartphones provided they have a high-quality camera (5 MP).[68]

Another type of smartphone-based microscope directly using the integrated flash can be found.[69] The components are 3D printed from electronic files and assembled with an additional mobile phone camera lens. It exploits the principle of using a camera lens from a smartphone, which is reverse mounted to another smartphone, increasing the spatial resolution and a large field of view.[70] The whole device is clipped over a standard smartphone.

Using a smartphone to view a histology or cytology slide allows diagnostic procedure, but is also telediagnostic and provides potentially automated analysis with dedicated software. A whole slide imaging system has been carried out with a smartphone using a conventional microscope equipped with a smartphone adapter and a specific application.[71] It brings perspective for low-cost cell analysis and potentially complete blood cell count in species whereby automated techniques are impaired by the nucleus of erythrocytes and thrombocytes.

Blood analysis has been explored with smartphones, including biochemistry markers, such as glucose, cholesterol, hemoglobin, or vitamin D levels.[72–76] At the moment, such analysis requires specific additional modules, which makes it possible but less practical compared with a standard analyzer. Development of these technologies is recent and will probably evolve significantly in the future.

ACKNOWLEDGMENTS

The author would like to thank Mikel Sabater for his proof review of this paper.

REFERENCES

1. Thomairy NA, Mummaneni M, Alsalamah S, et al. Use of smartphones in hospitals. Health Care Manag (Frederick) 2015;34(4):297–307.
2. Rosser BA, Eccleston C. Smartphone applications for pain management. J Telemed Telecare 2011;17(6):308–12.
3. Ozdalga E, Ozdalga A, Ahuja N. The smartphone in medicine: a review of current and potential use among physicians and students. J Med Internet Res 2012; 14(5):e128.
4. Kulendran M, Lim M, Laws G, et al. Surgical smartphone applications across different platforms: their evolution, uses, and users. Surg Innov 2014;21(4): 427–40.
5. Sun GC, Chen XL, Hou YZ, et al. Image-guided endoscopic surgery for spontaneous supratentorial intracerebral hematoma. J Neurosurg 2017;127(3):537–42.
6. Hirata M, Watanabe R, Koyano Y, et al. Using a motion sensor-equipped smartphone to facilitate CT-guided puncture. Cardiovasc Intervent Radiol 2017;40(4): 609–15.
7. Gregoski MJ, Mueller M, Vertegel A, et al. Development and validation of a smartphone heart rate acquisition application for health promotion and wellness telehealth applications. Int J Telemed Appl 2012;2012:696324.
8. Coppetti T, Brauchlin A, Muggler S, et al. Accuracy of smartphone apps for heart rate measurement. Eur J Prev Cardiol 2017;24(12):1287–93.
9. Ho CL, Fu YC, Lin MC, et al. Smartphone applications (apps) for heart rate measurement in children: comparison with electrocardiography monitor. Pediatr Cardiol 2014;35(4):726–31.
10. Kang SH, Joe B, Yoon Y, et al. Cardiac auscultation using smartphones: pilot study. JMIR Mhealth Uhealth 2018;6(2):e49.
11. Ramanathan A, Zhou L, Marzbanrad F, et al. Digital stethoscopes in paediatric medicine. Acta Paediatr 2019;108(5):814–22.
12. Kraus MS, Gelzer AR, Rishniw M. Detection of heart rate and rhythm with a smartphone-based electrocardiograph versus a reference standard electrocardiograph in dogs and cats. J Am Vet Med Assoc 2016;249(2):189–94.
13. Vezzosi T, Buralli C, Marchesotti F, et al. Diagnostic accuracy of a smartphone electrocardiograph in dogs: comparison with standard 6-lead electrocardiography. Vet J 2016;216:33–7.
14. Vezzosi T, Sgorbini M, Bonelli F, et al. Evaluation of a smartphone electrocardiograph in healthy horses: comparison with standard base-apex electrocardiography. J Equine Vet Sci 2018;67:61–5.
15. Smith J, Heller M, Smith F, et al. Use of an Alivecor Heart Monitor for Heart rate and rhythm evaluation in domestic goats. Paper presented at: ACVIM conference, Denver, June 8–11, 2016.
16. Yaw TJ, Kraus MS, Ginsburg A, et al. Comparison of a smartphone-based electrocardiogram device with a standard six-lead electrocardiogram in the Atlantic bottlenose dolphin (Tursiops truncatus). J Zoo Wildl Med 2018;49(3):689–95.
17. Savarese AS, Locatelli CL, Maurizi NM, et al. Comparative Analysis of a Portable Smartphone-Based Electrocardiograph (D-Heart®) Versus Standard 6-Leads Electrocardiograph in the Canine Patient. Paper presented at: 27th ECVIM-CA Congress, St Julian, September 14–16, 2017.
18. Lord RK, Shah VA, San Filippo AN, et al. Novel uses of smartphones in ophthalmology. Ophthalmology 2010;117(6):1274–1274.e3.

19. Haddock LJ, Kim DY, Mukai S. Simple, inexpensive technique for high-quality smartphone fundus photography in human and animal eyes. J Ophthalmol 2013;2013:518479.

20. Kanemaki N, Inaniwa M, Terakado K, et al. Fundus photography with a smartphone in indirect ophthalmoscopy in dogs and cats. Vet Ophthalmol 2017; 20(3):280–4.

21. Espinheira Gomes F, Ledbetter E. Canine and feline fundus photography and videography using a nonpatented 3D printed lens adapter for a smartphone. Vet Ophthalmol 2019;22(1):88–92.

22. Chen DZ, Tan CW. Smartphone imaging in ophthalmology: a comparison with traditional methods on the reproducibility and usability for anterior segment imaging. Ann Acad Med Singapore 2016;45(1):6–11.

23. Xu X, Ding W, Wang X, et al. Smartphone-based accurate analysis of retinal vasculature towards point-of-care diagnostics. Sci Rep 2016;6:34603.

24. Wu AR, Fouzdar-Jain S, Suh DW. Comparison study of funduscopic examination using a smartphone-based digital ophthalmoscope and the direct ophthalmoscope. J Pediatr Ophthalmol Strabismus 2018;55(3):201–6.

25. Hakimi AA, Lalehzarian SP, Lalehzarian AS, et al. The utility of a smartphone-enabled ophthalmoscope in pre-clinical fundoscopy training. Acta Ophthalmol 2019;97(2):e327–8.

26. Balland O, Russo A, Isard PF, et al. Assessment of a smartphone-based camera for fundus imaging in animals. Vet Ophthalmol 2017;20(1):89–94.

27. Bastawrous A, Giardini M, Bolster NM, et al. Clinical validation of a smartphone-based adapter for optic disc imaging in kenya. JAMA Ophthalmol 2016;134(2): 151–8.

28. Giardini ME, Livingstone IA, Jordan S, et al. A smartphone based ophthalmoscope. Conf Proc IEEE Eng Med Biol Soc 2014;2014:2177–80.

29. Korbel RT. Disorders of the posterior eye segment in raptors—examination procedures and findings. In: Lumeij JT, Remple D, Redig P, editors. Raptor biomedicine III. Lake Worth (FL): Zoological Education Network; 2000. p. 179–93.

30. Lahiri BB, Bagavathiappan S, Jayakumar T, et al. Medical applications of infrared thermography: a review. Infrared Phys Tech 2012;55(4):221–35.

31. Kanazawa T, Nakagami G, Goto T, et al. Use of smartphone attached mobile thermography assessing subclinical inflammation: a pilot study. J Wound Care 2016; 25(4):177–80, 182.

32. Hilsberg-Merz S. Infrared thermography in zoo and wild animals. In: Fowler ME, Miller ER, editors. Zoo and wild animal medicine current therapy. Saint Louis (MI): Saunders Elsevier; 2008. p. 20–33.

33. Hurley-Sanders JL, Bowman KF, Wolfe BA, et al. Use of thermography and fluorescein angiography in the management of a Chilean flamingo with avascular necrosis of the wing. J Avian Med Surg 2012;26(4):255–7.

34. Moe RO, Bohlin J, Flo A, et al. Effects of subclinical footpad dermatitis and emotional arousal on surface foot temperature recorded with infrared thermography in turkey toms (Meleagris gallopavo). Poult Sci 2018;97(7):2249–57.

35. Duncan AE, Torgerson-White LL, Allard SM, et al. An evaluation of infrared thermography for detection of Bumblefoot (Pododermatitis) in penguins. J Zoo Wildl Med 2016;47(2):474–85.

36. Beaufrere H. Infrared thermography of the distal avian pelvic limb. Paper presented at: Exoticscon, Atlanta, September 23–27, 2018.

37. Zhao Y, Xin H, Dong B. Use of infrared thermography to assess laying-hen feather coverage. Poult Sci 2013;92(2):295–302.

38. Jerem P, Herborn K, McCafferty D, et al. Thermal imaging to study stress non-invasively in unrestrained birds. J Vis Exp 2015;105:e53184.

39. Polit M, Rzasa A, Rafajlowicz W, et al. Infrared technology for estrous detection in Chinchilla lanigera. Anim Reprod Sci 2018;197:81–6.

40. Turner TA, Waldsmith J, Marcella K, et al. 2016. Available at: https://aathermology.org/organization-2/guidelines/veterinary-guidelines-for-infrared-thermography/. Accessed November 22, 2018.

41. Fraiwan L, AlKhodari M, Ninan J, et al. Diabetic foot ulcer mobile detection system using smart phone thermal camera: a feasibility study. Biomed Eng Online 2017;16(1):117.

42. Peleki A, da Silva A. Novel use of smartphone-based infrared imaging in the detection of acute limb ischaemia. EJVES Short Rep 2016;32:1–3.

43. Lin PH, Saines M. Assessment of lower extremity ischemia using smartphone thermographic imaging. J Vasc Surg Cases Innov Tech 2017;3(4):205–8.

44. Jaspers MEH, Carriere ME, Meij-de Vries A, et al. The FLIR ONE thermal imager for the assessment of burn wounds: reliability and validity study. Burns 2017;43(7):1516–23.

45. Xue EY, Chandler LK, Viviano SL, et al. Use of FLIR ONE smartphone thermography in burn wound assessment. Ann Plast Surg 2018;80(4 Suppl 4):S236–8.

46. Pereira N, Valenzuela D, Mangelsdorff G, et al. Detection of perforators for free flap planning using smartphone thermal imaging: a concordance study with computed tomographic angiography in 120 perforators. Plast Reconstr Surg 2018;141(3):787–92.

47. Avidan A, Shaylor R, Levin PD. Smartphone assisted laryngoscopy: a new technique to overcome light failure in a laryngoscope. Anesth Analg 2013;117(5):1262–3.

48. Bang JY, Hawes R, Fockens P, et al. Development of an endosonography app: a smart device for continuous education. Gastrointest Endosc 2015;81(5):1299–300.

49. Rappaport KM, McCracken CC, Beniflah J, et al. Assessment of a smartphone otoscope device for the diagnosis and management of otitis media. Clin Pediatr (Phila) 2016;55(9):800–10.

50. Erkkola-Anttinen N, Irjala H, Laine MK, et al. Smartphone otoscopy performed by parents. Telemed J E Health 2019;25(6):477–84.

51. Schoettker P, Corniche J. The AirView study: comparison of intubation conditions and ease between the Airtraq-AirView and the king vision. Biomed Res Int 2015;2015:284142.

52. Lee DW, Thampi S, Yap EP, et al. Evaluation of a smartphone camera system to enable visualization and image transmission to aid tracheal intubation with the Airtraq((R)) laryngoscope. J Anesth 2016;30(3):514–7.

53. Brant JA, Leahy K, Mirza N. Diagnostic utility of flexible fiberoptic nasopharyngolaryngoscopy recorded onto a smartphone: a pilot study. World J Otorhinolaryngol Head Neck Surg 2018;4(2):135–9.

54. Zhou ZQ, Zhao X, Xiang HB. Awake tracheal intubation using combination of an Airtraq((R)) optical laryngoscope with smartphone and video flexible endoscope: a case report. Am J Nucl Med Mol Imaging 2018;8(3):153–8.

55. Sohn W, Shreim S, Yoon R, et al. Endockscope: using mobile technology to create global point of service endoscopy. J Endourol 2013;27(9):1154–60.

56. Yoon R, Capretz T, Patel RM, et al. Global survey of a novel smartphone mobile endoscopy system. J Endourol 2018;32(5):451–4.

57. Liu H, Akiki S, Barrowman NJ, et al. Mobile endoscopy vs video tower: a prospective comparison of video quality and diagnostic accuracy. Otolaryngol Head Neck Surg 2016;155(4):575–80.

58. Mistry N, Coulson C, George A. endoscope-i: an innovation in mobile endoscopic technology transforming the delivery of patient care in otolaryngology. Expert Rev Med Devices 2017;14(11):913–8.

59. Quimby AE, Kohlert S, Caulley L, et al. Smartphone adapters for flexible Nasolaryngoscopy: a systematic review. J Otolaryngol Head Neck Surg 2018;47(1):30.

60. Liu YF, Kim CH, Bailey TW, et al. A prospective assessment of nasopharyngolaryngoscope recording adaptor use in residency training. Otolaryngol Head Neck Surg 2016;155(4):710–3.

61. Divers SJ. Making the difference in exotic animal practice: the value of endoscopy. Vet Clin North Am Exot Anim Pract 2015;18(3):351–7.

62. Maetani TH, Schwartz C, Ward RJ, et al. Enhancement of musculoskeletal radiology resident education with the use of an individual smart portable ultrasound device (iSPUD). Acad Radiol 2018;25(12):1659–66.

63. Miller JP, Carney MJ, Lim S, et al. Ultrasound and plastic surgery: clinical applications of the newest technology. Ann Plast Surg 2018;80(6S Suppl 6):S356–61.

64. Kim J, Kim S, Jeon S, et al. A longitudinal study investigating cervical changes during labor using a wireless ultrasound device. J Matern Fetal Neonatal Med 2018;31(13):1787–91.

65. Chen Y, Zheng H, Zang Z, et al. Real-time ultrasound-guided percutaneous nephrolithotomy using newly developed wireless portable ultrasound: a single-center experience. Surg Innov 2018;25(4):333–8.

66. Tapley A, Switz N, Reber C, et al. Mobile digital fluorescence microscopy for diagnosis of tuberculosis. J Clin Microbiol 2013;51(6):1774–8.

67. D'Ambrosio MV, Bakalar M, Bennuru S, et al. Point-of-care quantification of blood-borne filarial parasites with a mobile phone microscope. Sci Transl Med 2015; 7(286):286re284.

68. Skandarajah A, Reber CD, Switz NA, et al. Quantitative imaging with a mobile phone microscope. PLoS One 2014;9(5):e96906.

69. Orth A, Wilson ER, Thompson JG, et al. A dual-mode mobile phone microscope using the onboard camera flash and ambient light. Sci Rep 2018;8(1):3298.

70. Switz NA, D'Ambrosio MV, Fletcher DA. Low-cost mobile phone microscopy with a reversed mobile phone camera lens. PLoS One 2014;9(5):e95330.

71. Yu H, Gao F, Jiang L, et al. Development of a whole slide imaging system on smartphones and evaluation with frozen section samples. JMIR Mhealth Uhealth 2017;5(9):e132.

72. Yang J. Blood glucose monitoring with smartphone as glucometer. Electrophoresis 2019;40(8):1144–7.

73. Sun K, Yang Y, Zhou H, et al. Ultrabright polymer-dot transducer enabled wireless glucose monitoring via a smartphone. ACS Nano 2018;12(6):5176–84.

74. Oncescu V, Mancuso M, Erickson D. Cholesterol testing on a smartphone. Lab Chip 2014;14(4):759–63.

75. Edwards P, Zhang C, Zhang B, et al. Smartphone based optical spectrometer for diffusive reflectance spectroscopic measurement of hemoglobin. Sci Rep 2017; 7(1):12224.

76. Vemulapati S, Rey E, O'Dell D, et al. A quantitative point-of-need assay for the assessment of vitamin D3 deficiency. Sci Rep 2017;7(1):14142.

Advances in Exotic Animal Clinical Pathology

Sarah Alberton, DMV, IPSAV[a], Claire Vergneau-Grosset, DMV, IPSAV, CES, DACZM[b],
Noémie Summa, DMV, IPSAV, DACZM[b],*

KEYWORDS

- Clinical • Pathology • Review • Advances • Reptiles • Small mammals • Avian

KEY POINTS

- Various novel reference intervals have been published in recent years regarding multiple avian, small mammal, fish, reptile, and amphibian species.
- The effect of specific diseases and environmental factors on hematological, biochemical, acute phase protein, and novel biomarker results has been studied in many exotic species.
- The use of mobile applications is proving useful as a tool in veterinary clinical pathology (eg, in the case of blood smear analysis).

INTRODUCTION

Significant advances have been made in the recent years in exotic animal clinical pathology, including birds, mammals, fish, reptiles, and amphibians, ranging from new techniques and assistance from smart phone applications to the development of more accurate reference intervals. Although increasing numbers of articles are being published on hematology, biochemistry, and blood gas reference intervals, clinicians should be aware that the American Society for Veterinary Clinical Pathology guidelines are less strict regarding the minimal number of individuals required in zoologic medicine species. Indeed, only 20 to 40 species may be sampled to establish a reference interval. In addition, clinicians should remember that reference intervals established in ectotherm species only apply to specific environmental conditions, in addition to the usual restriction regarding variation between different laboratory techniques. Exotic animal clinical pathology is an expanding field of research, and it is the authors' hope to nurture ideas for new research projects through this review of the recent literature and newly available techniques that might find applications in zoologic medicine.

Disclosure Statement: No conflict of interest to report.
[a] Bird and Exotic Animal Department, Laval Veterinary Center, 4530 Highway 440, Laval, Quebec H7T 2P7, Canada; [b] Service de Médecine Zoologique, Université de Montréal, 3200 Rue Sicotte, Saint-Hyacinthe, Québec J2S 2M2, Canada
* Corresponding author.
E-mail address: noemie.summa@umontreal.ca

ADVANCES IN AVIAN CLINICAL PATHOLOGY

Avian hematology is a rapidly evolving field. However, many technical factors can affect the results, such as the technique used to obtain cell counts.[1] Hematology manual cell counting techniques have been compared in some *Strigiformes* species.[2] Significant differences in results between phloxine B technique, Natt and Herrick technique, and estimation from blood smear were observed.[2] This study confirms that method-specific reference intervals should be used when interpreting avian hematology results.[2] Other factors of variation in avian hematology include patient age and sex. Rather than using a single generic reference interval, specific reference intervals considering the patient status are becoming increasingly available. For instance, the effects of age on blood parameters were reported in bald eagles (*Haliaeetus leucocephalus*), in which a decrease in white blood cell count and an increase in total protein concentration were observed as age increased, as reported in other species. Increases in red blood cells, relative heterophil counts and ß-globulin protein fraction, and a decrease in albumin:globulin ratio were also observed.[3]

Interestingly, an automated avian blood cell counting technique has been reported, using high-throughput image cytometry. Although this method showed promise in cell identification, it was not consistent with results using traditional manual techniques. Further research regarding this alternative are needed.[4] Another recent advance regarding avian hematology is the ability to identify cellular types via specific antibodies. For example, an application of this technique was the recent discovery that the host cells of *Leucocytozoon sabrazesi* are in fact in thrombocytes in chickens, while previous studies suggested host cells were leukocytes.[5] *Leucocytozoon* spp. (**Fig. 1**A) is a hemoparasite commonly found in the blood of wild birds from various species. This research highlights the need of further research using cellular identification via specific antibodies for this parasite in different avian species, as well as possibly with other common avian hemoparasites such as hemoproteus (**Fig. 1**B).

Recently, thromboelastography has been evaluated in birds to detect coagulation disorders (**Fig. 2**).[6,7] Overall, healthy Amazon parrot profiles were compatible with hypocoagulable dog profiles.[6] Thus, results of this test should not be overinterpreted in birds. In addition, substantial interspecies variations were highlighted among avian species, and caution should be taken when interpreting thromboelastography results in birds.[7]

Although these techniques have been known for some time, the use of acute-phase proteins and plasma protein electrophoresis in avian medicine is also a developing field. In birds, proteins from the alpha- and beta-globulin fractions are acute-phase

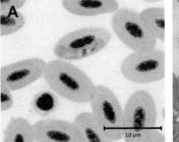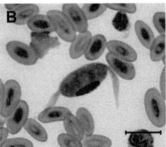

Fig. 1. Hemoparasites observed in the blood film of a wild red-tailed hawk (*Buteo jamaicensis*) stained with Diff quik: (*A*) *Hemoproteus spp.* in an erythrocyte. (*B*) *Leucocytozoon spp.*

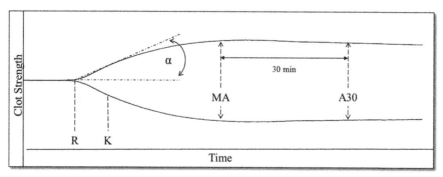

Fig. 2. A representative thromboelastograph from a Hispaniolan Amazon parrot (*Amazona ventralis*). R: reaction time. K: coagulation time. MA: maximum amplitude. A30: Clot strength 30 minutes after maximum amplitude. α angle: rapidity of fibrin cross-linking. (*From* Keller KA, Sanchez-Migallon Guzman D, Acierno MJ, et al. Thromboelastography values in hispaniolan amazon parrots (*Amazona ventralis*): a pilot study. J Avian Med Surg 2015;29:174-80; with permission.)

proteins, whereas gamma-globulins are typically raised in case of chronic inflammation.[8,9] Alpha-lipoprotein, Alpha1-antitrypsin, haptoglobin when present, and alpha2-macroglobulin, migrate with the alpha-globulin fractions while fibronectin, transferrin, and fibrinogen migrate with the beta-globulin fraction.[10] Often a prealbumin fraction is observed in birds,[8] which can be more prominent than albumin in some avian species such as budgerigars (*Melopsittacus undulates*) and monk parakeets (*Myiopsitta monachus*).[9] Conversely, a prealbumin peak is normally absent in Gray parrots (*Psittacus erithacus*), chickens (*Gallus gallus domesticus*),[9] and ostriches (*Struthio camelus*)[11] among others. Beta-globulins are the major globulin fraction in birds, while gamma-globulins are lower than in mammals.[9] Transferrin, which migrates in the beta-globulin fraction, is a positive major acute-phase protein in birds, whereas it is a negative acute-phase protein in mammals.[12] As a result, acute inflammation in birds causes an increase of the beta-globulin fraction, while the beta-globulin fraction is mainly elevated with chronic inflammation in mammals.[9] Reference intervals for plasma electrophoresis protein fractions and haptoglobin have recently been established for American Flamingos (*Phoenicopterus ruber*) among others.[13] This study established a correlation between pododermatitis scores and albumin results, which suggests this parameter may be a marker for pododermatitis, among other causes of inflammation.[13] In studies attempting to establish a correlation between diseases and electrophoretic pattern, control groups are often omitted to focus on case series; therefore protein electrophoresis specificity is seldom evaluated.[10,14,15] The main drawback of electrophoresis is indeed low specificity. A statistical association between decreased prealbumin concentration and aspergillosis has been previously reported in *Falconidae* in a study including a control group.[16] Expression of acute-phase protein in different tissues has recently been described in chickens.[17] Clinical pathologic changes following experimental infection with avian bornavirus have also been studied in African Gray parrots. A study including only 6 individuals showed no signs of acute-phase reaction on plasma protein electrophoresis at early stages of infection. An increase in gamma-globulin fraction 10 weeks after infection and the detection of bornavirus antibodies were correlated with recovery from clinical disease in a few individuals. Because of the small number of individuals and the lack of statistically significant results, further studies are needed.[18]

Due to the high prevalence of atherosclerosis in psittacine birds and in certain other avian species, an increasing number of studies is available regarding lipid panels. Lipid panel reference intervals have been established in Amazon parrots (*Amazona ventralis*).[19,20] Exercise has been shown to increase HDL-C in 12 Amazon parrots with naturally occurring hypercholesterolemia, similar to studies in people.[21] The increase of high density lipoprotein cholesterol (HDL-C) was transient in this study, which may be due to reduced participation in flight sessions within the exercised group over time.[22] A recent study conducted in 6 macaws (*Ara macao*) aimed to observe the effect of increased dietary fructose intake on lipid profiles, as a diet rich in fructose has been associated with cardiovascular disease in people.[23,24] There were no significant differences in lipid panel results following daily administration of a fructose solution for 5 days. However, low density lipoprotein (LDL) levels tended to decrease following the initial removal of fruits in the diet for a month and to subsequently increase 3 months after returning to their original diet in 4 macaws. Although no significant effect was demonstrated, this study suggests potential effects of dietary fructose on dyslipidemia. This raises the question of whether macaws under human care should be provided with high amounts of fruits in their diets. It may be relevant to evaluate the effect on lipid panel with higher amounts of fructose and longer periods of administration in future studies.[25]

Regarding blood biochemistry, equipment requiring minimal blood volumes and new biochemistry parameters is becoming available. For instance, ionized calcium can be measured at patient-side by portable analyzers. Reference intervals for ionized calcium have been published in birds (**Table 1**). The use of various handheld glucometers has been studied in Hispaniolan Amazon Parrots. A specific veterinary glucometer and multiple human meters (colorimetric and amperometric) were investigated. Results were in poor agreement,[26] and glycemia was often underestimated by the glucometers[27] when compared with laboratory analyzer results. The use of blood glucose meters in psittacine birds is therefore not recommended at this point. Diagnosing kidney injury is often difficult in avian patients because of the lack of sensitivity of uric acid plasmatic concentration. The tubular function parameter N-acetyl-b-D-glucosaminidase (NAG) has potential to improve kidney dysfunction detection.[28] An increase in plasma NAG and a severe increase in urine NAG were reported after gentamicin administration in pigeons (*Columba livia domestica*).[29] Serum and urine NAG activity were also studied in Hispaniolan Amazon parrots receiving meloxicam at a standard dosage. No significant changes were detected.[30] Further investigations are needed regarding this parameter. The utility of SDMA (symmetric dimethylarginine), a recently developed glomerular filtration marker, has not been studied in birds to date. Of note, other techniques are more sensitive to evaluated renal function, such as glomerular filtration rate evaluation and endoscopy-guided renal biopsy.[31]

ADVANCES IN MAMMALIAN CLINICAL PATHOLOGY

Reference intervals for blood biochemistry and hematology have been published in rabbits (*Oryctolagus cuniculus*),[41,42] chinchillas (*Chinchilla lanigera*),[43,44] guinea pigs (*Cavia porcellus*),[44,45] ferrets (*Putorius furo*),[46,47] African pygmy hedgehogs (*Atelerix albiventris*),[48] prairie dogs (*Cynomys sp.*),[49–51] hamsters (*Cricetinae sp.*),[52] gerbils (*Gerbillinae sp.*),[52] domestic mice (*Mus musculus*),[52] and recently for the first time in pet rats (*Rattus norvegicus*),[53] as well as urinalysis in some of these species (**Table 2**).[41,52,54–58] As previously explained, most of these papers extrapolated these reference ranges from small population numbers, which does not allow one to account adequately for physiologic variations, such as age and sex. For example, in the recent

Table 1
Reference values for total calcium, and ionized calcium in various exotic species, compared with canine values

Species	Units	Dog (Canis lupus familiaris)[32]	Ferret (Mustela putorius furo)[33]	Rabbit (Oryctolagus cuniculus)[34]	Guinea Pig (Cavia porcellus)[35]	African Gray Parrot (Psittacus erithacus)[36]	Green Iguana (Iguana iguana)[37]	Ball Python (Python regius)[38]	Tortoises (Testudo spp.)[39]	Map Turtle (Graptemys spp.)[40]
Total calcium	mg/dL	9–11.5	8–11.8	11.9–13.9	7.8–10.5	8.2–20.2	8–11	10.4–19.3	11.8–13.3	8.5–12.5
	mmol/L	2.2–3.8	2–2.9	2.98–3.48	2–2.6	2.1–5.1	2–2.8	2.6–4.8	2.95–3.32	2.1–3.1
Ionized calcium	mg/dL	5–6	4.4–5.2	6.4–7.2	5.2–6.8	2.4–2.5	5.6–6.4	6.8–7.6	4.8–6	4.2–4.6
	mmol/L	1.2–1.5	1.09–1.25	1.57–1.83	1.3–1.7	0.59–0.63	1.4–1.6	1.7–1.9	1.2–1.5	1.06–1.14

Table 2
Common urinalysis reference values in exotic companion animals

Parameters	Rabbit[41,54,55]	Chinchilla[56]	Ferret[57,58]	Rodents[52]
Volume (mL/24 h)	Large breeds: 20–350 Average breed 130		24.9 ± 14.3	Gerbils: 1 few drops – 4 Hamster: 5.1–8.4 Mouse: 0.5–2.5 Rat: 13–23
USG (mean)	1.003–1.036	1.014 to >1.060	Male: 1.034–1.070 Female: 1.026–1.060	Hamster: 1.060 Mouse: 1.034 Rat: 1.022–1.050
Average pH	8.2	8.5	Male: 6.0 Female: 6.1	Hamster: 8.5 Mouse: 5.0 Rat: 5–7
TP (g/L)	/	0.462 ± 0.203	Male: 0.068 ± 0.06 Female: 0.066 ± 0.03	Mice: Proteinuria in males Rat: <0.3
Dipstick analysis (% of positive sample in study group)	Trace protein	False positive for protein, up to 4 +	• False positive for trace blood (41%) • Trace protein (80%), higher prevalence in males • Bilirubin 1+ (16%)	/
Sediment analysis	• Calcium carbonate crystals • Occasional leukocytes • Occasional albumin in young rabbit	• Amorphous crystal • Squamous and/or transitional cells • Debris		/

study in pet rats, sex had a significant effect in 10 of the evaluated parameters.[53] Therefore, caution should be applied when interpreting small exotic mammal blood-work results. Of note, Kurloff cells are a leukocyte type, observed in guinea pigs and capybaras (*Hydrochoerus hydrochaeris*) (**Fig. 3**). They contain a single reticulated eosinophilic cytoplasmic inclusion, made of a mucopolysaccharide, and can represent 1% or 2% of the leukocyte count.[45] The exact origin and function of these cells are unknown. They may act as natural killer cells in the general circulation or as protectors of fetal antigen in the placenta, because their numbers can increase under the influence of increased estrogens.[45]

Primary and secondary hyperaldosteronisms have been well described in the veterinary literature; however, published data on these conditions remain scarce in exotic species. Serum aldosterone concentration measurements showed a wide variability among healthy and sick ferrets (n = 78), from 0.02 to 283.9 pg/mL, with 24% of the ferrets having a serum aldosterone concentration above 18 pg/mL.[59] Thus, a high aldosterone concentration should not be considered diagnostic of primary hyperaldosteronism in ferrets, as in other mammals. Although healthy ferrets tended to have lower aldosterone concentration than diseased ferrets, a cut off of 7.6 pg/mL differentiated them with a limited sensitivity of 72.7% and specificity of 73.2%.[59] These results warrant caution when interpreting serum aldosterone concentration in this species.

Similarly, assessment of thyroid function has been challenging in exotic species because of the lack of published data. Reference ranges for thyroid hormones have now been published in guinea pigs,[60,64] ferrets,[46] prairie dogs,[61] and recently in pet rabbits[62,63] (**Table 3**). In one study, the mean value of plasma total thyroxine concentration was significantly lower in sick rabbits, compared with healthy individuals, in favor of an euthyroid sick syndrome in this species similar to what is described in dogs and cats.[62] Therefore, this should be taken into account when interpreting total thyroxine concentration in diseased rabbits.

Knowledge about vitamin D metabolism is expanding in small mammals. A recent study documented oral absorption of dietary vitamin D in sugar gliders (*Petaurus breviceps*) but questioned vitamin D's role in dietary calcium absorption in this

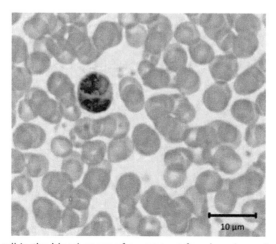

Fig. 3. A Kurloff cell in the blood smear of a pregnant female guinea pig (*Cavia porcellus*), Wright-Giemsa stain.

Table 3
Available reference ranges in plasma thyroid hormones concentrations in exotic species

Species	N	Techniques	TT4 (nmol/L) Mean ± SD, [Range]	fT4 (pmol/L) Mean ± SD, [Range]	TT3 (nmol/L) Mean ± SD, [Range]	fT3 (pmol/L) Mean ± SD, [Range]
Pet rabbit[62]	56	CLIA	[0.8–3.7]			
Rabbits[63]	36–48	RIA eD	35.7 ± 9.6 [18–59]	50.7 ± 16.1 [9–40] 22.9 ± 7.0 [21–80]	0.46 ± 0.13 [0.3–0.7]	6.8 ± 2.4 [1.7–12.4]
Laboratory and pet guinea pigs[60,64]	40 109	CLIA EIA	[14.2–66.9] [29.1–74.9]	16.2–26.1	0.60–0.68	2.84–3.35
Ferrets[46]	94	CLIA	[15.9–42.0]			
Prairie dogs[61]	31	EIA	57.8 ± 30.8 [7.2–103]			

Abbreviations: CIA, chemiluminescence immunoassay; eD, ultrasensitive radioimmunoassay; EIA, enzyme immunoassay; fT, free plasma triiodothyronine concentration; fT4 free plasma thyroxine concentration; N, number of animals included in the study; RI, radioimmunoassay; SD, standard deviation; TT, total plasma triiodothyronine concentration; TT4, plasma total thyroxine concentration.

species.[65] Ionized calcium reference intervals have been published in a few species (see **Table 1**). In lagomorphs and rodents, lack of exposure to UVB and vitamin D deficiency have been hypothesized as a contributing factor to poor bone quality and possibly dental disease.[66] Studies about the effect of artificial UVB radiation on dentistry in small exotic mammals do not all concur.[67] In a terminal prospective study over a 6-month period in 15-week-old New Zealand rabbits (n = 12) and acromelanic albino Hartley guinea pigs (n = 12), prolonged exposure to artificial UVB light sources led to a statistically significant increase in serum 25-hydroxyvitamin D3 concentrations that were sustained overtime compared with the control group, without significant detrimental health effects.[68,69] These findings were similar to previous research in guinea pigs,[70] rabbits,[71] and chinchillas.[72] An increased bilateral corneal thickness was also found in guinea pigs supplemented with UVB compared with those provided ambient light, but this abnormality was not observed in rabbits.[68] No difference in the bone mineral density of the skulls between groups was noted after 6 months. Although daily requirements for vitamin D in small exotic mammals have not been clearly determined, these findings highlight the need for additional research to determine if there is a correlation between disease and plasmatic vitamin D levels in these species.

ADVANCES IN FISH CLINICAL PATHOLOGY

Hematology reference intervals have been published for a variety of fish species.[73] Of note, certain articles report hematology reference values because of the low number of individuals sampled, as recommended by the American Society for Veterinary Clinical Pathology (ASVCP) guidelines.[74,75] A technical difficulty regarding fish hematology is the tendency of fish cells to quickly distort and lyse on smears. In addition, smears should be preserved in a dry location, as any contamination with salt water will result in cell lysis. A possible technique to avoid cell degradation is to store blood with a 1:5 dilution of 10% formaldehyde.[76] In lymphocytic species, the use of the Natt and Herrick technique has been recommended.[77]

Environmental parameters, stocking density, and nutritional status have been shown to significantly affect these values, as exemplified in wild-caught and aquarium-housed lake sturgeon (*Acipenser fulvescens*) and in white-spotted bamboo sharks (*Chiloscyllium plagiosum*), where specimens displayed different reference intervals in an observational study.[73,78] In addition, restraint techniques and phlebotomy site have also been shown to influence hematology results.[79] In contrast, parasitic infestation in wild-caught pike (*Esox lucius*) has been shown to influence hematology results only marginally, with a significant increase of mean corpuscular volume among all hematologic parameters investigated in a case-control study.[80] These findings highlight that blood tests may not be sensitive or specific in fish and should be further investigated to confirm their clinical relevance. Other conditions may cause hematologic changes with significant hematologic changes associated with cyprinid herpesvirus 2 infection in 10 moribund Prussian carp (*Carassius gibelio*),[81] trematode experimental infection in bluegill (*Lepomis macrochirus*),[82] and inflammatory leukograms associated with traumatic wounds of the claspers in white-spotted bamboo sharks.[77] Of note, sharks from this population also showed lower packed cell volumes associated with increased stocking density.[78] Clinicians should remain cautious when extrapolating clinical pathology interpretations from domestic mammal clinical pathology results in fish. Overall, environmental factors should be considered carefully when interpreting fish hematology.

Fish biochemistry reference intervals have also been published.[83–85] Recent studies have evaluated tissular distribution of various enzymes in the red lionfish (*Pterois volitans*)[86] and in the crevalle jack (*Caranx hippos*).[87] Of note, aspartate aminotransferase was found most prevalent in the heart muscle and liver.[87] No reliable marker of renal disease has been determined to date. Thus, it would be relevant to investigate SDMA correlation with renal disease, with the exception of aglomerular fish species such as syngnathidae. Fish biochemistry has recently been shown to be useful to highlight muscle damage associated with certain handling techniques; for example, electro-immobilization is associated with increased creatinine kinase and lactate concentrations compared with fish anesthetized with MS-222.[88]

ADVANCES IN AMPHIBIAN AND REPTILIAN CLINICAL PATHOLOGY

Amphibian and reptilian hematology is an area that would be benefit from technical advances to enable a better understanding of cell function. Immunohistochemistry has been used to differentiate reptile blood cells with a similar morphology, and it is now well established that stain uptake varies among species.[89–92] To assess whether biochemical parameters commonly measured in mammalian panels can be extrapolated to amphibians, the presence of enzymes in various tissues has been recently examined in Cuban tree frogs (*Osteopilus septentrionalis*),[93] as traditionally performed.[8] In addition to these older techniques, new techniques such as microarrays have been used to investigate the effect of feeding on intracellular components, for instance in the intestine of Burmese pythons (*Python bivittatus*).[94] Some findings of these research studies may be clinically applicable in the future. Bench analyzers requiring only a few drops of blood have also enabled the determination of reference intervals in smaller reptilian and amphibian species. Biochemistry and hematology or packed cell volume reference intervals have been recently published for axolotls (*Ambystoma mexicanum*)[95] and tiger salamanders (*Ambystoma tigrinum*)[96] among amphibians, and common chameleons (*Chamaeleo chamaeleon*),[97] panther chameleons (*Furcifer pardalis*),[98] Gila monsters (*Heloderma suspectum*),[99] crested geckos (*Correlophus ciliates*),[100] and leopard geckos (*Eublepharis macularius*) (**Fig. 4**) among others.[101] It is of particular interest to note that azurophils can be observed in high percentages, up to 17%, in healthy chameleons (*Chameleo sp.*).[97] These additional specific reference intervals will contribute to improve reptile medicine.

Although previously questioned by certain authors,[102] hematology and biochemistry are key components of health assessment in reptiles. Ionized calcium reference intervals have been published in a few species (see **Table 1**). Clinicians should remain cautious in their interpretation of these tests, as environmental parameters and common lymph contamination may affect results.[102] However, certain patterns are well established. Gravid female lizards typically display increased values for total calcium, phosphorus, alanine aminotransferase, total protein, albumin, and uric acid. These biochemical modifications can also be noted in cases of reproductive disorders.[103] Determination of the plasma total protein concentration is also helpful in reptile medicine. For instance, hypoalbuminemia and hyperglobulinemia were present in red-eared sliders (*Trachemys scripta elegans*) experimentally infected with a frog virus 3-like ranavirus in a prospective study.[104] It is noteworthy that agreement between point-of-care (iStat, Abaxis) and laboratory analyzers varies depending on the analyte in reptiles.[105] Thus establishing specific reference intervals for these analyzers would be relevant.

Regarding newer blood markers, cardiac troponin is detectable in the cardiac tissue of snakes.[106] However, its use for screening of cardiac disease in reptile is still questionable at this point.[92] The marker of glomerular filtration SDMA is currently under

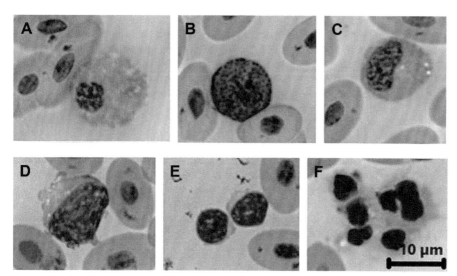

Fig. 4. Blood cells observed on blood smear of a leopard gecko (*Eublepharis macularius*) with Diff Quik stain. (*A*) Heterophil. (*B*) Eosinophil. (*C*) Monocyte. (*D*) Large lymphocyte. (*E*) Small lymphocyte. (*F*) Thrombocytes, which can be easily confused with small lymphocytes.

investigation in chelonians. Few studies have investigated the value of bile acids in reptiles. Reference intervals have been published in green iguanas (*Iguana iguana*),[107] crested geckos,[100] and leopard geckos, among others.[101] Bile acids have also been shown to increase certain case reports (eg, in a green iguana with a cholangiocarcinoma[108] and in a Pacific gopher snake [*Pituophis catenifer*] with a mycobacterial cholecystitis).[109] Expected concentrations of vitamin D metabolites have been described in Hermann tortoises (*Testudo hermanni*),[110] leopard geckos,[111] and Burmese pythons.[112] The use of fibrinogen as marker of acute inflammation is controversial in chelonians. Reference intervals have been recently established in ornate box turtles (*Terrapene ornata ornata*).[113] However, red-eared sliders (*Trachemys scripta elegans*) infected by ranavirus did not show increased fibrinogen despite acute inflammation, but these turtles were kept at 22°C.[114] Expected results and variations for plasma protein electrophoresis have been established recently in green iguanas.[99] Regarding coagulation tests, reference intervals have recently been established for thromboelastography in sea turtles.[115,116]

Various studies have evaluated osmolality in reptiles, including alligators,[117] bearded dragons (*Pogona vitticeps*),[118] loggerhead sea turtles (*Caretta caretta*),[119] and corn snakes (*Pantherophis guttatus*)[120] among others. Overall, osmolality is variable among reptile species, and species-specific formulas should be used to calculate osmolality based on ions concentrations. Sea turtle and corn snake normal osmolarity is higher than that of domestic mammals,[120] while it is similar to dogs in some lizards[118] and lower in alligators.[117] Although this information allows for more accurate interpretation of blood gas values, it is also relevant to choose appropriate fluids in reptiles and can be a prognostic factor in sea turtle rehabilitation.[119]

FUTURE PERSPECTIVES

On a final note, health-based mobile applications are common and considered useful in human patient care.[121] The relevance of these applications for veterinarians and clinical pathologists should not be ignored. Examples that are useful to exotic pet veterinarians are white blood cell count and differential counters such as blood counter.[122] With the increasing potential of cell phones, automated cell recognition is becoming more realistic, and recent studies have investigated phone imaging quality parameters that should improve progress in this direction.[123] Many more examples of cell phone applications exist and deserve to be investigated.

SUMMARY

Specific knowledge on exotic animal clinical pathology has been historically limited when compared with its small animal counterpart. However, important progress has been made in recent years. Many more hematology, biochemistry, and novel marker reference intervals have been established for exotic species. Novel techniques, biomarkers, and clinical changes related to disease have been described in avian, mammal, fish, reptile, and amphibian species. The use of mobile applications has even been suggested to be useful in this field.

REFERENCES

1. Beaufrère H, Ammersbach M. Variability and limitations in clinical avian hematology. In: Speer BL, editor. Current therapy in avian medicine and surgery. St Louis (MO): Elsevier; 2016. p. 467–78.
2. Ammersbach M, Beaufrère H, Gionet Rollick A, et al. Laboratory blood analysis in strigiformes-part I: hematologic reference intervals and agreement between manual blood cell counting techniques. Vet Clin Pathol 2015;44:94–108.
3. Jones MP, Arheart KL, Cray C. Reference intervals, longitudinal analyses, and index of individuality of commonly measured laboratory variables in captive bald eagles (*Haliaeetus leucocephalus*). J Avian Med Surg 2014;28:118–26.
4. Beaufrere H, Ammersbach M, Tully TN Jr. Complete blood cell count in psittaciformes by using high-throughput image cytometry: a pilot study. J Avian Med Surg 2013;27:211–7.
5. Zhao W, Liu J, Xu R, et al. The gametocytes of *Leucocytozoon sabrazesi* infect chicken thrombocytes, not other blood cells. PLoS One 2015;10:e0133478.
6. Keller KA, Sanchez-Migallon Guzman D, Acierno MJ, et al. Thromboelastography values in hispaniolan Amazon parrots (*Amazona ventralis*): a pilot study. J Avian Med Surg 2015;29:174–80.
7. Strindberg S, Nielsen TW, Ribeiro AM, et al. Thromboelastography in selected avian species. J Avian Med Surg 2015;29:282–9.
8. Lumeij JT. Avian clinical biochemistry. In: Kaneko JJ, Harvey JW, Bruss ML, editors. Clinical biochemistry of domestic animals. San Diego (CA): Academic Press; 2008. p. 839–72.
9. Melillo A. Applications of serum protein electrophoresis in exotic pet medicine. Vet Clin North Am Exot Anim Pract 2013;16:211–25.
10. Briscoe JA, Rosenthal KL, Shofer FS. Selected complete blood cell count and plasma protein electrophoresis parameters in pet psittacine birds evaluated for illness. J Avian Med Surg 2010;24:131–7.
11. Black PA, Macek M, Tieber A, et al. Reference values for hematology, plasma biochemical analysis, plasma protein electrophoresis, and *Aspergillus* serology in elegant-crested tinamou (*Eudromia elegans*). J Avian Med Surg 2013;27:1–6.
12. Cray C. Biomarkers of inflammation in exotic pets. J Exot Pet Med 2013;22(3):245–50.

13. Delk KW, Wack RF, Burgdorf-Moisuk A, et al. Acute phase protein and electrophoresis protein fraction values for captive American flamingos (*Phoenicopterus Ruber*). J Zoo Wildl Med 2015;46:929–33.

14. Lanzarot MP, Montesinos A, San Andres MI, et al. Hematological, protein electrophoresis and cholinesterase values of free-living nestling peregrine falcons in Spain. J Wildl Dis 2001;37:172–7.

15. Villar D, Kramer M, Howard L, al Het. Clinical presentation and pathology of sarcocystosis in psittaciform birds: 11 cases. Avian Dis 2008;52:187–94.

16. Kummrow M, Silvanose C, Di Somma A, et al. Serum protein electrophoresis by using high-resolution agarose gel in clinically healthy and *Aspergillus* species-infected falcons. J Avian Med Surg 2012;26:213–20.

17. Marques AT, Nordio L, Lecchi C, et al. Widespread extrahepatic expression of acute-phase proteins in healthy chicken (*Gallus gallus*) tissues. Vet Immunol Immunopathol 2017;190:10–7.

18. Hogemann C, Richter R, Korbel R, et al. Plasma protein, haematologic and blood chemistry changes in African grey parrots (*Psittacus erithacus*) experimentally infected with bornavirus. Avian Pathol 2017;46:556–70.

19. Michelle Ravich CC, Hess Laurie, Kristopher L. Arheart. Lipid panel reference intervals for Amazon parrots (*Amazona* species). J Avian Med Surg 2014;28:7.

20. Vergneau-Grosset C, Polley T, Holt DC, et al. Hematologic, plasma biochemical, and lipid panel reference intervals in orange-winged Amazon parrots (*Amazona amazonica*). J Avian Med Surg 2016;30:335–44.

21. Vanhees L, Geladas N, Hansen D, et al. Importance of characteristics and modalities of physical activity and exercise in the management of cardiovascular health in individuals with cardiovascular risk factors: recommendations from the EACPR. Eur J Prev Cardiol 2012;19:1005–33.

22. Gustavsen KA, Stanhope KL, Lin AS, et al. Effects of exercise on the plasma lipid profile in Hispaniolan Amazon parrots (*Amazona ventralis*) with naturally occurring hypercholesterolemia. J Zoo Wildl Med 2016;47:760–9.

23. Kolderup A, Svihus B. Fructose metabolism and relation to atherosclerosis, type 2 diabetes, and obesity. J Nutr Metab 2015;15:823081.

24. Stanhope KL, Bremer AA, Medici V, et al. Consumption of fructose and high fructose corn syrup increase postprandial triglycerides, LDL-cholesterol, and apolipoprotein-B in young men and women. J Clin Endocrinol Metab 2011;96:1596–605.

25. Béland K, Desmarchelier M, Ferrell ST, et al. Impact of dietary fructose on the lipid profile in six macaws – a pilot study. Paper presented at: Joint EAZWV/AAZV/Leibniz-IZW Conf. Prague, Czech republic, October 6–12, 2018.

26. Acierno MJ, Schnellbacher R, Tully TN Jr. Measuring the level of agreement between a veterinary and a human point-of-care glucometer and a laboratory blood analyzer in Hispaniolan Amazon parrots (*Amazona ventralis*). J Avian Med Surg 2012;26:221–4.

27. Acierno MJ, Mitchell MA, Schuster PJ, et al. Evaluation of the agreement among three handheld blood glucose meters and a laboratory blood analyzer for measurement of blood glucose concentration in Hispaniolan Amazon parrots (*Amazona ventralis*). Am J Vet Res 2009;70:172–5.

28. Speer BL. Advances in clinical pathology and diagnostic medicine. In: Speer BL, editor. Current therapy in avian medicine and surgery. St Louis (MO): Elsevier; 2016. p. 461–530.

29. Wimsatt J, Canon N, Pearce RD, et al. Assessment of novel avian renal disease markers for the detection of experimental nephrotoxicosis in pigeons (*Columba livia*). J Zoo Wildl Med 2009;40:487–94.

30. Dijkstra B, Guzman DS, Gustavsen K, et al. Renal, gastrointestinal, and hemostatic effects of oral administration of meloxicam to Hispaniolan Amazon parrots (*Amazona ventralis*). Am J Vet Res 2015;76:308–17.

31. Scope A, Schwendenwein I, Schauberger G. Plasma exogenous creatinine excretion for the assessment of renal function in avian medicine–pharmacokinetic modeling in racing pigeons (*Columba livia*). J Avian Med Surg 2013;27: 173–9.

32. de Brito Galvao JF, Schenck PA, Chew DJ. A quick reference on hypercalcemia. Vet Clin North Am Small Anim Pract 2017;47:241–8.

33. Sarah A, Cannizzo MR, Tara M, et al. Parathyroid hormone, ionized calcium, and 25-hydroxyvitamin D concentrations in the domestic ferret (*Mustela putorius furo*). J Exot Pet Med 2017;26(4):294–9.

34. Warren HB, Lausen NC, Segre GV, et al. Regulation of calciotropic hormones in vivo in the New Zealand white rabbit. J Endocrinol 1989;125:2683–90.

35. Watson MK, Stern AW, Labelle AL, et al. Evaluating the clinical and physiological effects of long term ultraviolet B radiation on guinea pigs (*Cavia porcellus*). PLoS One 2014;9:e114413.

36. de Carvalho FM, Gaunt SD, Kearney MT, et al. Reference intervals of plasma calcium, phosphorus, and magnesium for African grey parrots (*Psittacus erithacus*) and Hispaniolan parrots (*Amazona ventralis*). J Zoo Wildl Med 2009;40: 675–9.

37. Dennis PM, Bennett RA, Harr KE, et al. Plasma concentration of ionized calcium in healthy iguanas. J Am Vet Med Assoc 2001;219:326–8.

38. Hedley J, Eatwell K. The effects of UV light on calcium metabolism in ball pythons (*Python regius*). Vet Rec 2013;173:345.

39. Eatwell K. Calcium and phosphorus values and their derivatives in captive tortoises (*Testudo* species). J Small Anim Pract 2010;51:472–5.

40. Hernandez-Divers SJ, Hensel P, Gladden J, et al. Investigation of shell disease in map turtles (*Graptemys* spp.). J Wildl Dis 2009;45:637–52.

41. Melillo A. Rabbit clinical pathology. J Exot Pet Med 2007;16(3):135–45.

42. Christopher MM, Hawkins MG, Burton AG. Poikilocytosis in rabbits: prevalence, type, and association with disease. PLoS One 2014;9:e112455.

43. Silva TdO, Kreutz LC, Barcellos LJG, et al. Reference values for chinchilla (*Chinchilla laniger*) blood cells and serum biochemical parameters. Ciência Rural 2005;35(3):602–6.

44. Quesenberry KE, Donnelly TM, Mans C. Biology, husbandry, and clinical techniques of guinea pigs and chinchillas. In: Ferrets, rabbits, and rodents. St Louis (MI): Elsevier saunders; 2012. p. 279–94.

45. Zimmerman K, Moore DM, Smith SA. Hematological assessment in pet guinea pigs (*Cavia porcellus*): blood sample collection and blood cell identification. Vet Clin North Am Exot Anim Pract 2015;18:33–40.

46. Hein J, Spreyer F, Sauter-Louis C, et al. Reference ranges for laboratory parameters in ferrets. Vet Rec 2012;171(9).

47. Smith SA, Zimmerman K, Moore DM. Hematology of the domestic ferret (*Mustela putorius furo*). Vet Clin North Am Exot Anim Pract 2015;18:1–8.

48. Okorie-Kanu CO, Onoja RI, Achegbulu EE, et al. Normal haematological and serum biochemistry values of African hedgehog (*Atelerix albiventris*). Comp Clin Path 2015;24:127–32.

49. Broughton G 2nd. Hematologic and blood chemistry data for the prairie dog (*Cynomys ludovicianus*). Comp Biochem Physiol Comp Physiol 1992;101:807.

50. Gardhouse SM, Eshar D, Bello N, et al. Venous blood gas analytes during iso-flurane anesthesia in black-tailed prairie dogs (*Cynomys ludovicianus*). J Am Vet Med Assoc 2015;247:404–8.

51. Wyre N, Eshar D. Serum bile acids concentration in captive black-tailed prairie dogs (*Cynomys ludovicianus*). Comp Clin Path 2016;25:47–51.

52. Lennox AM, Bauck L. Basic anatomy, physiology, husbandry, and clinical tech-niques. In: Ferrets, rabbits, and rodents. St Louis (MI): Elsevier saunders; 2012. p. 339–53.

53. Houtmeyers A, Duchateau L, Grünewald B, et al. Reference intervals for biochemical blood variables, packed cell volume, and body temperature in pet rats (*Rattus norvegicus*) using point-of-care testing. Vet Clin Pathol 2016; 45:669–79.

54. Jenkins JR. Rabbit diagnostic testing. J Exot Pet Med 2008;17(1):4–15.

55. Quesenberry KE. Basic approach to veterinary care. In: Ferrets, rabbits, and ro-dents. St Louis (MI): Elsevier saunders; 2003. p. 13–24.

56. Doss GA, Mans C, Houseright RA, et al. Urinalysis in chinchillas (*Chinchilla la-nigera*). J Am Vet Med Assoc 2016;248:901–7.

57. Eshar D, Wyre N, Brown D. Urine specific gravity values in clinically healthy young pet ferrets (*Mustela furo*). J Small Anim Pract 2012;53:115–9.

58. Esteves M, Marini R, Ryden E, et al. Estimation of glomerular filtration rate and evaluation of renal function in ferrets (*Mustela putorius furo*). Am J Vet Res 1994; 55:166–72.

59. Di Girolamo N, Fecteau K, Carnimeo A, et al. Variability of serum aldosterone concentrations in pet ferrets (*Mustela putorius furo*). J Am Vet Med Assoc 2018;252:1372–6.

60. Müller K, Müller E, Klein R, et al. Serum thyroxine concentrations in clinically healthy pet guinea pigs (*Cavia porcellus*). Vet Clin Pathol 2009;38:507–10.

61. Eshar D, Nau MR, Pohlman LM. Plasma thyroxine (T4) concentration in zoo-kept black-tailed prairie dogs (*Cynomys ludovicianus*). J Zoo Wildl Med 2017;48: 116–20.

62. Milena Thöle TB, Fehr M, Schmicke M. Plasma thyroxine levels in healthy and sick domestic rabbits (*Oryctolagus cuniculus*). Paper presented at: Exoticscon. Atlanta, September 22–27, 2018.

63. Joao Brandao MR, Tully T. Measurement of serum free and total thyroxine and triiodothyronine concentrations in rabbits. Paper presented at: Exoticscon. Port-land, August 27-September 1, 2016.

64. Fredholm DVCL, Johnston MS. Evaluation of precision and establishment of reference ranges for plasma thyroxine using a point-of-care analyzer in healthy guinea pigs (*Cavia porcellus*). J Exot Pet Med 2012;21(1):87–93.

65. Dierenfeld ES, Pernikoff D, Brewer P. Dietary vitamin D3 influence on serum 25-hydroxy vitamin D concentrations in captive sugar gliders (*Petaurus breviceps*). J Exot Pet Med 2018;27(4):48–52.

66. Harcourt-Brown F. Calcium deficiency, diet and dental disease in pet rabbits. Vet Rec 1996;139:567.

67. Thilliez N, Larrat S, Vergneau-Grosset C. Lack of association between exposure du natural sunlight and dental disease in French companion rabbits. J Vet Med Surg 2017;1:13–9.

68. Watson M, Stern AW, Labelle AL, et al. Evaluating the clinical and physiological effects of long term ultraviolet B radiation on guinea pigs (*Cavia porcellus*) and rabbits (*Oryctolagus cuniculus*). PLoS One 2014;9(12):e114413.

69. Watson MK, Mitchell MA, Stern AW, et al. Evaluating the clinical and physiological effects of long term ultraviolet b radiation on rabbits (*Oryctolagus cuniculus*). J Exot Pet Med 2018;28(1):43–55.

70. Sander SJ, Mitchell MA, Whittington JK, et al. Effects of artificial ultraviolet radiation on serum 25-hydroxyvitamin d3 concentrations in captive guinea pigs (*Cavia porcellus*). J Exot Pet Med 2015;24(4):464–9.

71. Emerson JA, Whittington JK, Allender MC, et al. Effects of ultraviolet radiation produced from artificial lights on serum 25-hydroxyvitamin D concentration in captive domestic rabbits (*Oryctolagus cuniculi*). Am J Vet Res 2014;75:380–4.

72. Rivas AE, Mitchell MA, Flower J, et al. Effects of ultraviolet radiation on serum 25-hydroxyvitamin D concentrations in captive chinchillas (*Chinchilla laniger*). J Exot Pet Med 2014;23(3):270–6.

73. DiVincenti L, Priest H, Walker KJ, et al. Comparison of select hematology and serum chemistry analytes between wild-caught and aquarium-housed lake sturgeon (*Acipenser fulvescens*). J Zoo Wildl Med 2013;44:957–64.

74. Harms C, Ross T, Segars A. Plasma biochemistry reference values of wild bonnethead sharks, *Sphyrna tiburo*. Vet Clin Pathol 2002;31:111–5.

75. Ferreira CM, Field CL, Tuttle AD. Hematological and plasma biochemical parameters of aquarium-maintained cownose rays. J Aquat Anim Health 2010; 22:123–8.

76. Arnold JE, Matsche MA, Rosemary K. Preserving whole blood in formalin extends the specimen stability period for manual cell counts for fish. Vet Clin Pathol 2014;43:613–20.

77. Alexander AB, Parkinson LA, Grant KR, et al. The hemic response of whitespotted bamboo sharks (*Chiloscyllium plagiosum*) with inflammatory disease. Zoo Biol 2016;35:251–9.

78. Parkinson LA, Alexander AB, Campbell TW. Variability in hematology of whitespotted bamboo sharks (*Chiloscyllium plagiosum*) in different living environments. Zoo Biol 2017;36:284–8.

79. Naples LM, Mylniczenko ND, Zachariah TT, et al. Evaluation of critical care blood analytes assessed with a point-of-care portable blood analyzer in wild and aquarium-housed elasmobranchs and the influence of phlebotomy site on results. J Am Vet Med Assoc 2012;241:117–25.

80. Fallah FJ, Khara H, Rohi JD, et al. Hematological parameters associated with parasitism in pike, *Esox lucius* caught from Anzali wetland. J Parasit Dis 2015;39:245–8.

81. Lu J, Lu H, Cao G. Hematological and histological changes in Prussian carp *Carassius gibelio* infected with cyprinid herpesvirus 2. J Aquat Anim Health 2016;28:150–60.

82. Calhoun DM, Schaffer PA, Gregory JR, et al. Experimental infections of bluegill with the trematode *Ribeiroia ondatrae (Digenea: cathaemasiidae)*: histopathology and hematological response. J Aquat Anim Health 2015;27:185–91.

83. Tripathi NK, Latimer KS, Burnley VV. Hematologic reference intervals for koi (*Cyprinus carpio*), including blood cell morphology, cytochemistry, and ultrastructure. Vet Clin Pathol 2004;33:74–83.

84. Palmeiro BS, Rosenthal KL, Lewbart GA, et al. Plasma biochemical reference intervals for koi. J Am Vet Med Assoc 2007;230:708–12.

85. Otway NM. Serum biochemical reference intervals for free-living sand tiger sharks (*Carcharias taurus*) from east Australian waters. Vet Clin Pathol 2015; 44:262–74.

86. Anderson ET, Stoskopf MK, Morris JA Jr, et al. Hematology, plasma biochemistry, and tissue enzyme activities of invasive red lionfish captured off North Carolina, USA. J Aquat Anim Health 2010;22:266–73.

87. Cutler D, Davis M, Stacy N, et al. Tissue enzyme activities in the crevalle Jack. Paper presented at: Joint EAZWV/AAZV/Leibniz-IZW Conference. Prague, Czech Republic, October 6–12, 2018.

88. Lamglait B, Lair S. Ethical considerations for electro-immobilization in adult brook trout (Salvelinus frontinalis). Paper presented at: Joint EAZWV/AAZV/Leibniz-IZW Conference. Prague, Czech Republic, October 6–12, 2018.

89. Alleman AR, Jacobson ER, Raskin RE. Morphologic, cytochemical staining, and ultrastructural characteristics of blood cells from eastern diamondback rattlesnakes (*Crotalus adamanteus*). Am J Vet Res 1999;60:507–14.

90. Martinez-Silvestre A, Marco I, Rodriguez-Dominguez MA, et al. Morphology, cytochemical staining, and ultrastructural characteristics of the blood cells of the giant lizard of El Hierro (*Gallotia simonyi*). Res Vet Sci 2005;78:127–34.

91. Perpinan D, Sanchez C. Morphology, cytochemisty staining and ultrastructual characteristics of blood cells from European pond turtles (*Emys orbicularis*) and the Mediterranean pond turtle (*Mauremys leprosa*). J Herpetol Med Surg 2009;19:119–27.

92. Feltrer Y, Strike T, Routh A, et al. Point-of-care cardiac troponin I in non-domestic species: a feasibility study. J Zoo Aq Res 2016;4(2):99–103.

93. Bogan JEJ, Mitchell MA. Characterizing tissue enzyme activities of Cuban tree frogs (*Osteopilus septentrionalis*). J Herpetol Med Surg 2017;27:22–8.

94. Secor SM. Evolutionary and cellular mechanisms regulating intestinal performance of amphibians and reptiles. Integr Comp Biol 2005;45:282–94.

95. Takami Y, Une Y. Blood clinical biochemistries and packed cell volumes in the Mexican axolotl (*Ambyostomma mexicanum*). J Herpetol Med Surg 2017;27: 104–10.

96. Brady S, Burgdorf-Moisuk A, Kass PH, et al. Hematology and plasma biochemistry intervals for captive-born California tiger salamanders (*Ambystoma californiense*). J Zoo Wildl Med 2016;47:731–5.

97. Eshar D, Ammersbach M, Shacham B, et al. Venous blood gases, plasma biochemistry, and hematology of wild-caught common chameleons (*Chamaeleo chamaeleon*). Can J Vet Res 2018;82:106–14.

98. Laube A, Pendl H, Clauss M, et al. Plasma biochemistry and hematology reference values of captive panther chameleons (*Furcifer pardalis*) with special emphasis on seasonality and gender differences. J Zoo Wildl Med 2016;47: 743–53.

99. Cooper-Bailey K, Smith SA, Zimmerman K, et al. Hematology, leukocyte cytochemical analysis, plasma biochemistry, and plasma electrophoresis of wild-caught and captive-bred Gila monsters (*Heloderma suspectum*). Vet Clin Pathol 2011;40:316–23.

100. Mayer J, Knoll J, Wrubel K, et al. Characterizing the hematologic and plasma chemistry profiles of captive crested geckos (*Rhacodactylus ciliatus*). J Herpetol Med Surg 2011;21:68–75.

101. Alberton S, Cojean O, Froment R, et al. Determination of leopard gecko (*Eublepharis macularius*) packed cell volume and plasma biochemistry reference

intervals and reference values. Paper presented at: Exoticscon conference. Atlanta, GA, September 22–27, 2018.

102. Sykes JM, Klaphake E. Reptile hematology. Vet Clin North Am Exot Anim Pract 2008;11:481–500.

103. Cuadrado M, Diaz-Paniagua C, Quevedo MA, et al. Hematology and clinical chemistry in dystocic and healthy post-reproductive female chameleons. J Wildl Dis 2002;38:395–401.

104. Moore AR, Allender MC, MacNeill AL. Effects of ranavirus infection of red-eared sliders (*Trachemys scripta elegans*) on plasma proteins. J Zoo Wildl Med 2014; 45:298–305.

105. Di Girolamo N, Ferlizza E, Selleri P, et al. Evaluation of point-of-care analysers for blood gas and clinical chemistry in Hermann's tortoises (*Testudo hermanni*). J Small Anim Pract 2018;59:704–13.

106. Bogan JEJ. Measuring cardiac troponin i in snake cardiac muscle: a pilot study. J Herpetol Med Surg 2017;27:127–9.

107. McBride M, Divers SJ, Koch TF, et al. Preliminary evaluation of pre- and postprandial 3-alphahydroxy bile acids in the green iguana (Iguana iguana). J Herpetol Med Surg 2006;16:129–34.

108. Wilson GH, Fontenot DK. Pseudocarcinomatous biliary hyperplasia in two green iguanas, I*guana iguana*. J Herpetol Med Surg 2004;14:12–8.

109. Kinney ME, Chinnadurai SKC, Wack RE. Cholecystectomy for the treatment of mycobacterial cholecystitis in a pacific gopher snake (Pituophis catenifer). J Herpetol Med Surg 2013;23:10–4.

110. Selleri P, Di Girolamo N. Plasma 25-hydroxyvitamin D(3) concentrations in Hermann's tortoises (*Testudo hermanni*) exposed to natural sunlight and two artificial ultraviolet radiation sources. Am J Vet Res 2012;73:1781–6.

111. Gould A, Molitor L, Rockwell K, et al. Evaluating the physiologic effects of short duration ultraviolet B radiation exposure in leopard geckos (*Eublepharis macularius*). J Herpetol Med Surg 2018;28:34–9.

112. Bos JH, Klip FC, Oonincx D. Artificial ultraviolet b radiation raises plasma 25-hydroxyvitamin d3 concentrations in Burmese pythons (*Python bivittatus*). J Zoo Wildl Med 2018;49:810–2.

113. Parkinson L, Olea-Popelka F, Klaphake E, et al. Establishment of a fibrinogen reference interval in ornate box turtles (*Terrapene ornata ornata*). J Zoo Wildl Med 2016;47:754–9.

114. Moore AR, Allender MC, Mitchell MA, et al. Evaluation of plasma fibrinogen concentration as a diagnostic indicator of inflammation in red-eared sliders (*Trachemys scripta elegans*). J Am Vet Med Assoc 2015;246:245–53.

115. Barratclough A. Baseline thromboelastography in Kemp's ridley (Lepidochelys kempii), green (Chelonia mydas) and loggerhead (Caretta caretta) sea turtles and its use to diagnose coagulopathies in cold-stunned Kemp's ridley and green sea turtles. Paper presented at: Annual conference of the Internation Association for Aquarium Animal Medicine. Long Beach, CA, May 19–23, 2018.

116. Barratclough A, Hanel R, Stacy NI, et al. Establishing a protocol for thromboelastography in sea turtles. Vet Rec Open 2018;5:e000240.

117. Nevarez JG, Acierno MJ, Angel M, et al. Determination of agreement between measured and calculated plasma osmolality values in captive-reared American alligators (*Alligator mississippiensis*). J Herpetol Med Surg 2012;22:36–41.

118. Dallwig RK, Mitchell MA, Acierno MJ. Determination of plasma osmolality and agreement between measured and calculated values in healthy bearded dragons (*Pogona vitticeps*). J Herpetol Med Surg 2010;20:69–73.

119. Camacho M, Quintana MP, Luzardo OP, et al. Metabolic and respiratory status of stranded juvenile loggerhead sea turtles (*Caretta caretta*): 66 cases (2008-2009). J Am Vet Med Assoc 2013;242:396–401.
120. Sanchez-Migallon Guzman D, Mitchell MA, Acierno M. Determination of plasma osmolality and agreement between measured and calculated values in captive male corn snakes (*Pantherophis guttatus guttatus*). J Herpetol Med Surg 2011; 21:16–9.
121. Pal S. Hematology on the move: how are mobile health apps helping patients?. 2016. Available at: https://www.ashclinicalnews.org/features/hematology-on-the-move-how-are-mobile-health-apps-helping-patients/. Accessed July 11, 2019.
122. Google Play. Blood counter. 2018. Available at: https://play.google.com/store/apps/details?id=com.ksoftapps.ta.diffrentialbloodcounter&hl=en_US. Accessed July 11, 2019.
123. Skandarajah A, Reber CD, Switz NA, et al. Quantitative imaging with a mobile phone microscope. PLoS One 2014;9:e96906.

Technological Advances in Herpetoculture

Tariq Abou-Zahr, BVSc, CertAVP(ZooMed), MRCVS[a],*,
Daniel Calvo Carrasco, LV, CertAVP(ZooMed), DECZM(Avian), MRCVS[b]

KEYWORDS

- Herpetoculture • Herpetology • Terrarium • Husbandry • Lighting • Record-keeping
- LED

KEY POINTS

- Technology plays an especially vital role in herpetoculture in comparison with other animal-keeping sectors because ectothermic animals rely so heavily on their environment to carry out basic physiologic functions.
- Controlling the environment appropriately is key to ensuring the health and welfare of the reptiles and amphibians being cared for.
- The authors predict there will be many more advances in herpetocultural technology in the years immediately following publication of this article.

INTRODUCTION

There is evidence that reptiles and amphibians have been kept in captivity in some capacity for centuries. For example, William Laud, Bishop of London, purchased a spur-thighed tortoise in 1625, according to historical records.[1] The serious and widely practiced keeping and breeding of reptiles and amphibians in captivity, however, has only really been taking place for approximately 50 years.[2] This means that the science of herpetoculture (the keeping of reptiles and amphibians in captivity) is relatively new and is evolving at a rapid rate. Standards of husbandry have continued to improve with every decade that has passed and, for many species, current science focuses on refining husbandry to improve their welfare in captivity, considering issues such as environmental enrichment.[3] It is interesting to consider that it was only a few decades previous that the focus was only on how to keep the animals alive.

Technology plays an especially vital role in herpetoculture in comparison with other animal-keeping sectors because ectothermic animals rely so heavily on their

Disclose Statement: The authors have nothing to disclose.
[a] Valley Vets, 180 Merthyr Road, Whitchurch, Cardiff CF14 1DL, UK; [b] Great Western Exotic Vets, Unit 10, Berkshire House, County Business Park, Shrivenham Road, Wiltshire, Swindon SN1 2NR, UK
* Corresponding author.
E-mail address: ta9797@my.bristol.ac.uk

Vet Clin Exot Anim 22 (2019) 387–396
https://doi.org/10.1016/j.cvex.2019.06.007
vetexotic.theclinics.com

environment to carry out basic physiologic functions. Controlling the environment appropriately is key to ensuring the health and welfare of the reptiles and amphibians in our care. The authors predict that there will be many more advances in herpetocultural technology in the years immediately following publication of this article. It is worthwhile for herpetoculturists and veterinarians to keep up to date with recent technological advances because many could potentially significantly improve the lives of the animals we care for. This article summarizes some of the technological advances and technological products that are currently relevant in herpetoculture.

LIGHTING AND HEATING

Infrared, visible, and ultraviolet (UV) radiation are all crucially important for the health and welfare of reptiles and amphibians. They must all be provided to an appropriate degree to captive animals.[4] The premise that captive reptiles and amphibians should be provided with a thermal gradient is long established.[5] However, it is now also recognized that a lighting gradient, for both UV and visible light, spanning from a bright area to a shaded area is also of great importance.[6] Several technological advances have been made over the last decade with regard to the provision of heat, UV, and visible light to captive reptiles and amphibians, and this continues to be a rapidly developing avenue within herpetoculture.

Visible Light

Visible light, although often not considered to have the same degree of importance as UV light, has significant psychological and behavioral effects on many species.[7] In the naturalistic terrarium, it is also essential for plant growth.

When considering the visible light emitted from a lamp, it is useful to be familiar with the relevant units of measurement. The total amount of visible light emitted by a lamp is measured in lumens. In a terrarium or vivarium situation, however, the lumen measure of a lamp does not necessarily indicate whether the enclosure will appear bright to the human eye. Perception of light by the human eye does not depend on the total amount of light but on the light that is incident on the vivarium or terrarium surfaces. The amount of light incident on a surface is termed illuminance, or lumens per square meter.[8] The overall color temperature of a lamp should also be considered. This is a measure of how accurately the lamp will display colors to the human eye. Color temperature is measured in degrees kelvin.[9] Warm, red hues are observed when blue light is filtered ($\sim 3000°$K). In the natural world this would often be seen at sunrise and sunset. Blueish hues are observed when red light is filtered ($\sim 10,000°$K), as when there is cloud cover.[9] Sunny daylight lies at approximately 6000°K.[9]

Photosynthetically active radiation (PAR) is the unit used to assess a lamp's efficiency at facilitating plant growth.[10] PAR measures the spectral range of solar radiation from 400 to 700 nm, which is the range that photosynthetic organisms can use for photosynthesis.[11] Too high or too low a PAR level may become a stress factor for plants, resulting in photoinhibition and disturbances in the function of the photosynthetic apparatus.[12] It is difficult to recommend a specific PAR for use in the vivarium or terrarium because there are thousands of different plant species that may be included in an enclosure, all of which have slightly different growing requirements. To complicate matters, it is usually the case that several different plant species are included in a single enclosure. Plants tend to use light in the blue (4–500 nm) or red (650–750 nm) spectra, with blue light being of high importance for leaves or stems and red light for flowering and fruiting.[13] A combination of blue-emitting and red-emitting lights, or full-spectrum lighting, is recommended. A digital PAR meter can be used to determine PAR levels at different heights within a vivarium or terrarium.[14] PAR varies according to the distance from the lamp and obstructions such as glass or leaves.

Although, historically, developments in terrarium lighting have focused predominantly on incandescent and fluorescent lamps, more recently there have been significant advances in terrarium light-emitting diode (LED) technology.

LEDs are 2-lead semiconductor positive-negative junction diodes that emit light when activated.[15] Compared with incandescent and fluorescent lamps, LED lights are a more energy-efficient lighting option, with excellent light penetration and a long lifespan.

LED is also more compact, allowing creation of several microclimates in the terrarium.

Although most LEDs emit visible light only, without any UV light, specialized LEDs have more recently been developed that emit UV radiation.[16] It has recently been demonstrated that ultraviolet B (UVB)-emitting LEDs are more efficient and effective for producing vitamin D3 in human skin compared with natural sunlight.[16] It has also been suggested that UVB-emitting LED lights can lead to higher plasma concentrations of 25-hydroxyvitamin D3 (activated vitamin D3) in captive inland bearded dragons (*Pogona vitticeps*) than standard fluorescent bulbs.[17] Although LED lights that emit a suitable UVB wavelength for reptiles or amphibians are not currently available to the mainstream reptile market, this is an area of current technological development and it seems inevitable that such lights will become available to reptile and amphibian keepers in the future.

LED lamps that are designed and manufactured for vivarium or terrarium use are available in several different forms:

- Horizontal screw-in LED lamps, such as the Arcadia Jungle Dawn compact LED lamps (Arcadia Products plc, 8 Center, Salbrook Road, Redhill, Surrey RH1 5GJ, UK), are widely popular for promoting plant growth within the terrarium. The Arcadia Jungle Dawn compact lamp is a full-spectrum LED lamp that emits light with a color temperature of 6500°K (approximately the color of natural sunlight) and has a wide beam angle of 120°. The lamps can be rotated up to 300°, allowing light to be directed toward a specific area within the terrarium, to maximize desired plant growth. Arcadia Jungle Dawn lamps are available in 3 sizes: 9 W (9-cm length), 13 W (11-cm length), and 22 W (27-cm length), for different sized enclosures. These lamps are particularly useful for spreading light over a wide area.
- Screw-in LED spotlights, such as the Arcadia Jungle Dawn LED High Power Spotlight (Arcadia Reptile, Ely, UK) or the Lucky Reptile LED Sun Spot (Lucky Reptile, Waldkirch, Germany) are high-powered LED lamps that have a much narrower beam angle compared with the horizontal lamps and project light over a greater distance. They are particularly useful in very high terrariums. At 40w, the Arcadia Jungle Dawn LED High Power Spotlight is among the most powerful LED lamp available to the herpetocultural market, producing very bright light. It features a 60° lenticular lens for focused light projection and an internal fan to prevent overheating. The brightness of the light is equivalent to a 300-W incandescent lamp, approximately 3500 lumens. Multiple LED spotlights can be used to provide multiple sunspots in very large enclosures, such as in zoologic park exhibits.
- Linear LED lamps, such as the Zoo Med Reptisun LED (Zoo Med Laboratories, Inc, CA, USA) have particularly high efficiency ratings, with a lower overall

running temperature in general than the previously mentioned LED lighting forms. They also have an extremely long diode lifespan in general, often in the region of 20,000 hours. Light is emitted over a reasonably large area but often with slightly focused individual LEDs. These lamps are often considered a good all-round option for many terrarium setups.

- The Skylight (Skylight, Warsaw, Poland) range of slim-line LED lamps has recently become extremely popular. These lamps are available from distributors in Europe and North America. Several models are available, all of which are plug-and-play and do not require a separate lamp holder as do some other lamps. Anecdotally, many keepers report exceptional plant growth with this range of LED lights. Technical specifications, including PAR and color temperature, vary according to model and readers are directed to the company for further information on its range of products.

Ultraviolet Light

In general, there are 4 types of lamps used to provide UVB to reptiles and amphibians: fluorescent tubes, compact fluorescent bulbs, mercury vapor lamps, and metal halide lamps.[18] Fluorescent tubes produce little heat and diffuse light and, for reptile and amphibian lamps, come in 2 broad sizes: T8 and T5. T8 lamps (the classic or normal output UVB lamps) have a 25.4-mm diameter, whereas T5 lamps have a 15.9-mm diameter. T5 lamps have a higher lumens-per-watt ratio than T8 lamps and are often designated as high-output UVB tubes, having the ability to produce much higher levels of UVB.[4,19] For species that require higher UV light, a sunbeam method of providing UVB is described. It requires the use of some mercury vapor, metal halide, and high-output T5 lamps that produce much higher levels of UVB than T8 fluorescent tubes.[4]

For very large enclosures, particularly where large animals (eg, land tortoises or crocodilians) are housed, especially in a zoologic setting, it can be challenging to project enough UVB over a great distance to span the entirety of the animals' bodies. The Arcadia Super Zoo T5 (Arcadia Products plc, 8 Center, Salbrook Road, Redhill, Surrey RH1 5GJ, UK) has a useable UVB range of greater than 10 feet from the unit, illuminating an area of nearly 8 square feet. It is marketed as the most powerful reptile UVB system on the market. The unit is made of solid aluminum, is fully waterproof, and features 6 T5 UVB tubes in a reflector unit, with different configurations available in terms of the UVB percentage of the tubes.[20] The system has been used for a variety of species, including Burmese pythons, which were reported to have higher levels of vitamin D3 following 310 days of exposure to UVB from this system.[21]

Until recently, guidance was almost nonexistent regarding suitable levels of UVB for different species of reptiles and amphibians. In 2016, the UV-Tool was published.[4] This document divides 254 species of reptile and amphibian into 4 zones of UVB exposure (Ferguson zones) based on UV index measurements. UV index is a standardized, unitless measurement of the amount of sunlight, based on induction of erythema in human skin.[22] The UV index can be measured using a solar meter, of which several models are available aimed specifically at the herpetocultural market. The Solartech Solarmeter 6.5 UV Index meter (Solartech Inc, Harrison Township, MI, USA) was used by Ferguson and colleagues[23] in their original research for the designation of Ferguson zones. The Solarmeter has had UV index measurements compared with data provided from a Bentham spectrometer, a very accurate sensor used for UV measurements and deviations of only plus or minus 5% were found, which is considered to be within the normal limits for scientific instruments.[24] This meter is considered suitable for measuring irradiance from sunlight and from a lamp at specific distances, and has become the instrument that forms the basis of the UV-Tool previously mentioned.[4]

HUMIDIFICATION

Many different factors have to be accounted for when humidity needs to be maintained within a specific range or level, including not only the water added via different methods to the controlled environment but also ventilation, temperature, surface exposure, and the permeability and water retention capacity of the substrate. Humidity levels can be also altered by modifying those parameters within the vivarium.

In almost all scenarios, a heating source is provided that promotes evaporation, creating a higher humidity content within the tank, which tends to be homogenized through ventilation of the room air. Consequently, this entails a regular water input requirement.

Apart from the more traditional water input methods, such as water bowls and manual water sprayers, there are several misting and fogging devices and continuous running water features that can be installed. Misting devices are probably the most popular method used to maintain humidity levels. These devices simulate the rainfall naturally encountered in tropical and subtropical habitats. They contain a diaphragm misting pump that is generally connected to 4-6mm diameter rubber pipes that terminate in misting nozzles. Available commercial brands include MistKing (Ontario, Canada), Lucky Reptile Super Rain products, and Exo Terra ([part of Rolf C Hagen], Montreal, Canada) Monsoon, among others. Occasionally, misting units are also equipped with seconds timers that, in regard to amphibian husbandry, mimic the short but intense regular tropical rainfall required for certain species. It is worth mentioning the digital timers that are also available in the market, such as those offered by MistKing, or some smart timers controlled by Wi-Fi or Bluetooth that can be managed with smartphone applications (apps). Fogger humidifiers, on the other hand, function with a slightly more complex mechanism. They consist of ultrasonic humidifiers, often submerged in water. These generate vibrations of high-frequency waves that lead to the formation of small water particles in suspension, creating the desired mist. The benefits of these fogging devices compared with other rain systems is that they distribute the water production further throughout the vivarium, which is not always achieved with the nozzle-tipped watering systems. There are a wide range of affordable brands; the authors recommend those that are specifically designed to be installed externally. If a fogging unit that functions within the terrarium is chosen, then complete immersion in water has to be constantly ensured to avoid injuries to any exposed animal. Finally, drip water systems or running water features are also valid humidity and hydration sources. Dripping water units tend to be suspended above the enclosure and are systems to consider in certain tree-dwelling reptiles and amphibians, in particular chameleons. Running water systems tend to be equipped with an internal or external pump that allows constant circulation of fresh water. The latter can serve as a drinking source for those species that are reluctant to drink from stagnant water and simultaneously increase humidity levels within the terrarium through evaporation. These running water systems are assembled with simple pipes and a pump. Depending on the size, they may also be equipped with external filters to ensure optimal quality water. On a side note, apart from ensuring adequate humidity levels through direct water sources, providing a small container with a wet towel during shedding time will supply a roughened surface that will help complete ecdysis.

WATER QUALITY

Evidence shows that the quality of the water is crucial for the wellbeing of herpetofauna. Take into account: humidity, drinking water, aesthetics, husbandry requirements, and bathing. Aquatic or semiaquatic conditions keep animals healthy. The authors recommend reverse osmosis water for misting and fogging devices. Tap water is not recommended owing to its chlorinated content and osmolarity characteristics. Also, it can stain the glass and obstruct pipes and nozzles. Rain water could be seen as more natural; however, it can contain harmful chemicals from environmental pollutants and inadequate collection methods.

Water quality gains true importance when aquatic species are kept. As in aquiculture, parameters to consider include pH, oxygen content, ammonia, nitrates, nitrites bacterial load, and temperature because these can disrupt an animal's homeostatic mechanisms, resulting in secondary infections. If feasible, well-established aquatic plants will tend to keep water quality parameters stable. Partial water changes are widely recommended on a regular basis. There are 3 main types of filtration mechanisms (biological, mechanical, and chemical) that are commonly included within filter units. Internal and external filters exist; the authors recommend external because it provides a higher filtration capacity without occupying internal terrarium space and is easier to maintain and drain when required. More recently, filters with built-in UV lights are available in which the water flows through a high UV index, reducing the bacterial load significantly.

MULTIPARAMETRIC AND INTEGRATED THERMOSTATS

Digital thermostats are currently available. Some not only allow temperature regulation but also offer control of other parameters, including circadian light-cycles and humidity levels. These devices include the traditional probes of thermostats and electronic hygrometers, which are integrated within an electronic device with a touchscreen, such as the Microclimate EVO thermostat. Additionally, these integrated electronic devices create graphs from registered parameters over a 24-hour time frame.

The Raspberry Pi is a series of small single-board computers developed in the United Kingdom to promote teaching of basic computer science in schools and in developing countries. They can be operated in different systems, including Raspbian (developed by the Raspberry Pi Foundation [Cambridge, UK]), a Debian-based Linux distribution for download, as well as third-party Ubuntu, Windows 10 IoT Core, RISC OS, and specialized media center distributions. Those affordable computers can be used with a minimal knowledge in programming to set up a Terrarium Controller. Instructions on how to set it up are available online (https://www.carnivorousplants. co.uk/resources/raspberry-pi-terrarium-controller/). Once programmed, it not only monitors and regulates temperature, humidity, and light but also logs data from its sensors to the *Internet-of-Things* data platform *ThingSpeak*, which offers real-time data visualization and alerts.

The next steps on this smart transformation are the integrated systems. One of the first commercially and still quite popular available integrated systems is Biopod (**Fig. 1**). One of the authors has first-hand experience with the use of this type of intelligent vivarium and a particular emphasis must be made concerning the remarkable plant growth that supplies a reliable and stable bioactive vivarium with multiple microhabitats.

These remote-controlled vivariums function by means of an app to access a cloud-based platform from which one can either choose an already established environment setting based on certain species or choose the custom mode, which allows manual adjustments on personal preference. The Biopod includes integrated misting, a ventilation system with air injection, a compact but powerful UVB-emitting cold cathode fluorescent lamp, an LED light panel, integrated heating that regulates both substrate and air temperatures, integrated sensors to monitor and regulate internal vivarium

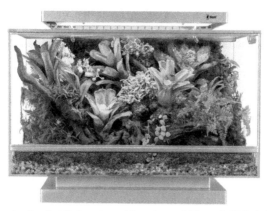

Fig. 1. Biopod Smart microhabitat system. (*Courtesy of* Biopods LLC, Lake Forest, IL; with permission.)

parameters (temperature, humidity, rainfall, and ventilation), and a high-definition camera to visualize the Biopod from any location via the app. Wi-Fi connectivity pairs the Biopod to the app and cloud server. Currently, there is a gradual emergence of more integrated systems that should be available in the near future.

The presence of integrated features with preestablished optimal environmental settings for certain species should aid those starting in herpetoculture to minimize the development of suboptimal conditions, and subsequently reduce chronic stress and immune depression in pet reptiles and amphibians, which overall will minimize morbidity and mortality.

A less considered factor is the addition of sounds and dynamic effects that simulate natural weather phenomenon such as thunderstorms. Although it may seem to be important only for design and aesthetics, rainfall is known to trigger reproductive behavior not only in amphibians but also reptiles and avian species. One of the authors, anecdotally, has observed increased reproductive behavior in captive behavior following thunderstorms or heavy rain.

There is a current trend to have bioactive tanks, basically creating a microhabitat composed not only of living plants but also of microfauna, including small invertebrates such as woodlice, springtails, and earthworms, among other detritivores. Literature is available on this topic.

Record-Keeping

In whichever system animals are kept, whether zoologic, laboratory, agricultural, or by private keepers, appropriate record-keeping is of high importance. Records have historically been kept using pen and paper in notebooks or on record cards to document activities such as feeding, shedding, defecating, ill health, deaths, and sales. In the zoologic sector, computerization of records started in the 1980s with the Animal Record Keeping System (ARKS), part of the International Species Information System (ISIS).[25] Private keepers have been slow to catch up; however, systems for computerized record-keeping in herpetoculture have started to gain traction. Reptile Scan (reptilescan.com) is an app-based system, which can be used by private keepers. Data are inputted into the system through via quick response (QR) codes. The app can be downloaded onto an iPhone, iPad, or Android device. A separate cloud-based Web app allows the keeper to input information about their animals into the collection (eg, identification, species, age, origin, cage number, photograph). A cage label, featuring a QR code unique to each animal, can then be downloaded and printed. When inputting a record, the camera on the keeper's iPhone, iPad, or Android smartphone or tablet is used to scan the QR code on the cage label. From here, records can be entered and recorded, including feeding, shedding, and medicating details; current length and weight; the sale or death of a specimen; and miscellaneous notes. PDF summaries of the records for an individual animal can be downloaded via the Web app and saved or printed. Data can also be saved from the Web app to Microsoft Excel. A backup of all Reptile Scan databases is performed every 24 hours and stored on Amazon S3 servers, which provide 99.999999999% durability (an average annual expected loss of 0.000000001% of objects). Reptile Scan is purchased for a 1-time fee, currently $24.99 (USD), making it quite affordable for most reptile or amphibian owners. A premium version of the app is available as an optional upgrade, which requires a monthly subscription fee and allows additional features, such as increased customizability of actions or categories within the app.

Ensuring suitable environmental parameters within an enclosure is also important to meet the welfare needs of captive reptiles and amphibians. For ectothermic animals such as reptiles and amphibians, ensuring suitable environmental temperatures and humidity levels in an enclosure is of paramount importance. The use of data loggers is becoming increasingly popular for monitoring reptile and amphibian environments in zoos, by private keepers, and in free-living animals.[26] The iButton (Maxim Integrated, San Jose, CA, USA) temperature and humidity logger is an example of a small, durable, standalone data logger that can be placed into the environment and will record data at a user-defined rate. They have been used in zoologic medicine and for enclosure monitoring but also for monitoring temperatures during the transportation of animals.[26] Data loggers have also been used for monitoring eggs during incubation, particularly in naturally occurring sea turtle nests and in aviculture.[26,27] Several potential herpetocultural apps for the use of data loggers exists and it is possible that this technology may become a mainstay of herpetoculture in the future.

Social Media

Social media has an integral part of modern day society. More information can be found in Nicola Di Girolamo's article, "Advances in Retrieval and Dissemination of Medical Information," this issue. In the last 10 to 15 years, the Internet has come to be the main source of information on husbandry for many reptile keepers, superseding a previous reliance on books and information gleaned at herpetocultural gatherings. In a study of 817 reptile keepers, 482 suggested that they use the Internet to find most of their reptile-keeping information.[28] The authors found more than 200 groups related to reptile-keeping and/or amphibian-keeping on Facebook. Several of these groups have more than 20,000 individual members. Such groups vary from generalist reptile-keeping groups to very specific groups discussing a single species or genus of reptile or amphibian. There are groups aimed at beginner reptile-keepers, as well as advanced keepers. One such Facebook group, Advancing Herp Husbandry, aims to promote best care, which is evidence-based when possible, and lists the promotion of new technologies in herpetoculture among its aims. There are also many online videos related to reptile-keeping. Indeed, a search for the keyword reptile on Google Videos produced more than 57,000,000 results. Although it can be considered very positive that so much readily accessible information is available to anybody involved in herpetoculture, and that new ideas can be disseminated quickly and widely, it must also be remembered that much of this content is not moderated or reviewed for accuracy or acceptability.

REFERENCES

1. Jacobson ER. Future directions in reptile medical education. J Vet Med Educ 2011;33(3). https://doi.org/10.3138/jvme.33.3.373.
2. Mitchell MA. History of exotic pets. In: Mitchell MA, Tully TN, editors. Manual of exotic pet practice. Philadelphia: W.B. Saunders; 2009. p. 1–3.
3. Rosier RL, Langkilde T. Does environmental enrichment really matter? A case study using the Eastern Fence Lizard, Sceloporus undulatus. Applied Animal Behaviour Science 2011;131(1-2):71–6.
4. Baines F, Chattell J, Dale J, et al. How much UVB does my reptile need? The UV-Tool, a guide to the selection of UV lighting for reptiles and amphibians in captivity. J Zoo Aquar Res 2016;4(1):42–63.
5. Peaker M. Some aspects of the thermal requirements of reptiles in captivity. Int Zoo Yearb 1969;9(1):3–8.
6. Adkins E, Driggers T, Ferguson G, et al. Ultraviolet light and reptiles, amphibians. J Herp Med Surg 2003;13(4):27–37.
7. De Vosjili P. Designing environments for captive reptiles & amphibians. Vet Clin North Am Exot Anim Pract 1999;2(1):43–68.
8. Meyer-Arendt J. Radiometry and Photometry: units and conversion factors. Appl Opt 1968;7(10):2081–4.
9. Brames H. Aspects of light and reptilian immunity. Iguana (IRCF) 2007;14(1):19–23.
10. Sultan SE. Phenotypic plasticity for plant development, function and life history. Trends Plant Sci 2000;5(12):537–42.
11. Sisson WB, Caldwell MM. Photosynthesis, Dark Respiration, and Growth of Rumex patientia L. Exposed to ultraviolet irradiance (288 to 315 nanometres) simulating a reduced atmospheric ozone column. Plant Physiol 1976;58:563–8.
12. Kalaji HM, Jajoo A, Oukarroum A, et al. The use of chlorophyll fluorescence kinetics analysis to study the performance of photosynthetic machinery in plants. In: Ahmad P, Saiema R, editors. Emerging technologies and management of crop stress tolerance: volume II - a sustainable approach. Cambridge (MA): Academic Press; 2014. p. 347–84.
13. Schuerger AC, Brown SC, Stryjewski EC. Anatomical Features of Pepper Plants (Capsicum annum L.) Grown under red light-emitting diodes supplemented with blue or far-red light. Ann Bot 1997;79(3):273–82.
14. Kühl M, Lassen C, Revsbech NP. A simple light meter for measurements of PAR (400 to 700 nm) with fiber-optic microprobes: application for P vs E_0(PAR) measurements in a microbial mat. Aquat Microb Ecol 1997;13:197–207.
15. LED. The American Heritage Society Dictionary. Boston (MA): Houghton Mifflin Company; 2005.
16. Kalajian TA, Aldoukhi A, Veronikis AJ, et al. Ultraviolet B light emitting diodes (LEDs) are more efficient and effective in producing vitamin D3 in human skin compared to natural sunlight. Sci Rep 2017;7:11489.
17. Cusack L, Rivera S, Lock B, et al. Effects of a light-emitting diode on the production of cholecalciferol and associated blood parameters in the bearded dragon (Pogona vitticeps). J Zoo Wildl Med 2017;48(4):1120–6.
18. Barten SL, Fleming GJ. Current herpetological husbandry and products. In: Mader DR, Divers SJ, editors. Current therapy in reptile medicine & surgery. St Louis (MO): Elsevier Saunders; 2014. p. 2–12.

19. HJ Imberti, Kiekhaefer DG, Wilhelm KL - US Patent 7,794,105, 2010 - Google Patents. Available at: https://patents.google.com/patent/US7794105B2/en. Accessed November 13, 2018.

20. Arcadia Reptile & Bird Australia, Arcadia super zoo T5. 2018. Available at: http://www.arcadia-aust.com.au/superzoot5-light-unit. Accessed November 18, 2018.

21. Bos JH, Fokko KC, Dennis GAB, et al. Artificial Ultraviolet B Radiation Raises Plasma 25-Hydroxyvitamin D_3concentrations In Burmese Pythons (*Python Bivittatus*). J Zoo Wildl Med 2018;49(3):810–2.

22. Vanicek K, Frei T, Litynska, et al. UV – Index for the Public. Available at: http://www.higieneocupacional.com.br/download/uv_index_karel_vanicek.pdf. Accessed November 12, 2018.

23. Ferguson GW, Brinker AM, Gehrmann WH, et al. Voluntary exposure of some western-hemisphere snake and lizard species to ultraviolet-B radiation in the field: how much ultraviolet-B should a lizard or snake receive in captivity? Zoo Biol 2010;29:317–34.

24. de Paula Corrêa M, Godin-Beekmann S, Haeffelin M, et al. Comparison between UV index measurements performed by research-grade and consumer products instruments. Photochem Photobiol Sci 2010;9:459–63.

25. Hayes KT. New developments in: the animal record system of the jersey wildlife preservation trust. Dodo J Jersey Wildl Preserv Trust 1991;(27):157–60.

26. Bailey T. The use of dataloggers in zoos, breeding projects, field studies and exotic animal practice. Proc Brit Vet Zool Soc spring meeting, 12-13 March, 2016, Chester Zoo.

27. Matsuzawa Y, Sato K, Sakamoto W. Seasonal fluctuations in sand temperature: effects on the incubation period and mortality of loggerhead sea turtle (*Caretta caretta*) pre-emergent hatchlings in Minabe, Japan. Marin Biol 2002;140(3):639–46.

28. Clark B. A report looking at the reptile keeping Hobby. 2013. Available at: http://www.fbh.org.uk/researchreport.pdf. Accessed November 21, 2018.

Technological Advances in Diagnostic Imaging in Exotic Pet Medicine

Graham Zoller, DMV, IPSAV (Zoological Medicine)[a],*, Harriet Hahn, DMV[b],
Nicola Di Girolamo, DVM, MS, PhD, DECZM (Herpetology)[c,1]

KEYWORDS

- Diagnostic imaging • X-rays • Ultrasound • CBCT • DEXA • Modality • Exotic
- Avian

KEY POINTS

- Technological advances in diagnostic imaging are rapidly developing, and modalities, such as cone beam computed tomography (CBCT), dual-energy x-ray absorptiometry (DEXA), and contrast-enhanced ultrasonography (CEUS), could have clinical interests in exotic pet medicine.
- CBCT is used mainly as a dental and maxillofacial imaging modality that provides fast acquisition of high-resolution images at a lower cost and with lower ionizing radiation levels compared with conventional computed tomography.
- DEXA is a quantitative imaging technique used to evaluate bone mineral content as well as fat mass and lean body mass, based on the absorption of x-rays emitted at high and low energies.
- CEUS relies on the administration of an ultrasound contrast agent to improve visualization of vessels and allow quantitative evaluation of the organ perfusion, which can be used to differentiate lesions with a similar appearance on conventional ultrasonography.
- Development of numerous diagnostic tools is associated with challenges concerning a decision to perform a specific test with a specific patient. Failure to use technological advances wisely could lead to potentially deleterious situations.

INTRODUCTION

Diagnostic imaging relies basically on the interpretation of the interaction of a form of energy with the body. Every modality requires emission of energy, such as x-rays, and

The authors have no commercial or financial conflicts of interest to declare. This study was not supported by a grant.
[a] Exotic Pet Department, Centre Hospitalier Vétérinaire Frégis, 43 Avenue Aristide Briand, Arcueil 94110, France; [b] Diagnostic Imaging Department, Centre Hospitalier Vétérinaire Frégis, 43 Avenue Aristide Briand, Arcueil 94110, France; [c] Tai Wai Small Animal and Exotic Hospital, 69-75 Chik Shun Street, Tai Wai, Sha Tin, New Territories, Hong Kong
[1] Center for Veterinary Sciences, Oklahoma State University, Stillwater, OK 74078.
* Corresponding author.
E-mail address: graham.zoller@gmail.com

magnetic, sonic, optical, or nuclear energies through the body, followed by detection of the changes in this energy by the body tissues and interpretation of the images obtained.[1] There has been no discovery of new diagnostic imaging energies in the past 2 decades.[2] Therefore, technological advances in diagnostic imaging rely mostly on the development of techniques related to generation and detection of energy waves as well as analysis of images. These advances aim at providing more accurate diagnosis and improving treatment of patients, while decreasing potential side effects.

Exotic pet diagnostic imaging is challenging because it requires precision, rapidity and high spatial resolution because of the small size of most patients and the need to reduce anesthesia time.[3] Among new technologies, cone beam computed tomography (CBCT), dual-energy x-ray absorptiometry (DEXA), and contrast-enhanced ultrasonography (CEUS) have been designed to overcome specific limitations and could be beneficial in the clinical management of exotic pets.

CONE BEAM COMPUTED TOMOGRAPHY
Historical Perspective

X-rays and radiography
X-rays were discovered in 1895 by physics professor Wilhem Röntgen, who realized that this new energy could go through the body to obtain a radiographic image.[4] Since then, radiography has been used increasingly and developed in medical diagnostic imaging.[5] Despite improvements in film emulsion, generator power, and development of digital imaging, however, conventional radiographs have inherent limitations due to the fact radiography is a planar 2-D projection. Such limitations include magnification, distortion, superimposition, and misrepresentation of structures.[6]

Computed tomography
In 1972, Sir Godfrey Hounsfield developed the first axial volumetric scanner to overcome these limitations and obtained a computed tomography (CT) scan of a human head.[7] The concept of CT image formation is that the internal structure of a complex object can be reconstructed if it is viewed from many different angles or projections. Basically, x-rays are emitted from a mobile gantry rotating around the patient and are detected on the opposite side after they have passed through the patient.[4] For each rotation, the level of attenuation is recorded and the shape and densities of the structures between the source and detectors are reconstructed, using specific algorithms for each slice. Acquisition of images has evolved from single-slice CT to multidetector CT (MDCT).[1]

Single-slice axial computed tomography Single-slice axial CT consisted in scanning single slices sequentially, with 1 x-ray tube and 1 detector. Once the first slice of the patient was scanned, the patient was transported for a scan increment and a second scan of the next slice was acquired; the procedure was repeated until the whole body area was scanned.[8] This mode is time consuming and has been largely replaced.

Helical computed tomography Helical scanning refers to systems in which continuous tube rotation is performed while the table moves simultaneously through the gantry. The x-ray tube describes a helical path around the object. The speed of the table motion relative to the rotation of the CT gantry is an important consideration, and the pitch is the parameter that describes this relationship. This technique improves the speed of acquisition and helps decrease motion artifacts. Helical CT can be single slice, dual slice, or multislice, depending on the maximum number of slice images generated by gantry rotation.[8]

The multislice CT scanner refers to a CT system equipped with a multiple-row detector array to simultaneously collect data at different slice locations. Image quality generally is improved with such devices, because of shorter scan times and thinner slices, leading to better contrast and spatial resolution. Although efficient, the use of MDCT can be limited because of its cost, limited access, and radiation dose consideration in human medicine. CBCT, therefore, was developed to overcome some of these limitations, while allowing better diagnosis and image guidance of operative and surgical procedures.[9]

Concept and Technology of Cone Beam Computed Tomography

CBCT, also known as cone beam volume CT or flat panel CT,[10] was developed in 1994 thanks to technological advances of high-quality detectors, adjustment of x-ray beam, and development of computers able to handle the computational complexity expected to reconstruct these images.[6]

X-ray tube

Beam geometry Similar x-ray tube technology is used for CBCT and MDCT.[11] Compared with conventional (or fan) beam CT, the x-ray beam of CBCT relies on a divergent pyramidal, or cone-shaped, source of ionizing radiation, directed through the middle of the area of interest onto an area of x-ray detectors on the opposite side[6] (**Fig. 1**). Typically, cone angle for CBCT is approximately 18°.[9]

Rotation of the x-ray tube Because CBCT exposure incorporates the entire field of view, only 1 rotational sequence of the gantry is necessary to acquire enough data for reconstruction.[12] The x-ray tube-detector system rotates totally (360°) or partially (from 180° to 360°)[13] around the patient During the rotation, multiple (from 150 to more than 600) sequential planar projection images of the field of view are acquired.[6]

Detectors

Because of the cone geometry of the beam, information in CBCT is acquired using an area detector instead of a row of detectors. CBCT exists thanks to the development of high-quality 2-D detector arrays able to meet the drastic constraints imposed by this method. The detector must be able to record x-ray photons and read off and send the signal to the computer, while being ready for the next acquisition, many hundreds of

A   **B**

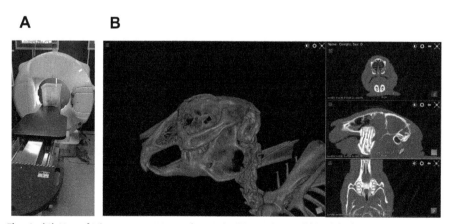

Fig. 1. (*A*) Use of Vimago system, a volumetric CT scan in a rabbit. (*B*) The images acquired can be visualized using volume rendering (on the left) or multiplanar reformated representation (transverse plane on the top right, sagittal plane on the right in the middle, and frontal plane on the bottom right). (Epica International, INC., San Clemente, CA).

times within a single rotation.[6] Earlier versions of CBCT used an image-intensifier tube/charge-coupled device as the area detector, but this technology could create distortion, and current CBCT technology typically uses a flat panel detector, which provides direct conversion of x-rays to a digital signal.[6]

Reconstruction

In CT, data obtained during acquisition must be processed to create the final image. This process is called reconstruction and is achieved differently between CBCT and conventional CT. In conventional CT, image slices are reconstructed individually and then stacked together to obtain a 3-D representation.[6] In CBCT, a 3-D volume must be reconstructed with a specific algorithm from several hundreds of 2-D projection data, containing more than 1 million pixels with 12 bits to 16 bits of data assigned to each pixel.[6] Development of CBCT was possible in the late 1990s thanks to improved computers capable of such a computational complexity.[6] Reconstruction time generally is longer than for conventional CT.

Display

CBCT images ultimately can be displayed and interpreted using multiplanar reformatted representation (oblique, curved, and cross-sectional views), volume rendering (especially maximal intensity projection), and panoramic view.[4]

Use in human and small animal medicine

CT is valuable in almost any case where radiography does not clearly define a lesion or the extent of it. Its use is most valuable in regions with complex anatomy, such as the skull, but it also can be used to guide intervention, such as biopsies or radiation therapy, or to obtain functional information through vascular studies. More specifically, from its physical properties, CBCT has most of its human and small animal applications in dental and maxillofacial imaging,[6] angiography,[14] mammography,[15] radiotherapy guidance,[16] and intraoperative imaging.[17]

Use in exotic pet medicine

Dental CBCT has been generally found superior to conventional CT when imaging the dentition of rabbits. Overall, tooth outline, pulp cavity, and germinal center were identified more easily on CBCT images. The most striking difference was the periodontal ligament significantly more visible on CBCT.[18] CBCT has been found helpful in diagnosing periodontal ligament space widening, premolar and molar malocclusion, apical elongation, coronal elongation, inflammatory tooth resorption, periapical lucency, moth-eaten pattern of lysis of the alveolar bone, ventral mandibular border contour changes, and missing teeth in a study involving 15 client-owned rabbits with clinical signs of dental disease. Except for coronal elongation, most of the lesions were not detectable on oral examination, which suggests that CBCT can be used to diagnose and plan treatment in dental disorders in rabbits.[19] CBCT has been used to evaluate bone healing in an experimental model of apical periodontitis in ferrets.[20]

Maxillofacial CBCT has been used in an experimental model on rabbits and rats to evaluate mandibular growth[21,22] or effectiveness of different treatments on bone regeneration.[23–25] It was able to reveal chronic osteoarthritis and condylar hypertrophy of the temporomandibular joint in rabbits.[26]

Oncology Although experimental, CBCT has been used in rabbits with implanted liver tumors for imaging-guided radiation therapy and has been proved more precise with the use of respiration-managed contrasted-enhanced CBCT.[27] Contrasted-enhanced CBCT accurately evaluates the volume of experimental liver tumors[28] as well as changes in the microenvironment of these tumors after radiation[29] and improves imaging guided radiation therapy.[30]

Advantages and Limits

Advantages

Practical advantages CBCT has emerged in veterinary medicine because of its lower cost, approximately 1/4 to 1/5 that of a conventional CT-scan,[6] and because of its installation ease compared to conventional CT-scan.[5] Indeed, CBCT does not require external cooling, is relatively small and operates on standard electrical supply.[5]

Image quality Regarding image production, CBCT offers multiple advantages such as:

- Scan time can be as short as 5 to 40 seconds,[4,18,31] which helps reducing motion artifacts, image unsharpness and distortion due to internal patient movements.
- CBCT delivers higher spatial resolution for high contrast objects than MDCT; this makes CBCT particularly interesting for exotic pet imaging, as it will allow visualization of small rabbits' teeth that would not be visible with conventional CT.[4,18,32]
- Collimation of the primary beam enables a reduction of X-ray radiation of the region of interest.[4,6] Subsequently, CBCT is associated with a dose reduction of 76.2% to 98.5% compared to conventional CT which is beneficial to reduce side effects in the patient.[33–36]

Limits

Contrast resolution It is important to realize that CBCT provides a relatively poor soft tissue contrast resolution because of its low radiation dose, its large amount of scattered radiation and the characteristics of flat panel detectors.[37,38] However, use of contrast media can improve soft tissue visualization.[39]

Image quality There is also limitation in image quality related to noise because of the detection of large amounts of scattered radiation.[4,40]

Artifacts Image artifacts are significantly more pronounced in CBCT.

Reconstruction time Routine use of CBCT is also limited by a greater delay between image acquisition and image display due to the complexity of the reconstruction algorithm. Reconstruction can require from 1 to 20 minutes depending on the number of images, the resolution expected and the reconstruction algorithm used.[6]

CT-number Hounsfield units values should be used with caution when measured on a CBCT because this modality produces different HU values for similar bony and soft tissue structures in different areas of the scanned volume.[41–43] Finally, CBCT detectors are not large enough in the axial direction to support full body scanning, but this is less a problem in exotic pets imaging. However, one of the most important factors limiting the use of CBCT is a poor access for veterinary patients. Hopefully, the recent development of portable scans using CBCT technology might overcome this limitation in a near future.[9]

DUAL-ENERGY X-RAY ABSORPTIOMETRY
Historical Perspective

Quantification of bone density using diagnostic imaging initially has been attempted using a phantom made from aluminum or ivory included in the field of view, as a means of calibration for radiographs.[44] Conventional x-rays require a bone loss of at least 40% to be detected.[45,46] In 1963, single-photon absorptiometry was developed.[47] With this technique, gamma rays emitted by a radioactive source of iodine or americium (with respective energies of 27 keV and 60 keV) would pass through 1 of the limbs of a patient immerged in a water bath, the water being used to simulate soft tissue. It thus was possible to calculate the amount of bone tissue in the scanned region by substracting photons attenuated by the soft tissue only from the photons attenuated by bone and soft tissue.[48] Because axial sites are not as easily immerged and soft tissue thickness is more variable, the simultaneous use of gamma rays with 2 different photon energies is required to distinguish soft tissue from bone. This technique, therefore, was designed as dual-photon absorptiometry and relied on emission of gamma rays with photon energies of 44 keV and 100 keV from gadolinium-153 to estimate total body composition, including bone mineral, fat and fat-free mass by means of calculations.[49] The use of a radioactive source was associated, however, with multiple drawbacks, including high costs associated with frequent replacement of the radioactive source due to natural decay, the potential hazards associated with radioactive sources, resolution limits, and a long scan time (20–40 minutes). To overcome these limitations, radioactive sources have been replaced with x-rays, which led to the respective development of single x-ray absorptiometry and DEXA in the late 1980s.[44,50]

Concept and Technology

Production of dual-energy x-rays

Like conventional x-ray, DEXA technology involves the use of an x-ray generator projecting a beam onto a detector through the body to determine fat mass (FM), lean mass (LM), and bone mineral content (BMC). It is basically different, however, because it uses 2 different low-dose energy x-rays, which are absorbed differently by bone and soft tissue.

The density profiles from these x-rays are used to calculate bone mineral density (BMD). Because the x-ray tube produces a beam that spans over a wide range of photon energies, different techniques have been developed to narrow the x-rays beam and produce 2 distinct photoelectric peaks.

Scanning methods

DEXA scan technology has evolved from pencil-beam densitometers with a rectilinear scanning fashion associated with long time of acquisition (5–10 minutes) to a fan beam technology in the early 1990. A wide-angle fan-beam x-ray source was first used with a set of detectors, which allowed scanning with a single sweep of the x-ray arm with a faster scan time (10–30 s) and better resolution but also a higher radiation dose and inherent magnification altering bone density measurements. In the early 2000s, a narrow fan beam has been introduced to offer a compromise between the former ones.[44,51–54]

Detectors

In DEXA technology, each x-ray energy is detected by a specific detector. Practically, this means that there are 2 detectors—the one on top sensitive to lower energy and the one underneath sensitive to higher energy. While the object is being scanned, each detector creates a 2-D image, one corresponding to the lower energy spectrum absorbency and the other capturing the higher-energy spectrum absorbency.[55]

Analysis of data and image generation

Bone mineral and soft tissue identification Dual-energy scanning is based on the principle that when an x-ray is projected through an object, some of the energy will be absorbed, while the remainder will pass through and will be detected on the other side. The degree of absorption depends on the initial x-ray intensity as well as a constant specific to the tissue (mass attenuation coefficient) and the mass of the tissue (or area density). For a given pixel, the radiation energy which is measured by the detector after the x-ray has been through the body will be converted into an areal density. While the area is being scanned, each pixel is analyzed to create a bone density image. After the acquisition, the machine software detects where bone edges begin and end. Finally, bone density is calculated for the specific bone in question. Because two energies are used in a DEXA scan, an estimate for the soft tissue absorption can be made in addition to that of the bones.[44]

Soft tissue differentiation between fat mass versus nonfat mass Although DEXA scan provides 3 body composition measurements (FM, LM, and BMC), it does not measure directly all 3 components. In a total body scan, approximately 40% to 45% of pixels contain bone; at this level, DEXA distinguishes bone from soft tissue (FM + LM). The remaining pixels, containing the pure soft tissue that is adjacent to bone, are used to calculate FM/LM ratio.[56–58]

Use in human and veterinary medicine

Body composition evaluated by DEXA scan has been validated by comparison with evaluation by chemical analysis both in humans and in animals.[59] DEXA scan is used mainly to evaluate BMD for the diagnosis of osteoporosis in humans, but it also has been used to diagnose Legg-Calve-Perthes disease in dogs[60] and secondary nutritional hyperparathyroidism in a cat.[61] Moreover, it also can be used in human medicine to evaluate the metabolic risk and cardiovascular risk, respectively, with the FM index,[62] and the visceral adipose tissue.[63] Other parameters that can be used include the appendicular LM index to diagnose sarcopenia[64] and evaluation of lipodystrophy in patients suffering from human immunodeficiency virus infection.

Use in exotic pet medicine

Validation studies DEXA provides accurate measurement of BMD and content when compared with chemical analysis in mice, rats, guinea pigs, and rabbits.[65–69] The use of DEXA scan has been validated in turkeys and chicken and was accurate and precise for determination of BMC and strength[70] as well as chemical composition.[71–73] It also has been validated in ruffed grouse (*Bonasa umbellus*), bobwhite quail (*Colinus virginianus*),[74] little stint (*Calidris minuta*), and various passerines.[75] The use of DEXA has been validated by comparison with ashes measurements in *Trachemys scripta*.[76] DXA estimates of body composition were highly correlated with chemical estimates for bone mass and lean tissue mass; however, DXA estimates were poorly correlated with chemical estimates for FM.[76]

Use in research

Small mammals In rabbits, DEXA has been used experimentally as a tool to evaluate osteoporosis after ovariectomy, glucocorticoid administration, or diet modification.[77,78] In guinea pigs, DEXA has been used mostly in experimental settings as a tool to evaluate the effect of different parameters on bone composition, such as UV-B radiation[79] or orchidectomy.[80]

Avian In avian medicine, DEXA has been used mainly in poultry production to select strains of chicken with higher bone density and to evaluate the effect of different parameters, such as activity, *Eimeria* spp infections, caponization, access to perch, and dietary factors on bone composition in chicken.[81–85] Although not validated, DEXA scan has been used in ostriches to evaluate BMC and BMD[86] and in blackcaps to evaluate body composition.[87]

Reptiles DEXA has been used to evaluate the effect of diet and/or environment on Hermann tortoises (*Testudo hermannii*) and leopard tortoises (*Stigmochelys pardalis*).[88,89]

Clinical use

DEXA has been used in a clinical setting to diagnose osteodystrophia fibrosa associated with nutritional secondary hyperparathyroidism caused by calcium-phosphorus imbalance in 2 guinea pigs.[90] A retrospective study has been performed in the green iguana (*Iguana iguana*) with or without naturally occurring metabolic bone disease and indicated that DEXA-scans could be used to study bone pathophysiology in reptiles.[91] Reference values for fat-free tissue mass, lean tissue mass, FM, ash mass, and total body water content have been provided for water snakes (*Nerodia rhombifer*) and healthy captive iguanas with a comparison to radiographic images.[92,93]

Advantages and Limits

Advantages

Compared with other techniques used to evaluate bone density, such as SPA, DPA, or quantitative CT, DEXA scans have several advantages, including[94]

- Better precision for measuring bone density. DEXA often is defined as the gold standard in diagnostic imaging of bone density and has the advantage of being a nondestructive technique compared with ash analysis.[75]
- Constant improvement in image quality as a result of better spatial resolution (from 1500 µm to approximately 300 µm)[94]
- Faster acquisition times (30 s) due to technical advances in scanning procedures[53,94]
- Low radiation dose. A DEXA scan of a human is equivalent to approximately less than 1 day of naturally occurring radiation.[44] A standard lung radiograph is associated with a radiation dose of 100 µSv in human medicine, whereas DEXA technology allows a radiation dose to the patient of approximately 3 µSv.[94]

When all these advantages are considered together, it seems that DEXA scans are able to provide images with a spatial resolution close to the ones obtained with conventional x-rays, with lower radiation and associated with the possibility to quantify bone density.[94]

Limits

DEXA is a projectional technique, which means that 3-D objects are analyzed as 2-D. This has 2 main drawbacks:

- DEXA provides an estimate of areal BMD in grams per square centimeter. This BMD is not a measure of volumetric density (in grams per cubic centimeter) because it provides no information about the depth of bone. In practice, this means that given 2 bones of identical volumetric BMD, the smaller bone have a lower areal BMD than the larger one because the difference in bone thickness. This limitation is known as size artifact.[44]
- DEXA measurements represent the sum of cortical and trabecular bone. Therefore, the influence of diseases or medications that differentially affect cortical versus trabecular bone may be obscured or difficult to detect by DEXA.[44]

Other artifacts, such as projection artifacts and bone detection limitations, can represent other weaknesses of this technology.

In veterinary medicine, the disadvantages of DEXA is a low accessibility, the initial expense, and the need for the subject to be motionless during the scanning procedure.[75] In exotic species, the lack of standardized normative data for most species also limits the clinical use of DEXA scan.[44]

CONTRAST-ENHANCED ULTRASONOGRAPHY
Historical Perspective

Inspired from sonar and radar technology developed during World War II, ultrasonography (US) became an established diagnostic tool in the early 1970s.[95] Conventional gray-scale US was first used to obtain structural information and Doppler US developed afterward to evaluate blood flow. Doppler US has a low signal-to-noise ratio, however, and its use, therefore, is limited to relatively large vessels, preventing evaluation of microvessels or perfusion.[96] Contrast agents for US have been developed to overcome this limitation and were introduced in 1996.[97] The use of CEUS can allow the visualization of perfusion characteristics of a lesion in vivo.[98]

Concept and Technology

Principles
Contrast US imaging consists in perfusion imaging. It requires a specific contrast media, contrast software, contrast-capable transducer, and intravenous access. The US contrast agent (UCA) is injected intravenously at the beginning of the procedure. These agents are strictly vascular agents, without any interstitial component. They contain microbubbles, which are highly reflective and elastic compared with normal tissue, resulting in a high backscatter signal from the vascular space[99] when administered into the vasculature,[100] and allow marked amplification of the signal from blood flow.[96] Unlike Doppler, contrast US is the assessment of perfusion—essentially to the level of the smallest capillaries in an organ or lesion.

Contrast agents
Five type of UCAs with different physical properties have been described in medical imaging: free gas bubbles (agitated saline), encapsulated gas bubbles (such as sulfur hexafluoride, air, or perfluorohexane), colloidal suspensions, emulsions, and aqueous solutions.[101] First-generation US contrast agents were associated with early breakdown of microbubbles, which limited the contrast effect. Second-generation UCAs, developed in 2001 and are still used, have allowed real-time evaluation.[97]

Use in human and veterinary medicine
Visualization of UCA in the vascular system provides information relative to vascular anatomy and allows characterization of hemodynamic parameters. Guidelines established in human medicine provide indications for abdominal CEUS to evaluate focal liver lesions and postoperative monitoring of focal liver, renal, and pancreatic lesions.[102] More recently, its use to differentiate inflammatory and neoplastic conditions, and furthermore benign versus malignant tumors, has been developed for various organs both in human and small animal medicine.[103–106]

CEUS can be used to differentiate, by the presence or absence of enhancement, the viable portion of a tumor from anecrotic portion in order to obtain targeted biopsy and avoid inconclusive histopathology.[97] Although rare to date, CEUS can be used to trigger short-pulsed diagnostic US to activate microbubbles containing chemotherapeutic agents, such as cisplatin near targeted cells,[107,108] to guide transcutaneous local injection of hemostatic agents[109] as well as radiofrequency ablation of the prostate.[110]

Use in exotic pet medicine

Use in normal animals Use of CEUS in exotic pet practice has been reported mostly in healthy animals. Sulfur hexafluoride has been used in micropigs to evaluate renal perfusion[111] and in a variety of birds, including Accipitriformes, Strigiformes, Psittaciformes, and Galliformes species to provide significant US contrast enhancement of the pecten oculi.[112] It also has been used in tortoise (*Testudo* spp), via the coccygeal vein, to evaluate cardiac anatomy and enabled a clearer distinction of the cardiac structure compared with contrast-free B-mode and color Doppler US.[113] In the green iguana (*Iguana iguana*), liver hemodynamics were determined with CEUS (**Fig. 2**).[114]

Clinical use Occasionally, CEUS has been used as an aid for diagnosis. Free air bubble has been used in avian cardiology to exclude a ventricular septal defect in a Moluccan cockatoo (*Cacatua moluccensis*).[115] CEUS also can differentiate between early-stage ovarian cancer and normal ovary in hens.[116] Finally, it also has been used to confirm naturally occurring liver lobe torsion in pet rabbits.[117]

Experimental use

Diagnostic purpose CEUS has been shown to be a valid technique in rabbits to evaluate microvessel density of VX2 lung peripheral tumor[118] and hepatic microcirculation after liver ischemia-reperfusion and to quantify the development of adventitial vasa vasorum associated with atherosclerosis.[119,120] CEUS has been studied mostly to evaluate

- Kidney disorders, including kidney ischemia-reperfusion injury,[121] acute renal failure,[122] and kidney after radiofrequency ablation[123]
- Liver disorders, such as liver fibrosis,[124,125] liver ischemia reperfusion injury,[126] hepatic vein outflow obstruction,[127] and VX2 liver cancer[128]
- Hyperplasic versus metastatic lymph nodes[129–132]
- Muscle crush injury,[133] quantitatively evaluating blood perfusion of injured peripheral nerves,[134] and detecting active bleeding of peritoneal artery[135] or femoral arteries[136]
- Testicles, such as from blunt scrotal trauma[137–139]

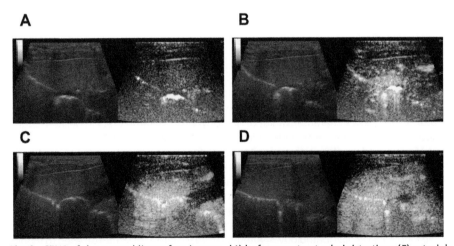

Fig. 2. CEUS of the normal liver of an iguana. (*A*) before contrast administration; (*B*) arterial phase 23 seconds after contrast administration; (*C*) parenchymal phase 80 seconds after contrast administration; and (*D*) venous phase 120 seconds after contrast administration. (*Courtesy of* Nicola Di Girolamo and Graham Zoller.)

Anecdotally, CEUS findings have been described in case of choroidal melanoma[140] and synovial pannus angiogenesis in an experimental model of arthritis[141] and could provide information for the diagnosis of these conditions. Sulfur hexafluoride has been found to be a suitable contrast agent, in New Zealand white rabbits, for rapid US diagnosis of experimentally induced thrombi in the aorta.[142]

Naked microbubbles associated with antibodies targeting specific markers have been developed to improve detection of specific lesions. For example, microbubbles targeting interleukin 18 or intercellular adhesion molecule - 1 have been used successfully to diagnose, respectively, atherosclerotic plaques[143] and ischemia-reperfusion injury.[144]

Therapeutic purpose In a rabbit experimental model, it has been shown that the combination of cisplatin, microbubbles, and US significantly delayed tumor growth compared with no treatment, cisplatin alone, or a combination of cisplatin and US.[107]

Advantages and Limits

Advantages
Practical advantages CEUS is a rapid, cost-effective, and noninvasive technique to evaluate perfusion both quantitatively and qualitatively. Compared with contrast-enhanced CT (CECT) or magnetic resonance imaging, CEUS allows continuous and real-time evaluation of contrast enhancement and it does not require sedation or anesthesia.[97,99]

Safety US contrast agents are excreted via the lung and bile after destruction of microbubbles and are safer compared with iodinated or gadolinium chelate contrast agents, which occasionally impair renal or thyroid function.[99] Moreover, there is no radiation compared with CT.[99]

Efficiency In specific clinical situations, sensibility and sensitivity of CEUS can be similar to that of CECT and contrast-enhanced magnetic resonance both in human and small animal medicine.[145–147] Compared with conventional ultrasound, CEUS has been found to provide more accurate measurements.[148]

Limits
Acquisition of images Similar to conventional US, CEUS is operator dependent and its use is limited when structures impairing the ultrasonic waves trajectory, such as air, bone, and metallic material, are present.[95] Moreover, unlike magnetic resonance imaging or CT modalities, CEUS lacks a panoramic view, and structures localized at more than 10 cm to 12 cm in depth can be more difficult to access. This should not be a major problem, however, in exotic pet medicine because most species generally are small.[99]

Side effects Although CEUS is considered a safe technique in human medicine, idiosyncratic hypersensitivity reaction have been described in humans.[97] In veterinary medicine, 2 out of 26 dogs developed anaphylactoid responses after administration of UCA containing human albumin,[149] but the technique is considered overall safe in cats and dogs.[150] In rabbits, auricular arterial damages composed of acute coagulation necrosis have been described after insonation of microbubbles, although this was observed only at exposure conditions (high mechanical index) above the Food and Drug Administration.[151] No side effects have been described in other exotic pet species where CEUS has been used.[112,115]

Fragility Unlike other imaging contrast media, ultrasound contrast media are micro-bubbles and therefore inherently fragile. These microbubbles are sensitive to mishandling, inadequate preparation or improper mechanical index of the ultrasound machine.[152]

Patient size Microbubbles contained in all ultrasound contrast media provide a signal which is maximal for a given diameter relatively to the frequency of the transducer. Commercially available ultrasound contrast media provide maximal signal with transducer used for large dogs. When the size of the patient decrease, a higher frequency will be used and thus the signal-to-noise ratio will decrease.[152]

SUMMARY

Initially limited to the evaluation of organ anatomy and pathology, medical imaging is a rapidly developing technique to assess physiology, pharmacology, and cellular or molecular biology and to assist therapeutic procedures.[98] These advances have been made possible thanks to various technological advances associated with improved image quality and decreased side effects. Such a rapid development of diverse techniques is promising in many ways and opens the field to numerous clinical applications, as described previously, for CBCT, DEXA and CEUS.

Improved accessibility, novelty, increased public demand, and realization of back-up examinations all can lead to the temptation of using these new imaging modalities excessively. Subsequently, development of technological advances should also raise questions on what makes a specific imaging modality indicated for a specific patient. Fundamentally, the use of new diagnostic methods depends on the added clinical value, which can be described as increased sensitivity, specificity, and cost effectiveness.[2,153] Therefore, the multiplication of imaging modalities can increase the finding of incidentalomas (ie, lesions without clinical signs), overdiagnosis (ie, diseases that may never cause clinical signs), and false-positive diagnoses (ie, wrong diagnoses) that potentially can lead to unnecessary interventions.[153,154]

One of the challenges associated with the development of new imaging techniques will be to understand how to use the right modality in the right patient. Studies, therefore, are needed to evaluate when these promising modalities are likely to (1) identify accurately a lesion in a patient given its clinical presentation and (2) have a beneficial impact on patient management.[155]

REFERENCES

1. Laal M. Innovation process in medical imaging. Proced Social Behav Sci 2013; 81:60–4.
2. Kuijpers F. The role of technology in future medical imaging. Med Mundi 1995; 40:181–9.
3. Brodbelt DC, Blissitt KJ, Hammond RA, et al. The risk of death: the confidential enquiry into perioperative small animal fatalities. Vet Anaesth Analg 2008;35(5): 365–73.
4. Venkatesh E, Elluru SV. Cone beam computed tomography: basics and applications in dentistry. J Istanb Univ Fac Dent 2017;51(3 Suppl 1):S102–21.
5. Johnson V. Diagnostic imaging: reflecting on the past and looking to the future. Vet Rec 2013;172(21):546.
6. Scarfe WC, Farman AG. What is cone-beam CT and how does it work? Dental Clin North Am 2008;52(4):707–30, v.

7. Goldman LW. Principles of CT and CT technology. J Nucl Med Technol 2007; 35(3):115–28 [quiz: 129–30].

8. Schwartz T, O'Brien R. CT acquisition principles. In: Saunders J, Stark T, editors. Veterinary computed tomography. Ames (IA): Wiley; 2011. p. 105–16.

9. Rohler D, Maniyedath A, Toth TL, et al. Comparison of Cone Beam CT (CBCT) vs. Multiple Detector CT (MDCT). 2015. Available at: http://www.dvmtoolbox. com/uploads/2/0/1/1/2011984/cbct_vs_mdct_rev_8.pdf. Accessed November 14, 2018.

10. Miles D, Danforth RA. A clinician's guide to understanding cone beam volumetric imaging (CVBI). Acad Dent Ther Stomatol 2007;1–13. Available at: https://www. yumpu.com/en/document/view/22671317/a-clinicians-guide-to-understanding-cone-beam-ineedcecom. Accessed June 25, 2019.

11. Pauwels R. What Is CBCT and How Does It Work?. In: Scarfe WC, Angelopoulos C, editors. Maxillofacial cone beam computed tomography: principles, techniques and clinical applications. Cham (Switzerland): Springer International Publishing; 2018. p. 13–42.

12. Orth RC, Wallace MJ, Kuo MD. C-arm cone-beam CT: general principles and technical considerations for use in interventional radiology. J Vasc Interv Radiol 2008;19(6):814–20.

13. Scarfe WC, Farman AG, Sukovic P. Clinical applications of cone-beam computed tomography in dental practice. J Can Dent Assoc 2006;72(1):75–80.

14. Robb RA. The dynamic spatial reconstructor: an X-Ray video-fluoroscopic CT scanner for dynamic volume imaging of moving organs. IEEE Trans Med Imaging 1982;1(1):22–33.

15. Chen B, Ning R. Cone-beam volume CT breast imaging: feasibility study. Med Phys 2002;29(5):755–70.

16. Cho PS, Johnson RH, Griffin TW. Cone-beam CT for radiotherapy applications. Phys Med Biol 1995;40(11):1863.

17. Cordemans V, Kaminski L, Banse X, et al. Accuracy of a new intraoperative cone beam CT imaging technique (Artis zeego II) compared to postoperative CT scan for assessment of pedicle screws placement and breaches detection. Eur Spine J 2017;26(11):2906–16.

18. Riggs GG, Arzi B, Cissell DD, et al. Clinical application of cone-beam computed tomography of the rabbit head: part 1 - normal dentition. Front Vet Sci 2016; 3:93.

19. Riggs GG, Cissell DD, Arzi B, et al. Clinical application of cone beam computed tomography of the rabbit head: part 2-dental disease. Front Vet Sci 2017;4:5.

20. Cotti E, Abramovitch K, Jensen J, et al. The influence of adalimumab on the healing of apical periodontitis in ferrets. J Endod 2017;43(11):1841–6.

21. Kim I, Duncan WJ, Farella M. Evaluation of mandibular growth using cone-beam computed tomography in a rabbit model: a pilot study. N Z Dent J 2012; 108(1):9–12.

22. Farias-Neto A, Martins AP, Figueroba SR, et al. Altered mandibular growth under functional posterior displacement in rats. Angle Orthod 2012;82(1):3–7.

23. Andrade Gomes do Nascimento LE, Sant'anna EF, Carlos de Oliveira Ruellas A, et al. Laser versus ultrasound on bone density recuperation after distraction osteogenesis-a cone-beam computer tomographic analysis. J Oral Maxillofac Surg 2013;71(5):921–8.

24. Alfotawei R, Naudi KB, Lappin D, et al. The use of TriCalcium Phosphate (TCP) and stem cells for the regeneration of osteoperiosteal critical-size mandibular

bony defects, an in vitro and preclinical study. J Craniomaxillofac Surg 2014; 42(6):863–9.

25. Zhou T, Yang HW, Tian ZW, et al. Effect of choukroun platelet-rich fibrin combined with autologous micro-morselized bone on the repair of mandibular defects in rabbits. J Oral Maxillofac Surg 2018;76(1):221–8.

26. Ahtiainen K, Mauno J, Ella V, et al. Autologous adipose stem cells and polylactide discs in the replacement of the rabbit temporomandibular joint disc. J R Soc Interf 2013;10(85):20130287.

27. Lock M, Jensen N, Kozak R, et al. PV-0376: Contrast-enhanced respiration managed cone-beam CT for image-guided intrahepatic radiotherapy. Radiother Oncol 2016;119:S175–6.

28. Pellerin O, Lin M, Bhagat N, et al. Comparison of semi-automatic volumetric VX2 hepatic tumor segmentation from cone beam CT and multi-detector CT with histology in rabbit models. Acad Radiol 2013;20(1):115–21.

29. Tang Q, Kim S, Clarkson R, et al. Sci-Sat AM(1): imaging-03: On-line dynamic contrast enhanced cone-beam CT for measuring. Med Phys 2008;35(7Part3): 3414–5.

30. Jensen NK, Stewart E, Lock M, et al. Assessment of contrast enhanced respiration managed cone-beam CT for image guided radiotherapy of intrahepatic tumors. Med Phys 2014;41(5):051905.

31. Hatcher DC. Operational principles for cone-beam computed tomography. J Am Dent Assoc 2010;141(Suppl 3):3s–6s.

32. Miracle AC, Mukherji SK. Conebeam CT of the head and neck, part 1: physical principles. AJNR Am J Neuroradiol 2009;30(6):1088–95.

33. Ludlow JB, Davies-Ludlow LE, Brooks SL. Dosimetry of two extraoral direct digital imaging devices: NewTom cone beam CT and Orthophos Plus DS panoramic unit. Dentomaxillofac Radiol 2003;32(4):229–34.

34. Schulze D, Heiland M, Thurmann H, et al. Radiation exposure during midfacial imaging using 4- and 16-slice computed tomography, cone beam computed tomography systems and conventional radiography. Dentomaxillofac Radiol 2004; 33(2):83–6.

35. Scaf G, Lurie AG, Mosier KM, et al. Dosimetry and cost of imaging osseointegrated implants with film-based and computed tomography. Oral Surg Oral Med Oral Pathol Oral Radiol Endod 1997;83(1):41–8.

36. Dula K, Mini R, van der Stelt PF, et al. Hypothetical mortality risk associated with spiral computed tomography of the maxilla and mandible. Eur J Oral Sci 1996; 104(5–6):503–10.

37. Schulze R, Heil U, Gross D, et al. Artefacts in CBCT: a review. Dentomaxillofac Radiol 2011;40(5):265–73.

38. Yu L, Vrieze TJ, Bruesewitz MR, et al. Dose and image quality evaluation of a dedicated cone-beam CT system for high-contrast neurologic applications. AJR Am J Roentgenol 2010;194(2):W193–201.

39. Kim MS, Kim BY, Choi HY, et al. Intravenous contrast media application using cone-beam computed tomography in a rabbit model. Imaging Sci Dent 2015; 45(1):31–9.

40. Endo M, Tsunoo T, Nakamori N, et al. Effect of scattered radiation on image noise in cone beam CT. Med Phys 2001;28(4):469–74.

41. Yamashina A, Tanimoto K, Sutthiprapaporn P, et al. The reliability of computed tomography (CT) values and dimensional measurements of the oropharyngeal region using cone beam CT: comparison with multidetector CT. Dentomaxillofac Radiol 2008;37(5):245–51.

42. Dillenseger JP, Matern JF, Gros CI, et al. MSCT versus CBCT: evaluation of high-resolution acquisition modes for dento-maxillary and skull-base imaging. Eur Radiol 2015;25(2):505–15.

43. Swennen GR, Schutyser F. Three-dimensional cephalometry: spiral multi-slice vs cone-beam computed tomography. Am J Orthod Dentofacial Orthop 2006; 130(3):410–6.

44. Crabtree NJ, Leonard MB, Zemel BS. Dual-energy X-ray absorptiometry. In: Sawyer AJ, Bachrach LK, Fung EB, editors. Bone densitometry in growing patients: guidelines for clinical practice. Totowa (NJ): Humana Press; 2007. p. 41–57.

45. Harris WH, Heaney RP. Skeletal renewal and metabolic bone disease. N Engl J Med 1969;280(4):193–202.

46. Johnston CC Jr, Epstein S. Clinical, biochemical, radiographic, epidemiologic, and economic features of osteoporosis. Orthop Clin North Am 1981;12(3): 559–69.

47. Cameron JR, Sorenson J. Measurement of bone mineral in vivo: an improved method. Science 1963;142(3589):230–2.

48. Cameron JR, Mazess RB, Sorenson JA. Precision and accuracy of bone mineral determination by direct photon absorptiometry. Invest Radiol 1968;3(3):141–50.

49. Peppler WW, Mazess RB. Total body bone mineral and lean body mass by dual-photon absorptiometry. I. Theory and measurement procedure. Calcif Tissue Int 1981;33(4):353–9.

50. Wahner HW, Dunn WL, Brown ML, et al. Comparison of dual-energy x-ray absorptiometry and dual photon absorptiometry for bone mineral measurements of the lumbar spine. Mayo Clin Proc 1988;63(11):1075–84.

51. Cole JH, Scerpella TA, van der Meulen MC. Fan-beam densitometry of the growing skeleton: are we measuring what we think we are? J Clin Densitom 2005;8(1):57–64.

52. Pocock NA, Noakes KA, Majerovic Y, et al. Magnification error of femoral geometry using fan beam densitometers. Calcif Tissue Int 1997;60(1):8–10.

53. Oldroyd B, Smith AH, Truscott JG. Cross-calibration of GE/Lunar pencil and fan-beam dual energy densitometers–bone mineral density and body composition studies. Eur J Clin Nutr 2003;57(8):977–87.

54. Bazzocchi A, Ponti F, Albisinni U, et al. DXA: technical aspects and application. Eur J Radiol 2016;85(8):1481–92.

55. Inspection EP. What is DEXA Technology and How Does it Measure Fat Content of Meat?. 2013. Available at: http://cdn2.hubspot.net/hub/20929/file-1563567081-pdf/docs/PLAN_-_Eagle_PI_-_White_Paper_-_What_is_DEXA_Technology_and_How_Does_it_Measure_Fat_Content_of_Meat.pdf?t=1437661657657. Accessed November 15, 2018.

56. Toombs RJ, Ducher G, Shepherd JA, et al. The impact of recent technological advances on the trueness and precision of DXA to assess body composition. Obesity (Silver Spring) 2012;20(1):30–9.

57. Pietrobelli A, Wang Z, Formica C, et al. Dual-energy X-ray absorptiometry: fat estimation errors due to variation in soft tissue hydration. Am J Physiol 1998; 274(5 Pt 1):E808–16.

58. Laskey MA. Dual-energy X-ray absorptiometry and body composition. Nutrition 1996;12(1):45–51.

59. Speakman JR, Booles D, Butterwick R. Validation of dual energy X-ray absorptiometry (DXA) by comparison with chemical analysis of dogs and cats. Int J Obes Relat Metab Disord 2001;25(3):439–47.

60. Isola M, Zotti A, Carnier P, et al. Dual-energy X-ray absorptiometry in canine legg-Calve-Perthes disease. J Vet Med A Physiol Pathol Clin Med 2005;52(8): 407–10.

61. Dimopoulou M, Kirpensteijn J, Nielsen DH, et al. Nutritional secondary hyperparathyroidism in two cats: evaluation of bone mineral density with dual-energy X-ray absorptiometry and computed tomography. Vet Comp Orthop Traumatol 2010;23(1):56–61.

62. Oliveros E, Somers VK, Sochor O, et al. The concept of normal weight obesity. Prog Cardiovasc Dis 2014;56(4):426–33.

63. Katzmarzyk PT, Greenway FL, Heymsfield SB, et al. Clinical utility and reproducibility of visceral adipose tissue measurements derived from dual-energy X-ray absorptiometry in White and African American adults. Obesity (Silver Spring) 2013;21(11):2221–4.

64. Fielding RA, Vellas B, Evans WJ, et al. Sarcopenia: an undiagnosed condition in older adults. Current consensus definition: prevalence, etiology, and consequences. International working group on sarcopenia. J Am Med Dir Assoc 2011;12(4):249–56.

65. Fink C, Cooper HJ, Huebner JL, et al. Precision and accuracy of a transportable dual-energy X-ray absorptiometry unit for bone mineral measurements in guinea pigs. Calcif Tissue Int 2002;70(3):164–9.

66. Norris SA, Pettifor JM, Gray DA, et al. Validation and application of dual-energy X-ray absorptiometry to measure bone mineral density in rabbit vertebrae. J Clin Densitom 2000;3(1):49–55.

67. Iida-Klein A, Lu SS, Yokoyama K, et al. Precision, accuracy, and reproducibility of dual X-ray absorptiometry measurements in mice in vivo. J Clin Densitom 2003;6(1):25–33.

68. Nagy TR, Prince CW, Li J. Validation of peripheral dual-energy X-ray absorptiometry for the measurement of bone mineral in intact and excised long bones of rats. J Bone Miner Res 2001;16(9):1682–7.

69. Castaneda S, Largo R, Calvo E, et al. Bone mineral measurements of subchondral and trabecular bone in healthy and osteoporotic rabbits. Skeletal Radiol 2006;35(1):34–41.

70. Zotti A, Rizzi C, Chiericato G, et al. Accuracy and precision of dual-energy x-ray absorptiometry for ex vivo determination of mineral content in turkey poult bones. Vet Radiol Ultrasound 2003;44(1):49–52.

71. Onyango EM, Hester PY, Stroshine R, et al. Bone densitometry as an indicator of percentage tibia ash in broiler chicks fed varying dietary calcium and phosphorus levels. Poult Sci 2003;82(11):1787–91.

72. Swennen Q, Janssens GP, Geers R, et al. Validation of dual-energy x-ray absorptiometry for determining in vivo body composition of chickens. Poult Sci 2004;83(8):1348–57.

73. Schreiweis MA, Orban JI, Ledur MC, et al. Validation of dual-energy X-ray absorptiometry in live White Leghorns. Poult Sci 2005;84(1):91–9.

74. Kim WK, Ford BC, Mitchell AD, et al. Comparative assessment of bone among wild-type, restricted ovulator and out-of-production hens. Br Poult Sci 2004; 45(4):463–70.

75. Korine C, Daniel S, van Tets IG, et al. Measuring fat mass in small birds by dual-energy x-ray absorptiometry. Physiol Biochem Zool 2004;77(3):522–9.

76. Stone MD, Arjmandi B, Lovern MB. Dual-energy x-ray absorptiometry (DXA) as a non-invasive tool for the prediction of bone density and body composition of turtles. Herpetol Rev 2010;41:36–42.

77. Baofeng L, Zhi Y, Bei C, et al. Characterization of a rabbit osteoporosis model induced by ovariectomy and glucocorticoid. Acta Orthop 2010;81(3):396–401.
78. Khandare AL, Suresh P, Kumar PU, et al. Beneficial effect of copper supplementation on deposition of fluoride in bone in fluoride- and molybdenum-fed rabbits. Calcif Tissue Int 2005;77(4):233–8.
79. Watson MK, Stern AW, Labelle AL, et al. Evaluating the clinical and physiological effects of long term ultraviolet B radiation on guinea pigs (Cavia porcellus). PLoS One 2014;9(12):e114413.
80. DeGuire JR, Mak IL, Lavery P, et al. Orchidectomy-induced alterations in volumetric bone density, cortical porosity and strength of femur are attenuated by dietary conjugated linoleic acid in aged guinea pigs. Bone 2015;73:42–50.
81. Aguado E, Pascaretti-Grizon F, Goyenvalle E, et al. Bone mass and bone quality are altered by hypoactivity in the chicken. PLoS One 2015;10(1):e0116763.
82. Fetterer RH, Miska KB, Mitchell AD, et al. The use of dual-energy X-ray absorptiometry to assess the impact of Eimeria infections in broiler chicks. Avian Dis 2013;57(2):199–204.
83. Muszynski S, Kwiecien M, Tomaszewska E, et al. Effect of caponization on performance and quality characteristics of long bones in Polbar chickens. Poult Sci 2017;96(2):491–500.
84. Enneking SA, Cheng HW, Jefferson-Moore KY, et al. Early access to perches in caged White Leghorn pullets. Poult Sci 2012;91(9):2114–20.
85. Baird HT, Eggett DL, Fullmer S. Varying ratios of omega-6: omega-3 fatty acids on the pre-and postmortem bone mineral density, bone ash, and bone breaking strength of laying chickens. Poult Sci 2008;87(2):323–8.
86. Krupski W, Tatara MR, Charuta A, et al. Sex-related differences of bone properties of pelvic limb and bone metabolism indices in 14-month-old ostriches (Struthio camelus). Br Poult Sci 2018;59(3):301–7.
87. Mizrahy O, Bauchinger U, Aamidor SE, et al. Availability of water affects renewal of tissues in migratory blackcaps during stopover. Integr Comp Biol 2011;51(3): 374–84.
88. Gramanzini M, Di Girolamo N, Gargiulo S, et al. Assessment of dual-energy x-ray absorptiometry for use in evaluating the effects of dietary and environmental management on Hermann's tortoises (Testudo hermanni). Am J Vet Res 2013; 74(6):918–24.
89. Fledelius B, Jorgensen GW, Jensen HE, et al. Influence of the calcium content of the diet offered to leopard tortoises (Geochelone pardalis). Vet Rec 2005; 156(26):831–5.
90. Schwarz T, Stork CK, Megahy IW, et al. Osteodystrophia fibrosa in two guinea pigs. J Am Vet Med Assoc 2001;219(1):63–6, 49.
91. Zotti A, Selleri P, Carnier P, et al. Relationship between metabolic bone disease and bone mineral density measured by dual-energy X-ray absorptiometry in the green iguana (Iguana iguana). Vet Radiol Ultrasound 2004;45(1):10–6.
92. Secor SM, Nagy TR. Non-invasive measure of body composition of snakes using dual-energy X-ray absorptiometry. Comp Biochem Physiol A Mol Integr Physiol 2003;136(2):379–89.
93. Greer LL, Daniel GB, Bartges JW, et al. Evaluation of bone mineral density in the healthy green Iguana, Iguana iguana: Correlation of dual energy x-ray absorptiometry and radiology. J Herpetological Med Surg 2006;16(1):4–8.
94. Gonzalez Rodriguez E, Favre L, Lamy O, et al. Imagerie par DXA: le couteau suisse multifonction ? Rev Med Suisse 2015;11:645–50.

95. Shung KK. Ultrasound: past, present and future. In: Van Toi V, Khoa TQD, editors. The third international conference on the development of biomedical engineering in vietnam. IFMBE Proceedings, vol. 27. Berlin: Springer; 2010. p. 10–3.
96. Greis C. Technology overview: SonoVue (Bracco, Milan). Eur Radiol 2004; 14(Suppl 8):P11–5.
97. Chung YE, Kim KW. Contrast-enhanced ultrasonography: advance and current status in abdominal imaging. Ultrasonography 2015;34(1):3–18.
98. Lee JS, Gleeson FV. Picture the future: emerging imaging modalities. Clin Med (Lond) 2014;14(Suppl 6):s95–9.
99. Ranganath PG, Robbin ML, Back SJ, et al. Practical advantages of contrast-enhanced ultrasound in abdominopelvic radiology. Abdom Radiol (NY) 2018; 43(4):998–1012.
100. Sontum PC. Physicochemical characteristics of Sonazoid, a new contrast agent for ultrasound imaging. Ultrasound Med Biol 2008;34(5):824–33.
101. Frinking PJA, Bouakaz A, Kirkhorn J, et al. Ultrasound contrast imaging: current and new potential methods. Ultrasound Med Biol 2000;26(6):965–75.
102. Claudon M, Dietrich CF, Choi BI, et al. Guidelines and good clinical practice recommendations for Contrast Enhanced Ultrasound (CEUS) in the liver - update 2012: a WFUMB-EFSUMB initiative in cooperation with representatives of AFSUMB, AIUM, ASUM, FLAUS and ICUS. Ultrasound Med Biol 2013;39(2): 187–210.
103. Piscaglia F, Nolsoe C, Dietrich CF, et al. The EFSUMB guidelines and recommendations on the clinical practice of contrast enhanced ultrasound (CEUS): update 2011 on non-hepatic applications. Ultraschall Med 2012;33(1):33–59.
104. Bargellini P, Orlandi R, Paloni C, et al. Contrast-enhanced ultrasonographic characteristics of adrenal glands in dogs with pituitary-dependent hyperadrenocorticism. Vet Radiol Ultrasound 2013;54(3):283–92.
105. Nakamura K, Takagi S, Sasaki N, et al. Contrast-enhanced ultrasonography for characterization of canine focal liver lesions. Vet Radiol Ultrasound 2010;51(1): 79–85.
106. Taeymans O, Penninck D. Contrast enhanced sonographic assessment of feeding vessels as a discriminator between malignant vs. benign focal splenic lesions. Vet Radiol Ultrasound 2011;52(4):457–61.
107. Sasaki N, Kudo N, Nakamura K, et al. Ultrasound image-guided therapy enhances antitumor effect of cisplatin. J Med Ultrason (2001) 2014;41(1):11–21.
108. Sasaki N, Kudo N, Nakamura K, et al. Activation of microbubbles by short-pulsed ultrasound enhances the cytotoxic effect of cis-diamminedichloroplatinum (II) in a canine thyroid adenocarcinoma cell line in vitro. Ultrasound Med Biol 2012;38(1):109–18.
109. Tang J, Lv F, Li W, et al. Contrast-enhanced sonographic guidance for local injection of a hemostatic agent for management of blunt hepatic hemorrhage: a canine study. AJR Am J Roentgenol 2008;191(3):W107–11.
110. Liu JB, Wansaicheong G, Merton DA, et al. Canine prostate: contrast-enhanced US-guided radiofrequency ablation with urethral and neurovascular cooling–initial experience. Radiology 2008;247(3):717–25.
111. Yi K, Ji S, Kim J, et al. Contrast-enhanced ultrasound analysis of renal perfusion in normal micropigs. J Vet Sci 2012;13(3):311–4.
112. Ferreira TAC, Fornazari G, Saldanha A, et al. The use of sulfur hexafluoride microbubbles for contrast-enhanced ocular ultrasonography of the pecten oculi in birds. Vet Ophthalmol 2018;00:1–7.

113. Prutz M, Hungerbuhler S, Lass M, et al. Contrast echocardiography for analysis of heart anatomy in tortoises. Tierarztl Prax Ausg K Kleintiere Heimtiere 2015; 43(4):231–7.
114. Nardini G, Di Girolamo N, Leopardi S, et al. Evaluation of liver parenchyma and perfusion using dynamic contrast-enhanced computed tomography and contrast-enhanced ultrasonography in captive green iguanas (Iguana iguana) under general anesthesia. BMC Vet Res 2014;10:112.
115. Zoller G, Guzman DS, Summa N, et al. Infundibular pulmonic stenosis in a moluccan cockatoo (cacatua moluccensis). J Avian Med Surg 2017;31(1):53–61.
116. Barua A, Bitterman P, Bahr JM, et al. Contrast-enhanced sonography depicts spontaneous ovarian cancer at early stages in a preclinical animal model. J Ultrasound Med 2011;30(3):333–45.
117. di Girolamo N, Nicoletti A, Selleri P, et al. Confirmation of naturally occurring liver lobe torsion in pet rabbits by means of contrast-enhanced ultrasound. Paper presented at: 15th Annual Conference of the Association of Exotic Mammals Veterinarians. Dallas, TX, September 23-28, 2017.
118. Xing J, He W, Ding YW, et al. Correlation between Contrast-Enhanced Ultrasound and Microvessel Density via CD31 and CD34 in a rabbit VX2 lung peripheral tumor model. Med Ultrason 2018;1(1):37–42.
119. Sun J, Liu K, Tang QY, et al. Correlation between enhanced intensity of atherosclerotic plaque at contrast-enhanced ultrasonography and density of histological neovascularization. J Huazhong Univ Sci Technolog Med Sci 2013;33(3): 443–6.
120. Li X, Zhang R, Li Z, et al. Contrast-enhanced ultrasound imaging quantification of adventitial vasa vasorum in a rabbit model of varying degrees of atherosclerosis. Sci Rep 2017;7(1):7032.
121. Li M, Luo Z, Chen X, et al. Use of contrast-enhanced ultrasound to monitor rabbit renal ischemia-reperfusion injury and correlations between time-intensity curve parameters and renal ICAM-1 expression. Clin Hemorheol Microcirc 2015;59(2):123–31.
122. Dong Y, Wang WP, Cao JY, et al. Quantitative evaluation of acute renal failure in rabbits with contrast-enhanced ultrasound. Chin Med J (Engl) 2012;125(4): 652–6.
123. Wu R, Xu FH, Yao MH, et al. Contrast-enhanced ultrasonography follow-up after radiofrequency ablation in normal rabbit kidney. Arch Med Sci 2013;9(4): 608–13.
124. Qiu T, Wang H, Song J, et al. Assessment of liver fibrosis by ultrasound elastography and contrast-enhanced ultrasound: a randomized prospective animal study. Exp Anim 2018;67(2):117–26.
125. Shin HJ, Chang EY, Lee HS, et al. Contrast-enhanced ultrasonography for the evaluation of liver fibrosis after biliary obstruction. World J Gastroenterol 2015; 21(9):2614–21.
126. Li H, Lu J, Zhou X, et al. Quantitative analysis of hepatic microcirculation in rabbits after liver ischemia-reperfusion injury using contrast-enhanced ultrasound. Ultrasound Med Biol 2017;43(10):2469–76.
127. Kim KW, Kim PN, Shin JH, et al. Acute outflow obstruction of hepatic veins in rabbits: quantitative analysis of hepatic perfusion with contrast-enhanced sonography. J Ultrasound Med 2011;30(5):635–42.
128. Xiang Z, Liang Q, Liang C, et al. The correlation of contrast-enhanced ultrasound and MRI perfusion quantitative analysis in rabbit VX2 liver cancer. Cell Biochem Biophys 2014;70(3):1859–67.

129. Cui Z, Gao Y, Wang W, et al. Evaluation of neck lymph node metastasis on contrast-enhanced ultrasound: an animal study. Clin Exp Otorhinolaryngol 2017;10(1):109–14.

130. Kogashiwa Y, Sakurai H, Akimoto Y, et al. Sentinel node biopsy for the head and neck using contrast-enhanced ultrasonography combined with indocyanine green fluorescence in animal models: a feasibility study. PLoS One 2015; 10(7):e0132511.

131. Zhang Y, Shi F, Li SM, et al. Intravenous contrast-enhanced ultrasound of metastatic lymph nodes in rabbit VX2 tongue carcinoma model. Zhonghua Er Bi Yan Hou Tou Jing Wai Ke Za Zhi 2012;47(6):503–6 [in Chinese].

132. Aoki T, Moriyasu F, Yamamoto K, et al. Image of tumor metastasis and inflammatory lymph node enlargement by contrast-enhanced ultrasonography. World J Radiol 2011;3(12):298–305.

133. Zhang CD, Lv FQ, Li QY, et al. Application of contrast-enhanced ultrasonography in the diagnosis of skeletal muscle crush injury in rabbits. Br J Radiol 2014; 87(1041):20140421.

134. Wang Y, Tang P, Zhang L, et al. Gray-scale contrast-enhanced ultrasonography for quantitative evaluation of the blood perfusion of the sciatic nerves with crush injury. Acad Radiol 2011;18(10):1285–91.

135. Zhou P, Xiang H, Zhou H, et al. Experimental study on retroperitoneal artery bleeding with contrast-enhanced ultrasound. J Emerg Med 2014;46(6): e167–72.

136. Luo W, Zderic V, Carter S, et al. Detection of bleeding in injured femoral arteries with contrast-enhanced sonography. J Ultrasound Med 2006;25(9):1169–77.

137. Jiang BL, Zhu PY, Zhao YX, et al. Establishment of an animal model of blunt scrotal trauma and evaluation of the lesion by conventional and contrast-enhanced ultrasonography. Zhonghua Nan Ke Xue 2014;20(7):624–9 [in Chinese].

138. Zhao YX, Huang HM, Liu YW, et al. Contrast-enhanced ultrasonography for detecting testicular perfusion in acute testis contusion in rabbits. Zhonghua Nan Ke Xue 2013;19(8):689–93 [in Chinese].

139. Chen L, Zhan WW, Shen ZJ, et al. Blood perfusion of the contralateral testis evaluated with contrast-enhanced ultrasound in rabbits with unilateral testicular torsion. Asian J Androl 2009;11(2):253–60.

140. Gao M, Tang J, Liu K, et al. Quantitative evaluation of vascular microcirculation using contrast-enhanced ultrasound imaging in rabbit models of choroidal melanoma. Invest Ophthalmol Vis Sci 2018;59(3):1251–62.

141. Jiang Y, Qiu L, Zhang L, et al. Noninvasive quantitative assessment of synovial pannus angiogenesis by contrast-enhanced gray-scale sonography in antigen-induced arthritis in rabbits. Acad Radiol 2011;18(3):359–68.

142. Vlasin M, Lukac R, Kauerova Z, et al. Specific contrast ultrasound using sterically stabilized microbubbles for early diagnosis of thromboembolic disease in a rabbit model. Can J Vet Res 2014;78(2):133–9.

143. Jiang ZZ, Liu XT, Ma CY, et al. Detection of atherosclerotic plaques in the rabbit aorta using ultrasound microbubbles conjugated to interleukin-18 antibodies. Med Sci Monit 2017;23:5446–54.

144. Xie F, Li ZP, Wang HW, et al. Evaluation of liver ischemia-reperfusion injury in rabbits using a nanoscale ultrasound contrast agent targeting ICAM-1. PLoS One 2016;11(4):e0153805.

145. Xie L, Guang Y, Ding H, et al. Diagnostic value of contrast-enhanced ultrasound, computed tomography and magnetic resonance imaging for focal liver lesions: a meta-analysis. Ultrasound Med Biol 2011;37(6):854–61.
146. Zhao DW, Tian M, Zhang LT, et al. Effectiveness of contrast-enhanced ultrasound and serum liver enzyme measurement in detection and classification of blunt liver trauma. J Int Med Res 2017;45(1):170–81.
147. You JS, Chung YE, Lee HJ, et al. Liver trauma diagnosis with contrast-enhanced ultrasound: interobserver variability between radiologist and emergency physician in an animal study. Am J Emerg Med 2012;30(7):1229–34.
148. Chu Y, Liu H, Xing P, et al. The morphology and haemodynamics of the rabbit renal artery: evaluation by conventional and contrast-enhanced ultrasonography. Lab Anim 2011;45(3):204–8.
149. Yamaya Y, Niizeki K, Kim J, et al. Anaphylactoid response to Optison(R) and its effects on pulmonary function in two dogs. J Vet Med Sci 2004;66(11):1429–32.
150. Seiler GS, Brown JC, Reetz JA, et al. Safety of contrast-enhanced ultrasonography in dogs and cats: 488 cases (2002-2011). J Am Vet Med Assoc 2013; 242(9):1255–9.
151. Zachary JF, Blue JP, Miller RJ, et al. Vascular lesions and s-thrombomodulin concentrations from auricular arteries of rabbits infused with microbubble contrast agent and exposed to pulsed ultrasound. Ultrasound Med Biol 2006; 32(11):1781–91.
152. O'Brien RT, Seiler GS. Clinical applications of contrast ultrasound. In: Penninck D, D'Anjou M-A, editors. Atlas of small animal ultrasonography. 2nd edition; 2000.
153. Black WC, Welch HG. Advances in diagnostic imaging and overestimations of disease prevalence and the benefits of therapy. N Engl J Med 1993;328(17): 1237–43.
154. Lamb CR. Veterinary diagnostic imaging: probability, accuracy and impact. Vet J 2016;215:55–63.
155. Weinstein S, Obuchowski NA, Lieber ML. Clinical evaluation of diagnostic tests. AJR Am J Roentgenol 2005;184(1):14–9.

Technological Advances in Exotic Pet Anesthesia and Analgesia

Jessica Comolli, DVM, LVT[a],
Dario d'Ovidio, DMV, MSc, SPACS, Dipl. ECZM (Small Mammal), PhD[b],
Chiara Adami, DMV, MRCVS, Dipl. ECVAA, Dipl. ACVAA, PhD[c],
Rodney Schnellbacher, DVM, Dipl ACZM[d,*]

KEYWORDS

- Anesthesia • Analgesia • Supraglottic airway devices • Endoscopic intubation
- Intermittent positive pressure ventilators • Blood pressure monitoring
- Regional nerve blocks

KEY POINTS

- Exotic animal anesthesia and analgesia have dramatically progressed over the past decade and continue to do so as more research and technologies develop.
- Technological advancements such as airway devices, endoscopic intubation techniques, positive intermittent pressure ventilators, and invasive and noninvasive blood pressure monitors have played a significant role in improving patient safety and the anesthetic outcomes of exotic animals.
- Even when performed by skilled operators, locating the nerves can be challenging in small exotic pets; in such cases, the use of an electrical nerve stimulator may be useful to confirm the correct identification of the target nerve.

INTRODUCTION

Exotic animal anesthesia and analgesia have dramatically progressed over the past decade and continue to do so as more research and technology develop. Technological advancements such as airway devices, endoscopic intubation techniques, positive intermittent pressure ventilators, and invasive and noninvasive blood pressure monitors have played a significant role in improving patient safety and the

Disclosure: The authors do not have any commercial or financial conflicts of interest with any of the technologies discussed in this article.
[a] Department of Small Animal Medicine and Surgery, Zoological Medicine Service, University of Georgia, 2200 College Station Rd, Athens, GA 30605, USA; [b] Via Cristoforo Colombo 118, Arzano, NA 80022, Italy; [c] Department of Clinical Sciences and Services, Royal Veterinary College - University of London, Hawkshead Lane, North Mymms, AL97TA Hatfield, UK; [d] Dickerson Park Zoo, Animal Health, 3043 North Fort, Springfield, MO 65803, USA
* Corresponding author.
E-mail address: rschnellbacher@springfieldmo.gov

anesthetic outcomes of exotic animals. Furthermore, technological devices such as nerve stimulators and ultrasonography have increased the accuracy and effectiveness of local anesthetic nerve blocks. With proper equipment and training, along with an adequate knowledge of the technologies available, exotic pet practitioners can successfully enhance their anesthetic and analgesic management of exotic patients.

ADVANCES IN AIRWAY MANAGEMENT

Airway management is vital during general anesthesia. The oropharyngeal anatomy and physiology of the rabbit makes intubation difficult. They have large incisors, a long and narrow dental arcade, fleshy tongue, and an acute angle between the mouth and the larynx. They are also predisposed to laryngospasm.[1–4] Multiple techniques (eg, blind orotracheal or nasotracheal intubation; otoscopic, laryngoscopic, or endoscopic intubation; laryngeal mask airway; supraglottic airway devices [SGADs]) have been used to manage the airway of rabbits.[1,4] Endotracheal intubation complications can occur in rabbits, including soft tissue swelling, arytenoid tears, tracheal stenosis, and even rupture. Laryngeal and tracheal damage can occur if multiple attempts at intubation are required.[3,5] These complications can be minimized by using SGADs and videoendoscopic intubation techniques.

V-GEL SUPRAGLOTTIC AIRWAY DEVICE

Recently, a rabbit-specific SGAD, the V-GEL, has been developed and is commercially available. The V-GEL is specifically designed to create a noninflatable, soft seal around the pharyngeal, laryngeal, perilaryngeal, and the upper esophageal structures. The soft contoured tip of the V-GEL is designed to enter the upper esophagus during placement to ensure gas flow is directed into the airways and to prevent aspiration. V-GEL masks are available in 6 sizes. The manufacturer recommends the use of the smallest size in rabbits weighing 0.6 to 1.5 kg and the largest size in rabbits weighing more than 4.5 kg. The devices can be used multiple times with up to 40 cleaning and autoclave sterilization cycles. For insertion, the preoxygenated rabbit must be fully anesthetized and placed in sternal recumbency with the head elevated and the tongue extended. The V-GEL must be lubricated with Docsinnovent lubricating spray or a sterile, water-based lubricating gel. Topical anesthetic spray should be lightly applied to the larynx. After 30 to 90 seconds, the V-GEL should be inserted into the oropharynx until either resistance is encountered or the incisors are within 1 to 2 cm of the device's fixation tabs. When correctly inserted, the V-GEL is designed to enter the upper esophagus during anesthesia to ensure gas flow is directed into the airway. Placement must be confirmed with a capnograph and by respiratory movement of the reservoir bag. The authors recommend visualization of multiple rectangular waveforms to ensure accurate positioning. If waveforms are not observed, the V-GEL should be repositioned slightly rostrally or caudally. After correct placement, the rabbit's head should be lowered gently, avoiding any movement of the V-GEL. The V-GEL should then be secured with umbilical tape or veterinary cotton cling, making sure to place the knot on the ventral surface of the device. A training video is available from the manufacturer at http://docsinnovent.com/training/rabbit-v-gelV-GelTM (Fig. 1).

Multiple studies have been performed showing that the V-GEL SGAD is quick and easy to place in rabbits compared with intubation techniques.[6–12] Placement could be achieved clinically in more than 90% of rabbits evaluated.[9,10] Depending on studies, placement time range from 13 to 302 seconds.[9,12]

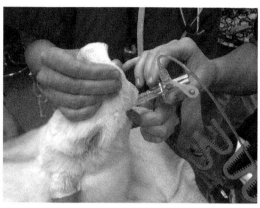

Fig. 1. SGAD (V-GEL) intubation in a New Zealand white rabbit using a sidestream capnograph. (Jorgensen Labs, Loveland, CO.) (*Courtesy of* S. Divers, BVetMed, DZooMed, Dip. ECZM(Herp), Dip. ECZM(ZHM), Dip. ACZM, FRCVS.)

However, lingual cyanosis was encountered as well as gastric inflation, insertion difficulties caused by inadequate anesthetic depth, or dental condition in less than 5% of the cases.[9,10] Manual adjustment was recommended to resolve the lingual cyanosis.[9] In 1 study using computed tomography (CT) to determine the correct V-GEL placement, results showed that, in 85% of the cases (6 out of 7 rabbits), the V-GELs were incorrectly placed with the tip of the V-GEL deviating ventrally into the laryngeal vestibule rather than into the upper esophagus, which caused a reduction in airway flow. In the same study, no significant differences were noted in any vital parameters or blood gases between animals.[11] In another CT study, only 50% (5 out of 10 rabbits) of the V-GELs were placed correctly with the tip of the SGAD in the esophagus. In 3 of the 5 cases in which the V-GEL was correctly placed, moderate or severe laryngeal compression with mucus accumulation was observed.[12] The rabbits weighed between 4.7 and 5.4 kg and the R5 and R6 V-GEL sizes were used. The manufacturer recommends the use of size R6 in rabbits weighing more than 4.5 kg; however, this study suggested that the R5 and R6 V-GELs were too large for New Zealand white rabbits.[12] Furthermore, the study found that 40% of the V-GEL devices were not positioned sufficiently caudal, resulting in the tip not reaching the esophagus.[12] It also showed that 10% of the V-GELs were inserted into the lumen of the larynx, and 20% of V-GELs were slightly tilted.[12] Transient hypoxemia was noted in half of the rabbits in which the V-GEL partially compressed the larynx or was inserted into the lumen of the larynx.[12] This finding may be verified endoscopically where the epiglottis or the arytenoid cartilage is compressed (**Fig. 2**).

Comparison between spontaneous and mechanical ventilation in V-GELs with other intubation techniques (laryngeal mask, face mask, and endotracheal intubation [cuff inflated to 20 cm H_2O]) showed that, for spontaneous ventilation, no leakage greater than 25% of the tidal volume was observed for any of the intubation techniques.[12] In contrast, for mechanical ventilation at pressures of 6 to 16 cm H_2O, 44% of the V-GEL group had significant leakage (>25% of the animal's tidal volume at a pressure of 6 cm H_2O).[12] At high pressures of 16 cm H_2O, 66% of the V-GEL group had no leakage noted.[12] Compared with other intubation devices, V-GELs leaked at a significantly higher pressure than face and laryngeal masks but at a significantly lower pressure than endotracheal tubes.[12] No leakage occurred for any rabbits in the endotracheal intubation group at pressures of 16 cm H_2O.[12] The volume of gastric distention was

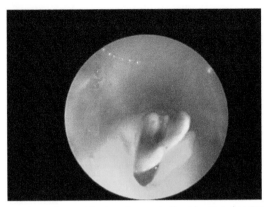

Fig. 2. V-GEL placement can be verified endoscopically. Abnormal V-GEL placement where the epiglottis and arytenoid cartilage are compressed. (*Courtesy of* M. Huynh, DVM, DipECZM (Avian), Dip. ACZM (Small mammals), Arcueil, France and Jorgensen Labs, Loveland, CO.)

measured via CT before and after positive pressure ventilation and no significant changes were noted in the V-GEL group.[12] Improper V-GEL placement could have led to the increased leakage observed.[12]

In a study comparing blind endotracheal tube placement with V-GEL placement, blind intubation resulted in significantly more damage to tracheal mucosa and submucosa.[13] Another study comparing endoscopic endotracheal intubation with V-GELs showed no significant difference in damage to the tracheal mucosa and submucosa.[8]

Proper V-GEL placement seems to be essential to ensuring good inhalant delivery and a good anesthetic outcome. Multiple studies have shown that, when properly placed, V-GELs are a useful tool for the intubation of spontaneously ventilating rabbits. More studies are needed to evaluate the oral/laryngeal anatomic differences of rabbit breeds and their effect on V-GEL placement and ventilation.

Furthermore, a prototype of V-GEL is currently under investigation for guinea pigs.[13] The guinea pig is a challenging species to intubate because of its small size and the existence of a palatal ostium, and the V-GEL may overcome this difficulty. A first prototype was designed but provoked hyperinflation of the stomach because of gas leakage and a stridor in an experimental trial (**Fig. 3**). Modification of this prototype allowed positive pressure ventilation in 2 guinea pigs with apparent success. Further developments are needed to ensure the safety of the device, but the first results are promising.

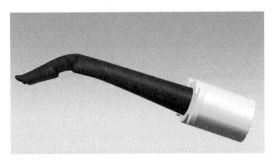

Fig. 3. A prototype of V-GEL for guinea pigs that is currently being researched. (*Courtesy of* DocsInnovent, Hemel Hempstead, UK.)

VIDEOENDOSCOPIC INTUBATION

Video endoscopic intubation is a noninvasive, simplistic, and effective technique. Videoendoscopic placement of endotracheal tubes seems to be a reliable and consistent method of intubation. Direct visualization seems to decrease the risk of trauma to the glottis that can be observed with other intubation methods. Endotracheal intubation is the gold standard for ventilatory support and protects the airway from aspiration. The authors recommend a 1.9-mm to 2.7-mm endoscope. The cost of the endoscope is the main disadvantage compared with other intubation techniques. Alternatively, some USB borescopes represent low-cost alternatives allowing video-assisted side-by-side intubation.[14] Those device are labeled as USB ear-cleaning endoscopes and have a diameter of 5.5 mm, which allows insertion in the mouth of a medium-sized rabbit.

Once general anesthesia has been induced, the endoscope should be carefully inserted into the mouth. The glottis and arytenoids should be directly visualized, and topical anesthetic spray applied. After 50 to 90 seconds, the endoscope can be advanced, during inspiration, through the glottis. The endotracheal tube can then be advanced further into the trachea (**Fig. 4**). Endoscopic visualization of the glottis allows proper placement while also assessing for trauma. If the endotracheal tube is too small to be placed over the endoscope, the tube can be passed beside it as it advances into the trachea. A study in 60 New Zealand white rabbits showed that, when using endoscopic intubation, all animals were intubated with no morbidity or mortality associated with the procedure. Intubation took between 30 and 120 seconds and no instances of esophageal intubation occurred. All animals underwent necropsy at 10 days or 30 days with no evidence of orotracheal injury observed.[15] In another study comparing videoendoscopic endotracheal intubation with SGAD V-GEL placement, it took significantly longer to endoscopically intubate rabbits, with a median time of

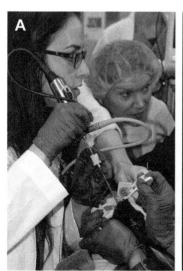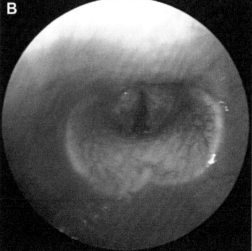

Fig. 4. (*A*) Endotracheal intubation using a 2.7-mm 30° rigid endoscope in a domestic rabbit. (*B*) Endoscopic visualization of the glottis and arytenoids prior to endoscpoc intubation. ([*B*] *Courtesy of* S. Divers, BVetMed, DZooMed, Dip. ECZM(Herp), Dip. ECZM(ZHM), Dip. ACZM, FRCVS.)

48 seconds (range, 20–126 seconds), compared with V-GEL, with a median place-ment time of 6 seconds (range, 2–20 seconds). Compared histologically at 4 days after initial anesthesia, there was no significant difference in the severity of inflammation, hemorrhage, and necrosis of the larynx or the trachea, and no identified trend in the distribution of lesions between the two techniques. Although the difference was not statistically significant, higher severity scores were observed for the larynx in the V-GEL group compared with the endotracheally intubated group.[8] Severity scores for the trachea were generally lower in the V-GEL group than the Endoscopic Endotra-cheal Intubation group.[8]

ADVANCES IN VENTILATION

Intermittent positive pressure ventilation (IPPV) through the use of mechanical ventila-tors has been a staple in treating apnea, hypoventilation, hypoxemia, ventilation-perfusion (V/Q) mismatch, and excessive breathing effort in both human and veterinary medicine. All general anesthetics can contribute to central respiratory depression, ultimately resulting in severe hypercapnia leading to acidemia, which may cause increased sympathetic stimulation. IPPV insufflates airways by pushing gas into the lungs, which improves tidal volume and gas exchange. Properly control-ling ventilation with a mechanical ventilator can increase the stability, control, and safety of anesthesia. Potential adverse effects in small animal medicine are decreased cardiac output, unintended respiratory alkalosis, gastric distention, and impairment of hepatic or renal function. Positive pressure ventilation may also result in pneumo-thorax, airway injury, alveolar damage, and ventilator-associated pneumonia.[16,17] IPPV is commonly used in small exotic mammals undergoing anesthesia for prolonged procedures or surgeries. The normal tidal volume of small mammals is between 10 and 20 mL/kg.[17] When using IPPV, the tidal volume for mechanical ventilation is usually slightly increased to compensate for pressure-mediated increases of the breathing system. In general, domestic small animal peak inspiratory pressures are recommen-ded to be 15 to 20 cm H_2O.[17–19] In patients that require smaller tidal volumes, an in-crease in respiratory rate may be needed to maintain appropriate minute ventilation.[17] Few studies in exotic mammals have been performed comparing IPPV and sponta-neous ventilation. A study in guinea pigs showed that mechanical ventilation at a tidal volume of 10 mL/kg at 20 breaths per minute resulted in stable compliance, normo-capnia, and normal acid-base balance. Blood gases of guinea pigs with spontaneous ventilation resulted in acidemia and hypercapnia.[20] In contrast, in a study of young rabbits that were ventilated with 20 cm H_2O peak airway pressure at a respiratory rate of 26 to 28 breaths per minute for 6 hours, 60% of the animals had pulmonary parenchymal damage and intra-alveolar edema. No animals showed hypoxia during the trial.[21] Caution is advised with increased pressures, and further study is needed. For small exotic mammalian species, the authors suggest using peak inspiratory pres-sures between 10 and 15 cm H_2O and tidal volumes between 10 and 20 mL/kg (Table 1).

In reptiles, because of the absence of a diaphragm and the reliance on skeletal mus-cle movement for respiration, it is recommended that animals be ventilated during anesthesia.[22–25] Reptiles can tolerate extended periods of oxygen shortage as well as pronounced metabolic acidosis during activity.[26] Functional lung (tidal) volumes vary greatly among reptile species (eg, 12.5 mL/kg in boa species and 45 mL/kg in slider turtle species). The lung capacities also seem to be much greater than those of mammals and may exceed 300 mL/kg, suggesting that there is a large functional reserve.[27] There is very little information on the effects of reptile mechanical ventilation

Table 1
Recommended tidal volumes and peak inspiratory pressures for mechanical ventilation of exotic animals

	Tidal Volume (mL/kg)	Peak Inspiratory Pressure (cm H_2O)
Small Exotic Mammals	10–20	10–15
Reptiles	15–30	4–10
Avian	10–20	4–10

concerning blood gases, and few studies have investigated specific reptilian ventilatory requirements. Nonetheless, because of reptile anatomy and physiology, it is generally recommended to use larger tidal volumes and lower frequency when ventilating reptiles.[28–30]

One study in fasted rattlesnakes compared spontaneous ventilation with mechanical ventilation with a tidal volume of 30 mL/kg at different respiratory rates. Ventilation at 1 breath per 90 seconds, 5 breaths per minute, and 15 breaths per minute resulted in hypocapnia, normocapnia, and hypercapnia, respectively. Mechanical ventilation caused a significant and proportional increase in mean arterial pressure (MAP). Unlike mammals, in which ventilation can decrease venous return, ventilation in reptiles, because of their lack of diaphragm, increases filling of the saccular caudal portion of the lungs, which increases venous return, cardiac output, and MAP.[31] Studies involving iguanas and varanid lizards showed that minute ventilation at 100 mL/kg (4 breaths per minute with a tidal volume of 25 mL/kg) lead to hypocapnia and respiratory alkalosis.[32,33] A patient's metabolism (environmental temperature and digestive state) should also be considered when ventilating reptiles. For example, in black racers, minute ventilation was 48 mL/kg at 30°C but was 6 mL/kg at 10°C.[34] In a study of fasted Burmese pythons, the minute ventilation was 27.8 mL/kg, but it was 118 mL/kg after feeding.[35] These studies suggest that metabolic requirements for reptiles may vary depending on the metabolic phase and time from the last meal, which should be considered during anesthesia and ventilation. The authors suggest the use of peak inspiratory pressures between 4 and 10 cm H_2O and tidal volumes between 15 to 30 mL/kg in reptiles (see **Table 1**).

Because of their unique anatomic and physiologic differences, birds do not have substantial functional residual capacity, defined as the volume of air remaining in the lungs at the end of expiration. Therefore, the physiologic effects of hypoventilation develop much more rapidly in birds than in mammals.[36]

Multiple studies of Gruiformes, Psittaciformes, Anseriformes, Galliformes, and Columbiformes have analyzed the effects of IPPV.[37–44] A study of cockatoos showed that birds with spontaneous breathing became metabolically acidotic soon after induction of anesthesia.[39] IPPV at 4 cm H_2O, at 12 breaths per minute, significantly reversed this acidosis.[39] Studies in sandhill cranes and Hispaniolan Amazon parrots showed that, compared with spontaneous respiration, mechanical ventilation provided a significant improvement in cardiovascular function and an increase in mean arterial blood pressure during anesthesia.[35,38] This higher blood pressure is thought to be caused by the lack of a diaphragm and increased venous return.[37,40] Some avian IPPV studies suggest not exceeding 12 to 20 cm H_2O to prevent barotrauma to the air sacs.[41,42] Ongoing research in psittacines has shown that a peak pressure of 4 to 5 cm H_2O provides adequate ventilation and normal venous blood gas values.[38] The authors suggest for avian species to use peak inspiratory pressures between 4 and 10 cm H_2O and tidal volumes between 10 and 20 mL/kg (see **Table 1**).

There are 2 main commercially available ventilators capable of handling the small but variable size of exotic animal patients. The Vetronics SAV04 ventilator is a pressure-cycled ventilator that can reliably give IPPV in patients ranging from 50 g to 12 kg. The maximum inspired pressure (MIP) can be set between 1 and 60 cm H_2O. This ventilator was designed to act as a typical nonrebreathing T-piece circuit until IPPV is activated. Once activated, the outflow valve in the circuit closes and gas continues to be directed into the patient through the endotracheal tube until the airway pressure reaches the MIP set point. Once reached, the outflow valve opens, and both fresh and inspired gas flows preferentially exit the animal and the circuit into the scavenging device. Breathing frequency can range between 1 and 120 breaths per minute by adjusting the expiration length from 0.1 to 60 seconds. The rate of inspiratory time depends on the rate of fresh gas flow and how quickly the set MIP can be attained.[27] As previously discussed, resistance and compliance of the respiratory system must be accounted for with pressure-cycled ventilators. If resistance and compliance are high, it is possible that an adequate tidal volume will not be delivered, even though the MIP has been met[17] (**Fig. 5**).

Hallowell EMC Anesthesia WorkStation is a time-cycled volume ventilator with an adjustable pressure safety limit. The only additional component necessary for immediate use is a vaporizer for the agent of the clinician's choice. This system is designed for animals between 150 g and 7 kg and can deliver tidal volumes up to 100 mL, at rates between 4 and 80 breaths per minute. It has a preset inspiratory-expiratory ratio of 1:2 and an adjustable pressure limit between 10 and 30 cm H_2O. As previously stated, when using a volume-cycled ventilator, operators must consider increased resistance and compliance of the airway in order to reduce instances of airway injury.[17]

ADVANCES IN BLOOD PRESSURE MONITORING

Blood pressure monitoring is a crucial component of patient care and has become a valuable clinical tool in small, large, and exotic animal anesthesia. Consistent hypotension can lead to renal failure, decreased hepatic metabolism, severe hypoxemia, neuromuscular complications, central nervous system abnormalities, and cardiac and respiratory arrest. Sudden, dramatic changes in blood pressure can indicate that cardiac arrest is imminent, which requires immediate action.[45,46]

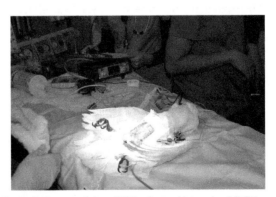

Fig. 5. An umbrella cockatoo receiving IPPV using a Vetronics SAV04 ventilator. (Vetronic Services, Devon, UK.) (*Courtesy of* S. Divers, BVetMed, DZooMed, Dip. ECZM(Herp), Dip. ECZM(ZHM), Dip. ACZM, FRCVS.)

Accurate determination of blood pressure is critical in any species and this can be evaluated through invasive and noninvasive techniques (**Table 2**). Invasive methods are considered the gold standard and have been found to more reliably correlate with systemic blood pressures. These methods require surgical or percutaneous placement of an arterial catheter and measurement through a pressure transducer. The disadvantage of obtaining direct blood pressure is that placement of the arterial line can be time consuming, technical, and difficult because of the anatomy and size of the patient. Potential complications consist of emboli, nerve or vessel damage, and ischemia. Moreover, frequent administration of heparin can lead to iatrogenic coagulation abnormalities, especially in smaller patients.[47]

Noninvasive methods rely on a system to detect blood flow under or past a pressurized cuff. Noninvasive techniques include Doppler sphygmomanometry, regular and high-definition oscillometric systems, and photoplethysmographic monitors. Multiple

Table 2			
Selected blood pressure reference range in exotic species			
Blood Pressures of Exotic Species			
Species	**SAP (mm Hg)**	**DAP (mm Hg)**	**MAP (mm Hg)**
Small Animal Exotic Mammals			
Rabbit	90–130[a]	80–90[a]	60–80[a]
Ferret	90–160 95–155[b]	50–90 51–87[b]	60–110 69–109[b]
Guinea pig	65–75 91.8–96.2[a,b]	44–52 47–50[a,b]	56–64 64[a] 61.9–65.3[a,b]
Rat	88–184	58–145	74–102
Avian			
Chicken	86–112	54–84	71–97
Sandhill crane	—	—	176–234
Amazon parrot	145–181 110.9–154.9	130–166 79.9–123.9	137–173 96.5–137
Cockatoo			139–147
Great horned owl	195–269[a]	153–203[a]	175–231[a]
Red-tailed hawk	169–271[a]	115–205[a]	145–229[a]
Bald eagle	181–207	145–171	—
Reptilian			
Red-eared turtle Greek tortoise	32.6–36 44.9–49.5	22.6–26.4 28.8–32.4	15–30
Green iguana	68–107[a] 40–50[a]	58–94[a]	58–95[a]
Monitor lizards	—	—	60–80
Mangrove snake	—	—	74[a]
Lowland copperhead	—	—	61[a]
Tiger snake	—	—	49
Yellow-lipped sea krait	—	—	36[a]

Abbreviations: DAP, diastolic arterial pressures; SAP, systolic arterial pressure.
[a] Blood pressure values are from awake animals.
[b] Blood pressure measurements that were noninvasive measurements.

factors can influence the accuracy and precision of the various noninvasive devices, including size and location of the cuff, hair density, patient movement, arrhythmias, anesthetic agents, and hemodynamic compromise.[45,46] Guidelines have been published by the Association for the Advancement of Medical Instrumentation (AAMI) for the evaluation of human blood pressure measurement devices, which set out the criteria to be tested against the accepted standards. AAMI guidelines recommend a mean difference of less than 5 mm Hg with a standard deviation of less than 8 mm Hg as an acceptable error when comparing noninvasive and direct blood pressure measurements.[48,49]

Multiple studies in rabbits, rats, and ferrets, have shown blood pressures similar to those of domestic mammals.[50–52] In the rabbit, highly reliable and accurate, direct arterial blood pressure measurements can be obtained using a 22-gauge to 24-gauge over-the-needle catheter placed in the central auricular artery. Normal ranges of blood pressures in rabbits consist of systolic arterial pressures (SAPs) between 90 and 130 mm Hg and diastolic arterial pressures (DAPs) between 80 and 90 mm Hg.[53] A study in anesthetized rabbits showed good agreement between noninvasive Doppler-measured arterial blood pressure of the forelimb and direct auricular arterial pressure, with Doppler measurement less than 80 mm Hg being a reliable indicator of arterial hypotension.[54] In another rabbit study comparing direct carotid with auricular arterial pressures, and direct auricular pressures with oscillometric thoracic limb blood pressures, the carotid and auricular direct pressures correlated well with each other, whereas only mean oscillometric hypotensive and normotensive pressures of the forelimb correlated with direct pressures.[55]

Normal direct arterial blood pressure ranges in ferrets consist of systolic pressures of 95 to 155 mm Hg, mean pressures of 69 to 109 mm Hg, and diastolic pressures of 51 to 87 mm Hg. The coccygeal artery is typically utilized using a 24-gauge catheter in a clinical setting; however, other sites, such as the carotid and femoral arteries, have also been reported. A study using high-definition oscillometric monitoring in hypotensive, normotensive, and hypertensive ferrets with cuff placements at the tail, forelimb, and hind limb, showed that high-definition oscillometry provided a reproducible, although less accurate, blood pressure measurement compared with direct blood pressure in normotensive ferrets.[52]

At present, there are only a few blood pressure studies that have been performed in guinea pigs, most likely because of the difficulty of arterial catheter placement. Guinea pig resting blood pressure is typically lower than in other small mammal exotic species, with normotensive pressure ranges consisting of aortic systolic pressures of 65 to 75 mm Hg, mean pressures of 56 to 64 mm Hg, and diastolic pressures of 44 to 52 mm Hg.[56] In one study, the average oscillometric blood pressure in awake animals consisted of a systolic blood pressure of 94.0 ± 2.2 mm Hg, mean blood pressure of 63.6 ± 1.7 mm Hg, and diastolic blood pressure of 48.4 ± 1.6 mm Hg. These pressures were similar to carotid direct blood pressures in anesthetized guinea pigs.[57]

Normal blood pressure in domestic rats is a systolic blood pressure between 88 and 184 mm Hg, a mean blood pressure of 74 to 102 mm Hg, and a diastolic blood pressure of 58 to 145 mm Hg. The central coccygeal artery, femoral artery, and carotid artery have all been used in various direct blood pressure studies.[51] An oscillometric study in which the cuff was placed on the tail showed good correlation between indirect systolic and mean blood pressures compared with carotid direct blood pressures in awake hypertensive and normotensive rats.[58]

Multiple studies on avian arterial blood pressure measurements have shown that arterial blood pressure in most avian species is significantly higher compared with that of mammals.[59–61] Bird arteries have a higher resilience, which may affect how quickly vessels respond to changes in cardiac output and resultant blood pressures.[62,63] Birds have a lower total peripheral resistance and a higher arterial pressure than mammals. Furthermore, they frequently have larger hearts, higher stroke volumes, and lower heart rates than mammals of corresponding body mass. These anatomic and physiologic differences ultimately allow sufficient cardiac output to meet their greater metabolic needs.[62,63]

Normal blood pressure values are higher in Psittaciformes, Gruiformes, Falconiformes, Accipitriformes, Strigiformes, and Galliformes (specifically turkeys) than in mammal and reptiles. Hispaniolan Amazon parrots anesthetized with 2.5% isoflurane were shown to have arterial systolic blood pressures of 132.9 ± 22.1 mm Hg, mean pressures of 116.9 ± 20.5 mm Hg, and diastolic pressures of 101.9 ± 22.0 mm Hg.[60] However, studies in Galliformes and Columbiformes showed blood pressures comparable with those of domestic mammals. A study in domestic chickens showed a normal arterial systolic blood pressure of 99 ± 13 mm Hg, mean blood pressure of 84 ± 13 mm Hg, and diastolic blood pressures of 69 ± 15 mm Hg.[64]

Noninvasive techniques have been reported to be inaccurate in psittacines compared with invasive blood pressure monitoring. A study performed on anesthetized Hispaniolan Amazon parrots showed poor agreement between noninvasive blood pressure measurement using the thoracic and pelvic limb compared with direct arterial blood pressures. This inaccuracy of noninvasive blood pressure could be a result of the higher heart rates and the inability of the indirect monitors to measure them.[60]

Unlike domestic mammals, there are only a few placement sites available for arterial catheterization in birds. For medium to large birds, the deep radial artery is the preferred site. However, for smaller birds (<200 g), the authors prefer catheterization of the superficial ulnar artery. For aquatic or long-legged birds, the cranial tibial or dorsal metatarsal arteries are acceptable choices for catheterization (**Fig. 6**). External carotid artery catheterization has also been reported. However, this is more invasive and requires a cut-down for visualization.[47]

Physiologic studies involving reptiles have revealed that resting blood pressures greatly vary with animal size, species, habitat, feeding, and external temperatures.[65] Blood pressures tend to be lower in chelonians with MAPs of 15 to 30 mm Hg.[66] A study in green iguanas reported systolic blood pressure ranges of 86 to 107 mm Hg, diastolic blood pressures ranges of 21 to 55 mm Hg, and mean blood

A   **B**

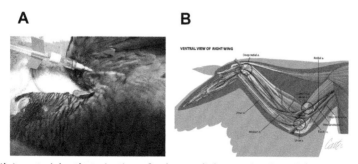

Fig. 6. (A) An arterial catheterization of a deep radial artery in Hispaniolan Amazon parrots for invasive blood pressure measurement. (B) Anatomy of an avian wing for the arterial catheterization of the deep radial and superficial ulnar artery. a., artery; n., nerve; v., vein. ([B] *Courtesy of* K. Carter.)

pressures ranges of 58 to 90 mm Hg.[67] Studies in some varanid lizards showed resting MAPs similar to those of mammals, ranging from 60 to 80 mm Hg.[68] Arboreal snakes have evolved with the highest blood pressures, with typical pressures between 40 and 70 mm Hg, compared with aquatic snakes with the lowest pressures, typically ranging between 20 and 30 mm Hg (see **Table 2**).[69] Temperature changes between 18°C and 33°C (64–91°F) have been shown to alter blood pressure in the black racer,[70] but not in the tiger snake.[71] Postural blood pressures in snakes have been shown to increase 3-fold to 4-fold after a meal.[72]

Cardiovascular physiology may contribute to unique challenges concerning accurate blood pressure measurement. In noncrocodilian species, the 3-chambered heart with 2 atria and 1 multichambered ventricle allows flow and pressure separation between chambers and intracardiac shunting. The extent to which shunting occurs when reptiles are anesthetized, and the effect of shunting on blood pressure and tissue perfusion, are unknown.

Noninvasive blood pressure measurements correlate poorly with direct arterial blood pressures in reptiles. Studies in green iguanas and boa constrictors have shown that commercially available oscillometric devices applied to the femoral artery and ventral coccygeal artery respectively are of limited value. Discrepancies between measured pressures could have been caused by cuff placement, noncompliant reptile skin/scales, size of the vessel, and the distance from the heart to the vessel.[73] Most reptilian direct blood pressure studies have used the carotid, the aortic arch, or the femoral artery for catheterization. At present, direct blood pressure measurements are rarely used in reptiles because of the necessity of a surgical cut-down for visualization and the lack of understanding of reptilian cardiovascular physiology.

ADVANCES IN REGIONAL NERVE BLOCKS

Locoregional anesthesia is gaining increasing popularity in exotic pet medicine. Although frequently reported, the use of blind techniques is not recommended because they may result in unintentional intraneural or intravascular injection, as well as in failure of the local anesthetic delivery in the targeted area. More reliable methods to deliver local anesthetics in the proximity of a target nerve structure rely on the use of either an electrical nerve stimulator (ENS) or an echograph, equipped with an appropriate ultrasonography probe, to locate the nerve or the group of nerves. The 2 techniques (the nerve stimulator–guided and the ultrasonography-guided nerve blocks) may be used either independently or in combination, for a double guidance.[74,75]

BASICS OF ELECTRICAL STIMULATION

An ENS is a power source that generates electrical impulses and is connected to an insulated, unipolar stimulating needle (**Fig. 7**). The needle insulation does not extend to the conductive tip, which is capable of transmitting electrical impulses to the anatomic target. A negative electrode is applied to the skin, usually proximal to the target nerve, in order to generate a circling current. If the needle is correctly positioned in the proximity of a motor nerve, the current of electrons generated by the ENS neutralizes the positive charge of the medium surrounding the resting nerve, generating an action potential. The depolarization of the motor fibers ultimately results in contraction of the muscles innervated by that nerve.[76,77] As stated by Coulomb's law, the current necessary to trigger a muscular response is directly proportional to the distance between the tip of the stimulating needle and the target anatomic structure, so the closer

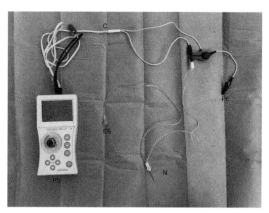

Fig. 7. A nerve stimulator (Stimuplex HNS12, B. Braun Melsugen AG) with all its components. C, connecting cable; ES, extension set (to syringe); N, stimulation needle; PE, positive electrode; PS, power source. (Braun-Medical Inc., Bethlehem, PA.)

the needle tip is to the nerve, the lower the electrical current (milliamps) necessary to elicit a muscular contraction.

The basic components of an ENS consist of a power source, a display (either digital or LCD [liquid crystal display]), an on-off switch, a microprocessor unit, an analog-digital converter, a unit for electrical measurement, and a constant-current generator equipped with a means of current regulation. The parameters that should be adjustable during needle advancement are the intensity of the generated current (milliamps), the frequency of the stimulation (Hertz) and the pulse width/duration of the electrical stimulus (milliseconds). The Sequential Electrical Nerve Stimulation (SENSe; B. Braun) technique is a peculiar stimulating pattern that applies 2 fixed 0.10-millisecond impulses followed by a third impulse, whose duration varies from 0.15 to 1 millisecond (**Fig. 8**). This sequence of stimuli allows the operator to detect a motor response before the needle tip reaches the perineurium, thus eliminating the need for constant adjustment of the current during needle advancement.

ELECTRICAL NERVE STIMULATOR–GUIDED NERVE BLOCKS

The cathode is connected to the insulated needle and the anode is applied to the patient's skin. The anatomic landmarks useful to locate the nerve to be blocked are identified and the area of interest is disinfected. The ENS is turned on and the initial stimulating current is set at 1.0 to 1.5 mA and 0.1 to 0.15 millisecond; or alternatively, the SENSe function can be used if available. At this point, the stimulating needle is inserted through the skin and advanced toward the target nerve until the desired muscular response is elicited. Thereafter, the current is decreased, first to 0.5 mA and then to 0.2 mA; if the lowest 0.2-mA current still elicits a response, intraneural injection is likely and therefore the needle should be withdrawn by a few millimeters. As an alternative technique, the minimum stimulating current (MSC) may be identified by reducing the current to zero and then by increasing it progressively until the muscular contractions reappear. An aspiration test should be performed to rule out intravascular needle location, followed by injection of the calculated volume of local anesthetic solution. The absence of resistance during injection serves as further confirmation that intraneural injection has not occurred.

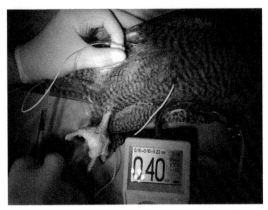

Fig. 8. Sequential electrical nerve stimulation (SENSe) technique (© B. Braun). Besides the 2 regular impulses of 0.1-millisecond duration used to locate the nerve, the stimulation pattern incorporates an additional stimulus, with a longer pulse duration and a 3-Hz stimulation. (Braun-Medical Inc., Bethlehem, PA.)

ULTRASONOGRAPHY-GUIDED NERVE BLOCKS

Ultrasonography is commonly used in both human and veterinary medicine to identify the nerves as well as the adjacent anatomic structures, namely blood vessels, bone, muscles, tendons, adipose tissue, and the eye globe.[74,77,78] The direct visualization of the needle allows its tip to be located as close as possible to the targeted nerve without causing iatrogenic damage of anatomic structures in the area of interest. In addition, the volume, and therefore the dose, of the local anesthetic can be minimized thanks to the real-time visualization of the spreading of the solution.[77] In exotic pets, the ultrasonography-guided blocks should be performed with echographers equipped with a linear transducer, ideally with frequencies ranging from 7 to 15 MHz to optimize the visualization of nerve structures.[78–81]

The ultrasonographic appearance of the tissues varies depending on several factors, such as size, degree of reflection and absorption of the ultrasound beam, and imaging performance of the medical ultrasonography equipment used. Nerves, tendons, and fascia typically seem as hyperechoic structures, whereas adipose and muscular tissues are hypoechoic (**Fig. 9**). The ultrasound beam should preferentially be perpendicular to the target nerve, because tissue echogenicity may vary depending on the angle of imaging.[82] Identification of the blood vessels is crucial to prevent inadvertent intravascular administration of local anesthetics, as well as to avoid hemorrhage and hematoma formation. In addition, because large arteries and veins are easily visible, they are often used as ultrasonographic landmarks to locate the target nerve. Blood is typically anechoic and the arteries can be distinguished from the veins owing to their thicker walls. The color Doppler allows clear identification of the blood flow and can be used to differentiate perineural vessels from nonvascular structures. The skeletal muscles show variable echogenicity and generally appear as hypoechoic layers surrounded by a hyperechoic fascia. The bones reflect the totality of the ultrasound beam and therefore appear as highly hyperechoic lines. Similarly, air is displayed as bright and hyperechoic on the ultrasonographic screen, because it reflects the ultrasound beam; its presence represents a challenging obstacle to the visualization of the adjacent organs.[74]

There are 2 main techniques of needle insertion during an ultrasonography-guided block. With the in-plane technique, the shaft of the needle is parallel to the long axis of

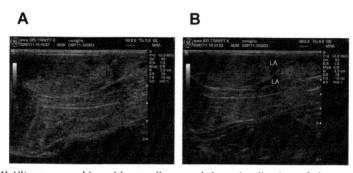

Fig. 9. (A) Ultrasonographic guidance allows real-time visualization of the needle while advancing it toward the sciatic nerve, (B) as well as the spread of the local anesthetic during and after the injection. The sciatic nerve (SN) appears as a hyperechoic structure. The local anesthetic (LA) appears as a hypoechoic pocket of fluid. Needle frequency (N) enables nerve stimulation at a distance. (*Courtesy of* G. Tranchese.)

the transducer, whereas with the out-of-plane technique the needle is perpendicular to it (**Fig. 10**). The in-plane technique is considered the safest and the easiest, especially for less experienced operators, because it allows visualization of the entire needle shaft, including the needle tip, as well as a comprehensive evaluation of the spatial relationship between the needle and the anatomic structures in the area of interest.[74,83]

One of the most important advantages of ultrasonography-guided techniques is the real-time visualization of the local anesthetic spread during the block.[84] When properly delivered, the anesthetic solution forms a black fluid ring around the nerve,

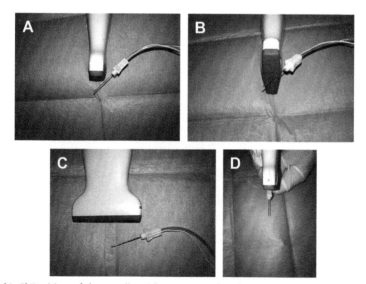

Fig. 10. (A, B) Position of the needle with respect to the ultrasonography probe for both the out-of-plane (C, D) and in-plane techniques for ultrasonography-guided nerve block. (*Courtesy of* L. Meomartino.)

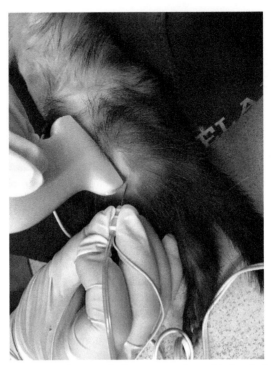

Fig. 11. Combined nerve stimulator and ultrasonography-guided technique (dual in-plane technique) for sciatic nerve block in a ferret before hind limb surgery. (*Courtesy of* L. Meomartino.)

called a doughnut sign, which confirms the perineural distribution of the solution and rules out its inadvertent intravascular injection.[83] Even when the anesthetic solution does not surround the entire section of the nerve, a successful blockade is still possible if sufficient surface of the nerve has been exposed to the liquid anesthetic solution.[85]

DUAL TECHNIQUE

The combined use of ENS and ultrasonography seems to help minimize the complications associated with both techniques, in both human and veterinary patients.[79,81] The so-called dual technique or dual guidance may improve the overall accuracy, reduce the time necessary to perform the block, and decrease the risk of iatrogenic damage (**Fig. 11**).[86] Even when performed by skilled operators, locating the nerves can be challenging in small exotic pets; in such cases, the use of an ENS may be useful to confirm the correct identification of the target nerve. When ultrasonography and ENS guidance are used in combination, it is advisable to set the ENS at the lowest frequency possible in order to minimize the movements within the ultrasonography image.[87]

REFERENCES

1. Wenger S. Anesthesia and analgesia in rabbits and rodents. J Exot Pet Med 2012;21:7–16.

2. Bateman L, Ludders JW, Gleed RD, et al. Comparison between facemask and laryngeal mask airway in rabbits during isoflurane anesthesia. Vet Anaesth Analg 2005;32:280–8.

3. Phaneuf LR, Barker S, Groleau MA, et al. Tracheal injury after endotracheal intubation and anesthesia in rabbits. J Am Assoc Lab Anim Sci 2006;45:67–72.

4. Johnson DH. Endoscopic intubation of exotic companion mammals. Vet Clin North Am Exot Anim Pract 2010;13:273–89.

5. Grint NJ, Sayers IR, Cecchi R, et al. Postanaesthetic tracheal strictures in three rabbits. Lab Anim 2006;40:301–8.

6. Uzun M, Kiraz HA, Ovali MA, et al. The investigation of airway management capacity of V-gelTM and cobra-PLA in anaesthetized rabbits. Acta Cir Bras 2015; 30:80–6.

7. Cruz ML, Sacchi T, Luna SP. Use of a laryngeal mask for airway maintenance during inhalation anaesthesia in rabbits. Vet Anaesth Analg 2000;27:115–6.

8. Schnellbacher R, Blas-Machado U, Quandt J, et al. Comparison between endotracheal intubation and supraglottic airway device in New Zealand white rabbits undergoing laparotomy. Proc Intern Conf Avi, Herp, Exot Mam Med. Paris, France, April 18–23, 2015. p. 388.

9. Eatwell K. Use of a novel airway device to maintain gaseous anaesthesia in rabbits (Oryctolagus cuniculus). Proc Intern Conf Avi, Herp, Exot Mam Med. Wiesbaden, Germany, April 20–26, 2013. p. 196.

10. Van Zeeland Y, Schoemaker N. Clinical use of a novel supraglottic airway device in rabbits. Proc Intern Conf Avi, Herp, Exot Mam Med. Wiesbaden, Germany, April 20–26, 2013. p. 192.

11. Engbers S, Larkin A, Rousset N, et al. Comparison of a supraglottic airway device (V-gelTM®) with blind orotracheal intubation in rabbits. Front Vet Sci 2017;10:49.

12. Wenger S, Müllhaupt D, Ohlerth S, et al. Experimental evaluation of four airway devices in anaesthetized New Zealand White rabbits. Vet Anaesth Analg 2017; 44:529–37.

13. Van Zeeland Y, Schoemaker N, Crotaz I. Development and use of a Supraglottic Airway Device in Guinea Pigs. Proc Exoticscon, Atlanta (Georgia), September 22–27, 2018. p. 781.

14. Yinharnmingmongkol C, Buranapim, N. Spend 10 dollars for visualize intubation technique in rabbits. Proc ICARE, London (United Kingdom), Apr 28–May 2, 2019. p. 356.

15. Tran HS, Puc MM, Tran JL, et al. A method of endoscopic endotracheal intubation in rabbits. Lab Anim 2001;35:249–52.

16. Hopper K, Powell L. Basics of mechanical ventilation for dogs and cats. Vet Clin North Am Small Anim Pract 2013;43:955–69.

17. Hartfield SM. Airway management and ventilation. In: Tranquilli WJ, Thurmon JC, Grimm KA, editors. Lumb and Jones' veterinary anesthesia and analgesia. 4th edition. Ames (IA): Blackwell Publ; 2007. p. 495–512.

18. Staffieri F, Franchini D, Carella GL, et al. Computed tomographic analysis of the effects of two inspired oxygen concentrations on pulmonary aeration in anesthetized and mechanically ventilated dogs. Am J Vet Res 2007;68:925–31.

19. Guarracino A, Lacitignola L, Auriemma E, et al. Which airway pressure should be applied during breath-hold in dogs undergoing thoracic computed tomography? Vet Radiol Ultrasound 2016;57:475–81.

20. Kluge R. Compliance, blood gases, and acid-base balance in guinea pigs artificially ventilated with different IPPV patterns. Acta Physiol Hung 1987;70:297–302.

21. John E, Ermocilla R, Golden J, et al. Effects of intermittent positive-pressure ventilation on lungs of normal rabbits. Br J Exp Pathol 1980;61:315–23.

22. Bennett RA. Anesthesia. In: Mader DR, editor. Reptile medicine and surgery. Philadelphia: WB Saunders; 1996. p. 241–7.

23. Perry SF. Lungs: Comparative anatomy, functional morphology, and evolution. In: Gans C, Gaunt AS, editors. Biology of the reptilia, Vol. 19. St Louis (MO): Morphology G. Society for the Study of Amphibians and Reptiles; 1998. p. 1–92.

24. Bertelsen MF. Squamates (snakes and lizards). In: West G, Heard D, Caulket N, editors. Zoo animal and wildlife immobilization and anesthesia. 2nd edition. Ames (IA): Blackwell Publ; 2014. p. 351–63.

25. Vigani A. Chelonia (tortoises, turtles and terrapins). In: West G, Heard D, Caulket N, editors. Zoo animal and wildlife immobilization and anesthesia. 2nd edition. Ames (IA): Blackwell Publ; 2014. p. 365–87.

26. Wang T, Smits AW, Burggren VW. Pulmonary function in reptiles. In: Gans C, Gaunt AS, editors. Biology of the reptilia, Vol. 19. St Louis (MO): Morphology G. Society for the Study of Amphibians and Reptiles; 1998. p. 297–374.

27. Hernandez-Divers S, Read M, Hernandez S. Reptile respiration and controlled ventilation during anesthesia. Proc Annu Conf Assoc Repti and Amphib Vet. Reno (NV), October 9–13, 2002. p. 145–7.

28. Heard D. Reptile anesthesia. Vet Clin North Am Exot Anim Pract 2001;4:83–117.

29. Schumacher J, Yelen T. Anesthesia and analgesia. In: Mader DR, editor. Reptile medicine and surgery. 2nd edition. Saint Louis (MO): Elsevier; 2006. p. 442–52.

30. Bertelsen MF. Squamates (snakes and lizards). In: West G, Heard D, Caulkett N, editors. Zoo animal and wildlife immobilization and anesthesia. Ames (IA): Wiley-Blackwell; 2007. p. 233–43.

31. Bertelsen MF, Buchanan R, Jensen HM, et al. Assessing the influence of mechanical ventilation on blood gases and blood pressure in rattlesnakes. Vet Anaesth Analg 2015;42:386–93.

32. Mosley C. Evaluation of Isoflurane and Butorphanol in the Green Iguana (Iguana iguana) [MSc Dissertation]. Guelph (Canada): Univ. Guelph; 2000.

33. Bertelsen MF, Mosley CA, Crawshaw GJ, et al. Minimum alveolar concentration of isoflurane in mechanically ventilated Dumeril monitors. J Am Vet Med Assoc 2005;226:1098–110.

34. Stinner J, Grguric M, Beaty S. Ventilatory and blood acid-base adjustments to a decrease in body temperature from 30 to 10 C in black racer snakes (Coluber constrictor). J Exp Biol 1996;199:815–23.

35. Secor SM, Hicks JW, Bennett AF. Ventilatory and cardiovascular responses of a python (Python molurus) to exercise and digestion. J Exp Biol 2000;203:2447–54.

36. Powell FL. Respiration. In: Whittow CG, editor. Sturkie's avian physiology. 5th edition. San Diego (CA): Academic Press Inc; 2000. p. 233–64.

37. Ludders JW, Rode J, Mitchell GS. Isoflurane anesthesia in sandhill cranes (Grus canadensis): minimal anesthetic concentration and cardiopulmonary dose response during spontaneous and controlled breathing. Anesth Analg 1989;68:511–6.

38. Edling TW, Degernes LA, Flammer K, et al. Capnographic monitoring of anesthetized African grey parrots receiving intermittent positive pressure ventilation. J Am Vet Med Assoc 2001;219:1714–8.

39. Chemonges S. Effect of intermittent positive pressure ventilation (IPPV) on acid base balance and plasma electrolytes during isoflurane anaesthesia in sulphur-crested cockatoos (Cacatua galerita galerita). Inter J Anim Vet Adv 2012;4:351–7.

40. Cornick-Seahorn JL, Smith JA, Tully TN, et al. Cardiopulmonary effects of controlled ventilation in isoflurane-anesthetized Hispaniolan Amazon Parrots. Vet Anaesth Analg 2000;27:111.

41. Carpenter JW, Mason DE. Use of heated, artificial ventilator in exotic animal anesthesia. Exot DVM 2001;3:15–7.

42. Curro TG. Anesthesia of pet birds: review article. Semin Avian Exot Pet Med 1998; 7:10–21.

43. Piiper J, Drees F, Scheid P. Gas exchange in the domestic fowl during spontaneous breathing and artificial ventilation. Respir Physiol 1970;9:234–345.

44. Touzot-Jourde G, Divers S, Trim C. Cardiopulmonary effects of controlled versus spontaneous ventilation in pigeons anesthetized for coelioscopy. J Am Vet Med Assoc 2005;9:1424–8.

45. Haskins SC. Monitoring the anesthetized patients. In: Tranquilli WJ, Thurmon JC, Grimm KA, editors. Lumb and Jones' veterinary anesthesia and analgesia. 4th edition. Ames (IA): Blackwell Publ; 2007. p. 409–99.

46. Hall LW, Clarke KW, Trim CM. Patient monitoring and clinical measurement. In: Adams JG, editor. Veterinary anaesthesia. Philadelphia: W.B. Saunders; 2001. p. 29–57.

47. Schnellbacher R, Cunha Da, Olson E, et al. Arterial catheterization, interpretation and treatment of arterial blood pressures and blood gases in birds. J Exot Pet Med 2014;23:129–41.

48. Association for the Advancement of Medical Instrumentation. American national standard for electronic or automated sphygmomanometers. ANSI/AAMI SP10-1987. Arlington (TX): AAMI; 1987. p. 25.

49. O'Brien E, Atkins N. A comparison of the BHS and AAMI protocols for validating blood pressure measuring devices: can the two be reconciled? J Hypertens 1994;12:1089–94.

50. Kurashina T, Sakamaki T, Yagi A, et al. A new device for indirect blood pressure measurement in rabbits. Jpn Circ J 1994;58:264–8.

51. Wang Y, Cong Y, Li J, et al. Comparison of invasive blood pressure measurements from the caudal ventral artery and the femoral artery in male adult SD and Wistar rats. PLoS One 2013;8:1–28.

52. van Zeeland YR, Wilde A, Bosman IH, et al. Non-invasive blood pressure measurement in ferrets (Mustela putorius furo) using high definition oscillometry. Vet J 2017;228:53–62.

53. Gillet CS. Select drug dosages and clinical reference data. In: Manning PJ, Ringerly DH, Newcomer CE, editors. The biology of the laboratory rabbit. 2nd edition. San Diego (CA): Academic Press Inc; 1994. p. 492–6.

54. Harvey L, Knowles T, Murison PJ. Comparison of direct and Doppler arterial blood pressure measurements in rabbits during isoflurane anaesthesia. Vet Anaesth Analg 2012;39:174–84.

55. Ypsilantis P, Didilis VN, Politou M, et al. A comparative study of invasive and oscillometric methods of arterial blood pressure measurement in the anesthetized rabbit. Res Vet Sci 2005;78:269–75.

56. Schmitz S, Henke J, Tacke S, et al. Successful implantation of an abdominal aortic blood pressure transducer and radio-telemetry transmitter in guinea pigs — Anaesthesia, analgesic management and surgical methods, and their influence on hemodynamic parameters and body temperature. J Pharmacol Toxicol Methods 2016;80:9–18.

57. Kuwahara M, Yagi Y, Birumachi Ji, et al. Non-invasive measurement of systemic arterial pressure in guinea pigs by an automatic oscillometric device. Blood Press Monit 1996;1:433–7.

58. Ikeda K, Nara Y, Yamori Y. Indirect systolic and mean blood pressure determination by a new tail cuff method in spontaneously hypertensive rats. Lab Anim 1991; 25:26–9.

59. Hawkins M, Wright B, Pascoe P, et al. Pharmacokinetics and anesthetic and cardiopulmonary effects of propofol in red-tailed hawks (Buteo jamaicensis) and great horned owls (Bubo virginianus). Am J Vet Res 2003;64:677–83.

60. Acierno MJ, da Cunha A, Smith J, et al. Agreement between direct and indirect blood pressure measurements obtained from anesthetized Hispaniolan Amazon parrots. J Am Vet Med Assoc 2008;233:1587–90.

61. Zehnder A, Hawkins M, Pascoe P, et al. Evaluation of indirect blood pressure monitoring in awake and anesthetized red-tailed hawks (Buteo jamaicensis): effect of cuff size, cuff placement, and monitoring equipment. Vet Anaesth Analg 2009;36:464–79.

62. Smith F, West N, Jones D. The cardiovascular system. In: Whittow C, editor. Sturkies avian physiology. 5th edition. San Diego (CA): Academic Press Inc; 1994. p. 141–223.

63. Büssow H. The wall structure of large arteries in birds, Investigations by light and electron microscopy. Z Zellforsch Mikrosk Anat 1973;142:263–88.

64. Naganobu K, Fujisawa Y, Ohde H, et al. Determination of the minimum anesthetic concentration and cardiovascular dose response for sevoflurane in chickens during controlled ventilation. Vet Surg 2000;29:102–5.

65. Bogan J. Ophidian cardiology—a review. J Herpetol Med Surg 2017;27:62–77.

66. Shelton G, Burggren W. Cardiovascular dynamic of chelonia during apnoea and lung ventilation. J Exp Biol 1976;64:323–34.

67. Chinnadurai SK, DeVoe R, Koenig A, et al. Comparison of an implantable telemetry device and an oscillometric monitor for measurement of blood pressure in anaesthetized and unrestrained green iguanas (Iguana iguana). Vet Anaesth Analg 2010;375:434–9.

68. Burggren W, Farrell A, Lillywhite HB. Vertebrate cardiovascular systems. In: Dantzler WH, editor. Handbook of physiology: comparative physiology (section 13). New York: Oxford University Press; 1997. p. 254–67.

69. Seymour RE. Scaling of cardiovascular physiology in snakes. Am Zool 1987;27: 97–109.

70. Stinner JN. Cardiovascular and metabolic responses to temperature in Coluber constrictor. Am J Physiol 1987;253:222–7.

71. Lillywhite HB, Seymour RS. Regulation of arterial blood pressure in Australian tiger snakes. J Exp Biol 1978;75:65–79.

72. Stinner JN, Ely DL. Blood pressure during routine activity, stress, and feeding in black racer snakes (Coluber constrictor). Am J Physiol 1993;264:79–84.

73. Chinnadurai SK, Wrenn A, DeVoe RS. Evaluation of noninvasive oscillometric blood pressure monitoring in anesthetized boid snakes. J Am Vet Med Assoc 2009;234:625–30.

74. Re M, Bianco J, Gomez de Segura IA. Ultrasound-guided nerve block anesthesia. Vet Clin North Am Food Anim Pract 2016;32:133–47.

75. Tsui BCH, Hopkins D. Electrical nerve stimulation for regional anesthesia. In: Boezaart AP, editor. Anesthesia and orthopaedic surgery. New York: McGraw-Hill; 2006. p. 249–54.

76. Urmey WF. Electrical nerve stimulation for regional anesthesia. Minerva Anestesiol 2006;72:467–71.
77. Marhofer P, Harrop-Griffiths W, Kettner SC, et al. Fifteen years of ultrasound guidance in regional anaesthesia: part 1. Br J Anaesth 2010;104:538–46.
78. Najman IE, Ferreira JZ, Abimussi CJ, et al. Ultrasound-assisted periconal ocular blockade in rabbits. Vet Anaesth Analg 2015;42:433–41.
79. d'Ovidio D, Noviello E, Nocerino M, et al. Application of brachial plexus block (BPB) in wild birds undergoing surgery of the wings. Proc. of the International Conference on Diseases of Zoo and Wild Animals (EAZWV). Verona, Italia, May 16–19, 2012. p. 23.
80. da Cunha AF, Strain GM, Rademacher N, et al. Palpation and ultrasound-guided brachial plexus blockade in Hispaniolan Amazon parrots (Amazona ventralis). Vet Anaesth Analg 2013;40:96–102.
81. Fonseca C, Server A, Esteves M, et al. An ultrasound-guided technique for axillary brachial plexus nerve block in rabbits. Lab Anim 2015;44:179–84.
82. Helayel PE, da Conceição DB, de Oliveira Filho GR. Ultrasound-guided nerve blocks. Rev Bras Anestesiol 2007;57:106–23.
83. Sites BD, Antonakakis JG. Ultrasound guidance in regional anesthesia: state of the art review through challenging clinical scenarios. Local Reg Anesth 2009; 2:1–14.
84. Griffin J, Nicholls B. Ultrasound in regional anaesthesia. Anaesthesia 2010; 65:1–12.
85. Latzke D, Marhofer P, Zeitlinger M, et al. Minimal local anaesthetic volumes for sciatic nerve block: evaluation of ED 99 in volunteers. Br J Anaesth 2010;104: 239–44.
86. Vassiliou T, Eider J, Nimphius W, et al. Dual guidance improves needle tip placement for peripheral nerve blocks in a porcine model. Acta Anaesthesiol Scand 2012;56:1156–62.
87. Raw RM, Read MR, Campoy L. Peripheral nerve stimulators. In: Campoy L, Read MR, editors. Small animal regional anesthesia and analgesia. 1st edition. Ames (IA): Wiley-Blackwell; 2013. p. 65–76.

Advances in Exotic Animal Osteosynthesis

Mikel Sabater González, LV, CertZooMed, DECZM (Avian)[a],*,
Daniel Calvo Carrasco, LV, CertAVP(ZM), DECZM (Avian)[b]

KEYWORDS

- Exotic pets • Orthopedics • Osteosynthesis • Plate • Graft • Intramedullary fixation

KEY POINTS

- Important advances have occurred in osteosynthesis of exotic pets.
- New materials, conformations, and even surgical techniques have been studied and used in laboratory animal models also considered as exotic pets.
- Exotic animal clinicians should be proactive and consider using this new equipment in order to improve the quality of the orthopedic treatments provided.
- However, the lack of sufficient studies supporting the utility of these materials and techniques requires clinicians to be critical about the outcome expectations when extrapolating their use in exotic pets.

INTRODUCTION

Exotic animal orthopedics has not incorporated the most recent progress made in small animal surgery or human medicine. This failure has been attributed to limited access to specialized equipment able to adapt to the anatomic particularities (eg, the small size of bones or their cortices) of exotic animals or the cost of this equipment. Another potential explanation may be related to the acceptance of the outcomes by surgeons experienced in exotic animal orthopedics, who have mastered traditional techniques to the point of achieving very good results and are therefore reluctant to try new techniques, or that inexperienced orthopedic surgeons prefer to continue using widely described techniques instead of innovating. Although minimally invasive osteosynthesis has been incorporated as a routinely used alternative in small animals, its use in exotic animals is still in its infancy. This article compliments the reviews of orthopedics in small mammals, birds, and reptiles published in the previous issue. In order to do so, it reviews relevant recent studies performed in laboratory animals about new orthopedic materials and techniques showing potential to become incorporated into the routine orthopedic treatment of exotic animals in the coming years. The results of these

Disclosure: The authors has nothing to disclose.
[a] Exoticsvet, Valencia 46015, Spain; [b] Wildfowl & Wetlands Trust, Slimbridge, Newgrounds Ln, Gloucester, GL2 7BT, UK
* Corresponding author.
E-mail address: exoticsvet@gmail.com

studies do not allow direct extrapolation to clinical cases because some relevant aspects, including specific anatomic particularities or long-term consequences for the species treated, were not studied and therefore further studies are warranted.

The development of new materials in combination with important technological advances in the manufacture of orthopedic equipment (eg, three-dimensional [3D] printing) in the last decade has widely expanded the number of possibilities available for veterinary orthopedic surgeons.

SMALL MAMMALS

Some small mammal species such as rabbits, Guinea pigs, mice and rats are animal models for the evaluation of orthopedic materials or techniques.[1]

The methods of internal fixation in humans and small animals have evolved towards 'biological osteosynthesis', which is based in the promotion of a biological favorable fracture environment, specially the preservation of periosteal vascular supply. Contrarily to traditional opens surgical approaches, a limited open approach is preferred. Fracture segments can be manipulated but disturbance of the fracture site should be minimized. Examples of these techniques are interlocking nails, plate-rod constructs, linear and hybrid linear-circular external skeletal fixation, and elastic plate osteosynthesis.[2] In comparison with traditional open fixation techniques, these methods result in shorter healing times, lower rates of failure and fewer complications.[2]

Advances in Intramedullary Bone Fixation

The development of intramedullary nailing (IMN) and interlocking compression nails (ICNs) has been an important advance in veterinary medicine. IMN stabilizes long bone fractures, transferring the load across the fracture site while maintaining the anatomic integrity of the bone.[3] In human medicine, this technique is considered the gold standard treatment of femoral shaft fractures.[3] ICNs provide interfragmentary compression at the fracture site and more axial and torsional stability in transverse and oblique fractures with fragments showing enough cortical contact than IMN, making this technique useful not only for acute long bone fractures but also for the treatment of osteotomies, and pseudoarthrosis.[3] A study comparing the use of titanium IMN and ICNs in experimental femoral shaft osteotomies in rabbits reported faster fracture healing with ICNs than IMN.[3] A custom-designed stainless steel intramedullary nail with interlocking system (RabbitNail, RISystem AG, Davos Platz, Switzerland) was used for the fixation of closed femoral fractures (midshaft femur fracture created by blunt force or femoral fractures created by transverse osteotomy) producing satisfactory bone healing in laboratory rabbits.[4] Thanks to technological advances, the size of orthopedic equipment is less of a limiting factor in the treatment of small patients. A good example of is the intramedullary titanium screw (length 18 mm, diameter 0.5 mm) consisting of a distal cone-shaped head (diameter 0.8 mm) and a proximal thread (nominal outer diameter 0.5 mm, length 4 mm) developed by AO Foundation (Research Implants Systems, Davos, Switzerland) to treat experimental femoral fractures in mice.[5]

Metallic pinning is not the only option for intramedullary long bone fixation. The combination of 3 bioresorbable nonmetallic (poly-L-lactide [PLLA]) woven tubes (Nipro Co., Ltd., Tokyo, Japan), a nonwoven polyhydroxyalkanoate fiber mat, and an injectable calcium phosphate cement (CPC) (Biopex-R, advanced type BPRad, HOYA Co., Ltd., Tokyo, Japan), was able to reinforce and stabilize distal femoral incomplete fractures in osteoporotic rabbits and provided better results in mechanical tests than the use of PLLA + CPC, CPC, or Kirschner wire.[6] Fish scale–derived bone pins used for the internal fixation of fractures of the radii in rabbits showed integration with the adjacent tissue and were surrounded by new extracellular matrix 8 weeks postplacement.[7] Another recently developed alternative to pins for the treatment of long bone fractures could be the IlluminOss System (IlluminOss Medical Inc., East Providence, RI) which comprises an inflatable balloon filled with photopolymerizable liquid monomer delivered percutaneously into the medullary canal.[8] This system has been used to stabilize fractures in humans.[9] In the femurs of rabbits, this system presented similar biocompatibility to Kirschner wires 1 year postimplantation.[8]

Advances in Plate/Screw Systems

New plate/screw systems have been studied and used within the last 15 years.

Titanium miniplates and screws are light, provide resistance to fatigue, are available in multiple designs, and are biocompatible.[10] Specific plate conformations, such as L-shaped and T-shaped plates designed for hand surgery in humans, have been considered useful for fractures with small fragments and anecdotally used in exotic animals.[11] Semitubular plates fit close to the bone and are ideal for extremities on which soft tissue coverage is reduced. However, they have not been frequently used in small animals. These plates are proportionally weaker than other alternatives, such as dynamic compression plates (DCPs).[11] One-third of tubular plates present a collar that prevents the screw head from protruding and secures plate-bone contact.[12]

The size of new plates is more and more reduced to adapt to the treatment of small patients. A good example of this is the intramedullary titanium locking plate with a cylindrical undersurface (length 7.75 mm, width 1.5 mm, thickness 0.7 mm) and the 4 microscrews developed by the AO Foundation (Research Implants Systems, Davos, Switzerland) to treat experimental femoral fractures in mice.[5]

Metal 3D printing is a manufacturing technique allowing the creation of bespoke conformations in a fast and accurate process. 3D printed titanium alloy plates fabricated by selective laser melting showed favorable biocompatibility in rabbits.[13] Allergenicity and lack of toxicity to implant extracts were previously tested in Guinea pigs and mice, respectively.[13]

In humans, bioresorbable polymers present fewer long-term complications than permanent metal plates; however, they are not suitable for many load-bearing applications.[14] A comparison of titanium miniplates and bioresorbable miniplates (Lactosorb, Biomet Microfixation, formerly W. Lorenz Surgical) in experimental mandibular osteotomies in rabbits showed faster bone healing in the group treated with titanium miniplates after 15 and 30 days but similar results after 60 days. The resorbable miniplates did not cause acute or chronic inflammatory reaction or foreign body reaction during the study period.[10] Biodegradable polymers, such as PLLA, PLG, and poly(lactic-co-glycolic acid) (PLGA) are currently used in humans.[15] Plates and screws made of PLGA tested in a rabbit mandible fracture model resulted in fracture healing 8 weeks postsurgery.[16] The use of resorbable 2-mm profile 4-hole miniplates (CPS Inion Ltd, Tampere, Finland) and 7-mm screws in rabbits undergoing mandibulotomies provided a fixation stable enough to allow immediate oral alimentation and callus formation after 1 and 3 months, showing a better adaptation of the bone to the miniplates and screws 3 months after implantation.[17] However, the use of biodegradable polymers presents some limitations related to their mechanical properties or their local inflammatory effects.[15] Alternatives such as magnesium alloys as degradable implants for orthopedic applications have therefore been studied.[15] The test of bioresorbable magnesium-based (MgYREZr alloy) screws containing rare earth elements located in the marrow cavity of the rabbit femur showed good biocompatibility and osteoconductivity (moderate bone formation with direct implant contact without a fibrous capsule) and no toxicity.[15] Absorbable magnesium alloys may provide enough strength for some orthopedic procedures. A study in a rabbit ulnar fracture model suggested that magnesium plates and screws provide stabilization to facilitate healing but, at the same time they degrade, they stimulate new bone formation.[14] Biocompatibility and a foreign body response for various magnesium endosseous implants have been shown in rabbits, Guinea pigs, and rats.[14,18]

Some research about the effect of other technological advances on the materials used in plate construction has been published. Nickel-titanium shape memory alloy plates can increase their stiffness with noninvasive transcutaneous electromagnetic induction heating. Rabbits with experimental tibial osteotomies treated with this type of plates healed but, despite electromagnetic induction heating induced shape memory effect in the group in which it was used, no significant differences were observed between the individuals treated with it or just treated with the plates.[19]

The advances in plate/screw fixation systems are not limited to the properties of the materials used. New concepts of osteosynthesis and new equipment designs are continuously incorporated into routine orthopedic practice.

Plate length selection depends on the location and the configuration of the fracture as well as its intended functional application. In elastic plate osteosynthesis, the rigidity of the construct is decreased by increasing the working length (length of the plate in the middle where no screws are placed). In this case, the plate length is chosen to be as long as possible expanding from metaphysis to metaphysis with only 2 to 3 screws in each fragment. The advantages of using longer bridging plates without placing screws in the center portion of the plate are supported by several biomechanical studies.[20]

Minimally invasive plate osteosynthesis, also known as percutaneous plating, is based in minimal surgical approaches; fracture reduction by using indirect reduction techniques; and the insertion of a plate through the incision made in the end of the fracture, which is advanced through an epiperiosteal tunnel and fixed with screws placed at the ends of the plate and, if required, through cutaneous incisions made over the screw holes.[21]

Compression plates allow the compression of bone segments using dynamic compression holes.[20] A wide range of plate designs, including DCPs, locking compression plates (LCPs), and limited contact DCPs (LC-DCPs), are commercially available for orthopedic surgeons. LCPs combine the use of conventional screws with locking head screws, increasing the versatility of screw placement. LCPs do not require the intimate contact between the plate and the underlying bone in all areas, because the screw locks on the plate, which results in the stabilization of the segments without the related compression caused by traditional plates, preserving therefore the periosteal vascularization. The use of LCPs has been reported in rabbits[22] (**Fig. 1**). LC-DCPs have a scalloped undersurface, which reduces the area of contact with the bone and results in a more even stress distribution within the plate.[11]

Grafts, Mesenchymal Stem Cells, Tissue Engineering And Endoprostheses

In human medicine, the gold standard for restoring bone defects is the autologous (same individual) bone graft but resorption, donor-site morbidity and insufficient donor sites restrict its use.[23] Additionally, allograft (same species), xenograft (different species) and artificial bone substitutes have been associated with relatively few complications.[23]

The bonding strength of cortical bone fragments to plates using common polymethyl methacrylate (PMMA) cement in rabbit calvarial bones (a non-load-bearing region) was assessed at two and twelve weeks post-implantation. Results suggested its potential use in those cases in which conventional techniques provide insufficient stability or are not feasible.[24] The use of a quick-setting hydroxyapatite cement (Mimix, Biomet Microfixation, formerly W. Lorenz Surgical, Jacksonville, FL, USA) with or

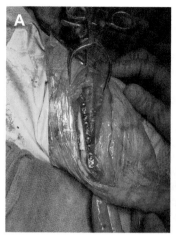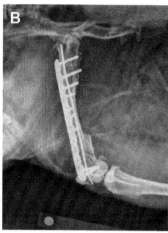

Fig. 1. (*A*) Intraoperative and (*B*) postoperative photographies showing a comminuted left distal femoral fracture with an intrarticular condylar fracture stabilized using a locking compression plate and pin fixation (cross pins and intramedullary pin) in a rabbit. (*Courtesy of* J. Brandao, LMV, MS, DECZM(Avian) and C. Blake, DVM, DACVS, Stillwater, OK).

without a resorbable polyglycolic acid plate (Lactosorb, Biomet Microfixation, formerly W. Lorenz Surgical) in critical size calvarial defects in rabbits resulted in the growth of new bone only into the periphery of the cement after six months in all specimens.[23] A different study reported that infrared laser phototherapy associated to hydroxyapatite grafts improved the healing of surgical tibial fractures treated with mini-plates in rabbits.[25]

Mesenchymal stem cells administration may be useful to induce osteogenesis at sites of periosteal distraction.[26] Additionally, tissue engineering in combination with stem cell research allowed the creation of new scaffolds for bone grafts. A tissue-engineered bone graft constructed with pre-vascularized β -tricalcium phosphate scaffold and mesenchymal stem cells significantly promoted the new bone regeneration and vascularization compared to non-vascularized tissue-engineered bone grafts in rabbits.[27] A scaffold of tetrapod-shaped alpha tricalcium phosphate granules (TB) combined with basic fibroblast growth factor (bFGF)-binding ion complex gel (f-IC gel), TB/f-IC gel, facilitated both neovascularization and new bone formation in segmental femoral defects of rabbits stabilized with a plate of polypropylene mesh cage.[28] However, there were no differences in the extent of neovascularization and new bone formation between the TB and TB/f (bFGF without binding ion complex gel) groups.[28] A graft consisting on decellularized trabecular bone (Tutobone®, Tutogen Medical GmbH and RTI Biologics, Neunkirchen, Germany) seeded with bone marrow mesenchymal stromal cells was used in combination or not with vessel to treat a humeral segmental defect model in rabbits for twelve weeks, resulting in callus formation in absence of graft bone formation or remodeling.[29]

Modular endoprostheses are commonly used in humans to reconstruct defects of the distal femur and proximal tibia after bone tumor resection.[30] Silver-coated endoprosthetic replacements (eg, Mutars system, Modular Universal Tumor And Revision System; implantcast, Buxtehude, Germany) of the diaphyseal femurs resulted in significant reduced infection rates without toxicological side effects when compared to non-silver coated prostheses according to a study performed in rabbits with surgical sites infected with *Staphyloccocus aureus*.[31]

The articular surface of the synovial joint in rabbits can regenerate after radical resection by implanting customized anatomical bio-scaffolds infused with collagen gel containing transforming growth factor β3 and without direct transplantation of stem cell progenitors.[32] In a rabbit primary surgery model, a titanium tibial plateau prosthesis was used to assess the stability of prosthetic fixation with and without the use of a bone substitute composed of calcium sulfate and hydroxyapatite at six and twelve weeks after surgery.[33] This study concluded that a bone substitute does not influence early prosthesis-bone interface but might provide improved mechanical support for the prosthesis during remodeling.[33] High-density nano-hydroxyapatite/polyamide prostheses with polyvinyl alcohol hydrogel humeral head surfaces were implanted after humeral head excisions in laboratory New Zealand rabbits and diagnostic imaging and histological results revealed excellent biocompatibility and biologic fixation of the prostheses without observed damage to the glenoid surface after three months of continuous functional motions.[34]

3D printing also facilitated the creation of titanium porous plates. The use of these plates embedding a gelatin scaffold accelerated bone repair in rabbit models of osteonecrosis of the femoral head.[35] Porous plates were studied in order to achieve more solid bone-implant interface.[36] Titanium-25 niobium alloy porous femoral stem prostheses placed in the medullary cavity of laboratory rabbits showed good biocompatibility and provides biological fixation between the bone and the implant.[36]

AVIAN
Advances In Intramedullary Bone Fixation

The use of the IlluminOss System, an already described alternative to pins for the treatment of long bone fractures in small mammals and humans, has been recently reported in a bird.[37]

Advances In Plate/Screw Systems

Plate fixation is becoming a more common therapeutic option for avian bone fractures (**Fig. 2**). Examples of this include the use of: a 4-hole, 1.5-mm T-plate and a 6-hole, 2.0-mm dynamic compression plate (DCP) placed side by side to stabilize a luxation affecting the coracoid-sternal articulation in a bald eagle (*Haliaeetus leucocephalus*), a locking compression plate system to treat a comminuted tarsometatarsal fracture with delayed union after 1 month of external coaptation in a bald eagle, a 2.0-mm

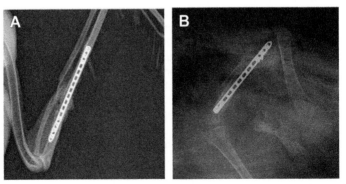

Fig. 2. (*A*) Use of an LCP plate to treat an ulnar fracture in a griffon vulture (*Gyps fulvus*). (*B*) Use of an LCP plate to treat a femoral fracture in a mute swan (*Cygnus olor*). *Courtesy of Minh Huynh.*

titanium miniplate to stabilize a mid diaphyseal fracture of the left tibiotarsus in a blue-and-yellow macaw (*Ara ararauna*), a miniplate to stabilize a simple, complete, spiral-third fractured right tibia in a goose (*Anser anser*), and a 14-hole, 2.7-mm locking plate fixed with 6 screws in a bicortical manner to stabilize a transverse, diaphyseal fracture of the distal third of the right tibiotarsus with a craniolateral displacement of the distal fragment in another goose.[38–42]

However, the use of plate fixation in individuals weighting less than 500g has been less commonly reported until the last ten years. The *ex vivo* biomechanical evaluation of pigeon (*Columba livia*) cadaver intact humeri and ostectomized humeri stabilized with caudally applied titanium 1.6 mm locking plate secured with locking screws (2 bicortical and 4 monocortical) or stainless steel 1.5 mm nonlocking plate constructs secured with bicortical nonlocking screws revealed that increased torsional strength may be needed before bone plate repair can be considered as the sole fixation method for avian species.[43]

Dorsal single plating of the ulna with a 6-hole maxillofacial miniplate in experimentally induced ulnar and radial fractures in pigeons did not result in adequate stabilization according to a study.[44] A posterior studied evaluated three miniplate systems (a 1.3 adaption plate, a limited contact system created with washers placed between a 1.3 mm adaption plate and the bone, and a 1.0 mm maxillofacial miniplate) to stabilize the ulna after provoking unilateral ulnar and radial fractures in pigeons, and concluded that best flight results (100%) were achieved with the 1.3 adaption plate, whereas the limited contact system resulted in a higher percentage of screw loosening (leading to failure in 33% of the cases), and all the maxillofacial miniplates bent.[45] A study evaluating the healing of unilateral ulnar and radial fractures after repair using two steel miniplate systems in pigeons concluded that both the 1.3-mm adaption plate and the 1.0-mm compression plate meet the requirements for avian osteosynthesis and can be recommended for fracture repair of the ulna or other long bones in birds weighing less than 500 g, and that the application of a figure-of-eight bandage might be beneficial in fracture healing.[46]

The evaluation of three titanium microplates (one with six holes and a central spacer, another with eight holes without a spacer in the center, and another with eight holes and a central spacer) for the treatment of tibiotarsal fractures in pigeons concluded that despite the complications related with their use, they are an option for tibiotarsal osteosynthesis in birds of medium size.[47]

Grafts

Autologous bone grafting techniques have been described in avian species. However, less information is available about the use of nonautologous bone grafts. The evaluation of allogeneic demineralized bone matrix (DBM) in the healing of long bone defects in a pigeon model concluded that it is osteogenic, biocompatible, and safe in orthopedic sites and is potentially useful in useful in avian bone grafting.[48]

REPTILES

The use of recently developed plates previously mentioned in reptiles is still anecdotal. A fracture of the ramus of the mandible in a boa constrictor (*Boa constrictor*) was stabilized with a plate and compression screws.[49] A fractured mandible in an adult American alligator was repaired with a 10 hole, 20 × 1.5 cm, titanium DCP formed to and placed on the lingual side of the mandible, and secured with nine 3.5 mm cortical screws, leaving one plate hole open over the fracture site.[50]

REFERENCES

1. Wancket LM. Animal models for evaluation of bone implants and devices: Comparative bone structure and common model uses. Vet Pathol 2015;52(5): 842–50.
2. Lewis DD. Minimally invasive fracture repair. Proceedings NAVC Conference, February 4–8, 2017, Orlando, FL, USA. p. 776–8.
3. Baki ME, Aldemir C, Duygun F, et al. Comparison of non-compression and compression interlocking intramedullary nailing in rabbit femoral shaft osteotomy model. Eklem Hastalik Cerrahisi 2017;28(1):7–12.
4. Yoshino O, Brady J, Young K, et al. Reamed locked intramedullary nailing for studying femur fracture and its complications. Eur Cell Mater 2017;34:99–107.
5. Histing T, Garcia P, Matthys R, et al. An internal locking plate to study intramembranous bone healing in a mouse femur fracture model. J Orthop Res 2010;28: 397–402.
6. Nishizuka T, Kurahashi T, Hara T, et al. Novel intramedullary-fixation technique for long bone fragility fractures using bioresorbable materials. PLoS One 2014;9(8): e104603.
7. Chou CH, Gen YG, Lin CC, et al. Bioabsorbable fish scale for the internal fixation of fracture: a preliminary study. Tissue Eng 2014;20(17):2493–502.
8. McSweeney AL, Zani BG, Baird R, et al. Biocompatibility, bone healing, and safety evaluation in rabbits with an IlluminOss bone stabilization system. J Orthop Res 2017;35(10):2181–90.
9. Gausepohl T, Pennig D, Heck S, et al. Effective management of bone fractures with the IlluminOss® photodynamic bone stabilization system: initial clinical experience from the European Union registry. Orthop Rev (Pavia) 2017;9:6988.
10. Hochuli-Vieira E, Gabrielli MAC, Pereira-Filho VA, et al. Rigid internal fixation with titanium versus bioresorbable miniplates in the repair of mandibular fractures in rabbits. Int J Oral Maxillofac Surg 2005;34:167–73.
11. Johnston SA, von Pfeil DJ, Déjardin LM, et al. Internal fracture fixation. In: Tobias KM, Johnston SA, editors. Veterinary surgery: small animal, 2 volume-set. St Louis (MO): Elsevier Saunders; 2012. p. 576–607.
12. Available at: www2.aofoundation.org. Accessed January 10, 2018.
13. Lin X, Xiao X, Wang Y, et al. Biocompatibility of bespoke 3D-printed titanium alloy plates for treating acetabular fractures. Biomed Res Int 2018;2018:2053486.
14. Chaya 2015a Chaya A, Yoshizawa S, Verdelis K, et al. *In vivo* study of magnesium plate and screw degradation and bone fracture healing. Acta Biomater 2015;18: 262–9.
15. Waizy H, Diekmann J, Weizbauer A, et al. In vivo study of a biodegradable orthopedic screw (MgYREZr-alloy) in a rabbit model for up to 12 months. J Biomater Appl 2014;28(5):667–75.
16. Park S, Kim JH, Kim IH, et al. Evaluation of poly(lactic-co-glycolic acid) plate and screw system for bone fixation. J Craniofac Surg 2013;24:1021–5.
17. Atali O, Gocmen G, Aktop S, et al. Bone healing after biodegradable mini-plate fixation. Acta Cir Bras 2016;31(6):364–70.
18. Chaya 2015b Chaya A, Yoshizawa S, Verdelis K, et al. Fracture healing using degradable magnesium fixation plates and screws. J Oral Maxillofac Surg 2015;73(2):295–305.
19. Müller CW, Pfeifer R, Meier K, et al. A novel shape memory plate osteosynthesis for noninvasive modulation of fixation stiffness in a rabbit tibia osteotomy model. Biomed Res Int 2015;2015:652940.

20. Chao P, Lewis DD, Kowaleski MP, et al. Biomechanical concepts applicable to minimally invasive fracture repair in small animals. Vet Clin Small Anim 2012; 42:853–72.
21. Lewis DD. Minimally invasive fracture repair. Proceedings NAVC Conference 2017; Orlando, FL, USA. p. 776–8.
22. Ueno H, Uto S, Seo K, et al. Usagi no kossetu: locking plate wo mochiita seihuku. J Exo Anim Pract 2016;8(1):56–64.
23. Ascherman JA, Foo R, Nanda D, et al. Reconstruction of cranial bone defects using a quick-setting hydroxyapatite cement and absorbable plate. J Craniofac Surg 2008;19(4):1131–5.
24. Smeets R, Endres K, Stockbrink G, et al. The innovative application of a novel bone adhesive for facial fracture osteosynthesis – *In vitro* and *in vivo* results. J Biomed Mater Res A 2013;101(7):2058–66.
25. Pinheiro ALB, Aciole GTS, Ramos TA, et al. The efficacy of the use of IR laser phototherapy associated to biphasic ceramic graft and guided bone regeneration on surgical fractures treated with miniplates: a histological and histomorphometric study on rabbits. Lasers Med Sci 2014;29:279–88.
26. Sato K, Haruyama N, Shimizy Y, et al. Osteogenesis by gradually expanding the interface between bone surface and periosteum enhanced by bone marrow stem cell administration in rabbits. Oral Surg Oral Med Oral Pathol Oral Radiol Endod 2010;110:32–40.
27. Wang L, Fan H, Zhang ZY, et al. Osteogenesis and angiogenesis of tissue-engineered bone constructed by prevascularized β–tricalcium phosphate scaffold and mesenchymal stem cells. Biomaterials 2010;31(36):9452–61.
28. Honnami M, Choi S, Liu I, et al. Repair of rabbit segmental femoral defects by using a combination of tetrapod-shaped calcium phosphate granules and basic fibroblast growth factor-binding ion complex gel. Biomaterials 2013;34(36): 9056–62.
29. Kaempfen A, Todorov A, Güven S, et al. Engraftment of prevascularized, tissue engineered constructs in a novel rabbit segmental bone defect model. Int J Mol Sci 2015;16:12616–30.
30. Bus MP, van de Sande MA, Fiocco M. What are the long-term results of MUTA-RS® modular endoprostheses for reconstruction of tumor resection of the distal femur and proximal tibia? Clin Orthop Relat Res 2017;475(3):708–18.
31. Gosheger G, Hardes J, Ahrens H, et al. Silver-coated megaendoprostheses in a rabbit model – an analysis of the infection rate and toxicological side effects. Biomaterials 2004;25:5547–56.
32. Lee CH, Cook JL, Mendelson A, et al. Regeneration of the articular surface of the rabbit synovial joint by cell homing: a proof of concept study. Lancet 2010;376: 440–8.
33. Zampelis V, Tägil M, Lidgren L, et al. The effect of a biphasic injectable bone substitute on the interface strength in a rabbit knee prosthesis model. J Orthop Surg Res 2013;8:25.
34. Guo Y, Gou J, Bai D, et al. Hemiarthroplasty of the shoulder joint using a custom-designed high density nano-hydroxyapatite/polyamide prosthesis with a polyvinyl alcohol hydrogel humeral head surface in rabbits. Artif Organs 2014;38(7):580–6.
35. Zhu W, Zhao Y, Ma Q, et al. 3D-printed porous titanium changed femoral head repair growth patterns: osteogenesis and vascularization in porous titanium. J Mater Sci Mater Med 2017;28:62.
36. Weng X, Yang H, Xu J, et al. *In vivo* testing of porous Ti-25Nb alloy serving as a femoral stem prosthesis in a rabbit model. Exp Ther Med 2016;12:1323–30.

37. Lierz M. IlluminOss®, a novel minimal invasive technique for fracture repair in birds, using light activated monomers. In: Proceedings ICARE Conference 2019. April 28-May 2. London, UK. 152.

38. Guzmán DS, Bubenik LJ, Lauer SK, et al. Repair of a coracoid luxation and a tibiotarsal fracture in a bald eagle (*Haliaeetus leucocephalus*). J Avian Med Surg 2007;21(3):188–95.

39. Montgomery RD, Crandall E, Bellah JR. Use of a locking compression plate as an external fixator for repair of a tarsometatarsal fracture in a bald eagle (*Haliaeetus leucocephalus*). J Avian Med Surg 2011;25(2):119–25.

40. Dal-Bó IS, Alievi MM, Silva LM, et al. Tibiotarsus osteosynthesis in blue-yellow-macaw (*Ara ararauna*) using titanium miniplate. Arq Bras Med Vet Zoo 2011; 63(4):1003–6.

41. Sá SS, Filho JC, Souza FS, et al. Osteosynthesis in tibiae fractures with mini plate, screws and cerclage wire in goose (*Anser anser*): case report. Acta Vet Bras 2012;6(1):61.

42. Slunsky P, Weiβ J, Haake A, et al. Repair of a tibiotarsal fracture in a Pomeranian goose (*Anser anser*) with a locking plate. J Avian Med Surg 2018;32(1):50–6.

43. Darrow BG, Biskup JJ, Weigel JP, et al. Ex vivo biomechanical evaluation of pigeon (*Columba livia*) cadaver intact humeri and ostectomized humeri stabilized with caudally applied titanium locking plate or stainless steel nonlocking plate constructs. Am J Vet Res 2017;78(5):570–8.

44. Christen C, Fischer I, von Rechenberg B, et al. Evaluation of a maxillofacial miniplate compact 1.0 for stabilization of the ulna in experimentally induced ulnar and radial fractures in pigeons (*Columba livia*). J Avian Med Surg 2005;19(5):185–90.

45. Gull JM, Saveraid TC, Szabo D, et al. Evaluation of three miniplate systems for fracture stabilization in pigeons (*Columba livia*). J Avian Med Surg 2012;26(4): 203–11.

46. Bennert BM, Kircher PR, Gutbrod A, et al. Evaluation of two miniplate systems and figure-of-eight bandages for stabilization of experimentally induced ulnar and radial fractures in pigeons (*Columba livia*). J Avian Med Surg 2016;30(2): 111–21.

47. Gouvea A, Meller M, Noriega V, et al. Titanium microplates for treatment of tibio-tarsus fractures in pigeons. Cienc Rural 2011;41(3):476–82.

48. Sanaei R, Abu J, Nazari M, et al. Evaluation of osteogenic potentials of avian demineralized bone matrix in the healing of osseous defects in pigeons. Vet Surg 2015;44:603–12.

49. Castro JLC, Santalucia S, Pachaly JR, et al. Mandibular osteosynthesis in a *Boa constrictor* snake. Semin Cienc Agrar 2014;35:911–8.

50. Mader D. Double repair of a fractured mandible in an adult American alligator (Alligator mississipiensis). In: Proceedings ICARE Conference 2019. April 28-May 2. London, UK. 168.

Technological Advances in Wound Treatment of Exotic Pets

Mikel Sabater González, LV, CertZooMed, DECZM (Avian)[a],[*],
Jörg Mayer, Dr med vet, MSc, DABVP (ECM), DECZM (Small Mammals), DACZM[b]

KEYWORDS

- Exotic pets • Skin wound healing • Negative pressure therapy • Laser therapy
- Skin grafts

KEY POINTS

- Technological advances have occurred in wound management of exotics pets.
- Some technologies, such as laser therapy, became widely available in veterinary medicine.
- Clinicians should be proactive and consider using this technology, when available.
- However, the lack of sufficient studies or confirmed evidence supporting the utility of these techniques requires the clinician to be critical about the outcome expectations when using them.

INTRODUCTION

Although most research about the use of technological advances for wound healing was performed in laboratory animals but oriented to human medicine, recent technological advances allowed its application not only to small animals but also to exotic pets.

This article reviews the literature available about some of these techniques (negative wound pressure therapy, photobiomodulation [laser therapy], electrical stimulation therapy [EST], therapeutic ultrasonography [TU], hyperbaric oxygen therapy [HBOT]) and other advances in wound management (skin expanders, xenografts, and bioengineered autologous skin substitutes) in exotic pet species.

NEGATIVE PRESSURE WOUND THERAPY

Negative pressure wound therapy (NPWT) is based on the controlled application of subatmospheric pressure evenly distributed across a wound bed within a closed environment.[1]

The authors have nothing to disclose.
[a] Exoticsvet, Valencia, Spain; [b] Department of Small Animal Medicine and Surgery, University of Georgia, Athens, GA, USA
* Corresponding author.
E-mail address: exoticsvet@gmail.com

vetexotic.theclinics.com

The wound should be clipped (margins of 3–5 cm when possible), cleansed (the last clean of the margins should be done with alcohol), debrided, and lavaged before the application of the NPWT dressing, normally under general anesthesia.[2] An aseptic technique should be maintained throughout the dressing application. An open-cell or reticulated polyurethane or polyvinyl alcohol foam dressing with a pore size ranging from 400 to 600 mm is placed over the wound and covered with a semiocclusive plastic adhesive film that adheres to the surrounding skin sealing it completely and creating a closed moist wound-healing environment.[1,2]

Although gauze and foam are equally effective at delivering negative pressure and creating mechanical deformation of the wound, the physical presence of polyurethane foam in wound dressings treated with NPWT provoked a 2-fold increase in vascularity when compared with the use of NPWR and an occlusive dressing without foam.[3,4]

Then, a suction tube connected to a collection reservoir and a suction pump is attached to the dressing. The pump pressure is programmed to apply negative pressures ranging from −75 to −150 mm Hg (−125 mm Hg is commonly used for open wounds).[1,5] Negative pressure pulls exudate through the foam into the collection reservoir and bathes the wound in tissue fluids from inside to outside, creating a healthy wound environment without maceration[6] (**Fig. 1**). NPWT can be applied continuously, cyclically, or intermittently.[7–9] Dressings are replaced every 48 to 72 hours, often just under sedation. Acute traumatic wounds typically require 1 to 3 dressing changes before a healthy bed of granulation tissue is observed.[2]

The exact mechanism of action of NPWT to promote wound healing is not yet completely understood. However, it is likely based on the modulation of cytokines to an anti-inflammatory profile, and mechanoreceptor and chemoreceptor-mediated cell signaling, resulting in angiogenesis, extracellular matrix remodeling, and deposition of granulation tissue[10–12] (**Table 1**).

Acute, subacute, and chronic wounds, flaps, and free grafts respond favorably to NPWT.[33–40] The prolonged time (up to 72 hours) between wound dressings compares favorably with the traditional daily wet-to-dry dressing for open wounds still in the inflammatory phase.[2]

In large complicated wounds, NPWT provides a "mechanical bridge" to reconstruction.[2] It also can be used to recruit skin preoperatively as a skin-stretching device and over closed surgical incisions to relieve tension and shear forces on the wound edges.[41] In relation to grafts, NPWT reduces seroma formation, and granulation tissue appears earlier in the interstices of the meshed graft, resulting in better early adhesion, faster closure of open meshes, and increased percentage of graft taken.[2]

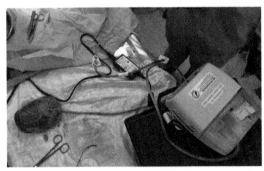

Fig. 1. Use of negative wound pressure therapy in a carapacial wound in a 3-toed box turtle (*Terrapene carolina triunguis*). (*Courtesy of* J. Brandão, LMV, MS, Dip. ECZM (Avian), Stillwater, Oklahoma.)

Table 1
Effects of negative pressure wound therapy

Increases vascularity	Provokes the synthesis of nitric oxide, which significantly increases wound vascularity[13]
	Correct blood perfusion provides nutrients (including oxygen), cells, and growth factors to the wound and enhances the removal of free radicals, carbon dioxide, and waste products[14]
	Improve delivery of antibiotics when administered[15]
Macrodeformations	Induce hyperperfusion and increased nutrient (including oxygen) delivery by traction forces over the deep layers
	Induce hypoperfusion and hypoxia, which promote endothelial angiogenesis and fibroplasia by the compression forces applied over the superficial layers[9,16,17]
	Following termination of NPWT, the hypoperfusion adjacent to the wound edge may turn into hyperperfusion, making intermittent or cyclical modes more effective at stimulating fibroplasia and neovascularization than the continuous one.[4,9,18–21]
Microdeformations	Activation of growth factor 1, which provokes myofibroblasts differentiation and production of granulation tissue by interaction between the foam and the surface of the wound[6]
Bacterial reduction	Controversial. Reductions, no difference or increases in the bacterial load on the wound have been reported[7,22–27]
Fluid drainage	May reduce edema (not demonstrated) but also alters the fluid composition of the wound and decreases the levels of cytokines, metalloproteinases, plasmin, thrombin, elastase, and other proteolytic enzymes, which negatively affect wound healing[1,6,28–31]
Nerve growth stimulation	Increases dermal and epidermal nerve fiber densities, substance P, calcitonin gene-related peptide, and nerve growth factor expression in full-thickness wounds of diabetic mice[32]

Contraindications for the use of NPWT include patients with coagulation disorders or its use over local malignancy, untreated osteomyelitis, exposed tendons, ligaments or nerves, unprotected organs, or anastomotic sites not well covered by a nonadherent polyethylene sheet or other suitable nonadherent material, hemorrhage, scar tissue covering necrotic tissue, unexplored fistulae, or wounds with potentially undetected connections with the chest or abdomen.[6,42]

Monitoring of the procedure is necessary because complications may occur. These complications include loss of suction, blood vessel damage, dislodging of hemostatic agents, coverage of devitalized tissue with granulation tissue, bony sequester, lack of response to therapy, and pain.[6]

Experience with NPWT in exotic, zoo, and wild animals is scarce and consists of research studies in laboratory animals and clinical observations described as case reports.

In rabbits, it promotes capillary blood flow velocity, increases capillary caliber and blood volume, stimulates endothelial proliferation and angiogenesis, narrows endothelial spaces, and restores the integrity of the capillary basement membrane of full-thickness ear skin defects.[18] Another study in rabbits showed that NPWT penetrates up to 0.4 mm into the wound tissue at the recommended −125 mm Hg pressure setting and no more than 1 mm into wound tissue at −200 mm Hg when using open-cell foam dressings.[43] In rats, NPWT resulted in accelerated wound closure rates, increased proangiogenic growth factor production, and improved collagen deposition when compared with control group (not treated with NPWT).[44] NWPT was used in a tiger with a not-adhering caudal superficial epigastric skin flap used to cover a defect over the hind limb, resulting in adhesion after 4 weeks.[45] It also was used in an Eastern black rhinoceros after a toe amputation due to progressive suppurative osteomyelitis.[46] In birds, NPWT has been successfully used in the management of extensive degloving traumatic wounds caused in the pelvic limb of a red-tailed hawk and a bald eagle.[1,47] In reptiles, reported cases are restricted to chelonians. It has been used in 8 gopher tortoises, 2 yellow-bellied sliders, an eastern box turtle, a Florida cooter, and a Florida chicken turtle that presented with trauma.[48] NPWT has also been reported in a Greek tortoise and 2 Aldabra tortoises after surgical debridement of deep and infected wounds in the carapace.[49–51] In one of the Aldabras, already receiving antibiotic treatment after debridement of a deep shell abscess and osteomyelitis of the carapace, NPWT was combined with a silver-impregnated bandage to enhance wound healing and control microbial contamination.[51] NWPT has also been used in a loggerhead sea turtle to manage a fistulous tract reaching the celomic cavity provoked by the insertion of a spotted eagle ray's spine in the left prefemoral fossa.[52]

PHOTOBIOMODULATION (LASER THERAPY)

Photobiomodulation is a photochemical process in which light (eg, laser) interacts with chromophores in cells, causing upregulation or downregulation of some biochemical processes. Wavelengths in the range from the violet (400 nm) to the near infrared (1100 nm) can result in photobiomodulation. When light interacts with a biological tissue, it can be absorbed, scattered (including reflection), and/or transmitted. The major chromophores that absorb light and prevent light penetration to target tissues are melanin, hemoglobin, and water. Melanin has a very high absorption, and therefore, dark skins absorb more light, especially for wavelengths less than 830 nm. Wavelengths from 600 nm (red end of the spectrum) to 1100 nm (near infrared end of the spectrum) are in the optimal range for penetrating into tissue.[53]

The mechanism of action of photobiomodulation is not yet completely understood and likely multifactorial. The most recognized mechanism involves the cytochrome c system. Nitric oxide binds reversibly to cytochrome c oxidase, the unit IV of the mitochondrial respiratory chain, inhibiting its activity. Light wavelengths between 500 and 1100 nm break those bonds, which result in a higher availability of nitric oxide (vasodilator signaling), production of a burst of reactive oxygen species (cytoprotective signaling), and ATP production (energy source for many cellular processes; eg, reduction of pain and inflammation, and tissue healing)[53–55] (Box 1).

Box 1
Effects of laser therapy

- Enhances leukocyte infiltration and macrophage activity[53,55]

- Promotes neovascularization,[53,55] promotes fibroblast and keratinocyte proliferation and production of growth factors that result in earlier wound epithelialization and greater tensile strength[53,55]

- Stimulates wound healing at distant locations[56,57]

- Reduces edema[58]

- Enhances fur regrowth[58]

- Potential pain relief[58]

A synergistic effect of laser and phthalocyanine-derived photosensitizer in a gel-based delivery system was observed for wound healing in a group of rats treated with laser when compared with the control group (not treated with the photosensitizer drug).[59]

The small size of many of the exotic and wildlife species requires the use of lower therapeutic doses than those used in larger species. This lower dosing is accomplished by adjusting the laser delivery mode (pulsed mode instead of continuous), power, or treatment duration.[58] Potential risks associated with the use of lasers include retinal damage (operators and patients should have their eyes protected; **Fig. 2**A, B), increased absorption in pigmented areas, tissue overheating, and stimulation and alteration of cellular activity (potentially detrimental in the case of neoplastic or infected tissue).[60] Treatment is not recommended over open fontanels, hemorrhagic tissue (as the increase in microcirculation and vasodilation may enhance bleeding), a pregnant uterus (although the use of laser in pregnant rats with preeclampsia is of benefit for the animal), some malignancies (although some studies suggest photobiomodulation may have an inhibitory effect on some cancerous tissue in mammals), or in patients receiving photosensitive medications.[53,58,61–63]

Although multiple doses (different wavelengths and powers) of laser therapy have been reported for different indications in different species, there is no consensus yet about the ideal parameters for tissue repair and pain relief. Doses reported in literature are frequently based on clinical experience (including single case reports) or research studies without a true control group (sometimes the "control group" consisted of nontreated wounds in animals receiving laser in other wounds), and because different methodologies have been used but rarely compared.

Effects of laser therapy in wounds of small mammals include enhancement of wound healing, reduction of edema, enhancement of fur regrowth, and potential pain relief.[58] Several experimental data are available in rat models.[56,64–67] In rats, low-level laser therapy reduced the intensity of the inflammatory reaction and induced switching of the leukocyte infiltration pattern (neutrophilic to lymphoplasmacytic infiltration), stimulated deposition and enhanced organization of collagen type III, and promoted angiogenesis when compared with nontreated rats.[64] A single laser treatment stimulates wound healing; however, no significant differences between control and

A   **B**

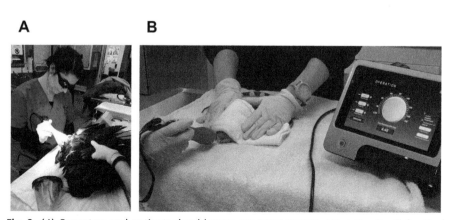

Fig. 2. (*A*) Operators and patients should wear eye protectors to prevent potential retinal damage when applying or looking at the laser beam. Photobiomodulation therapy in the extremity of a bald eagle (*Haliaeetus leucocephalus*) (*B*) and in an iguana (*Iguana* sp) presented for rostral erosions.

treated wounds were observed by day 14.[65] When different fluencies (10, 20, and 30 J/cm^2) were applied 3 times weekly, best results were obtained with 20 J/cm^2.[66] Another study reported that the combination of 685- and 830-nm wavelengths (10 J/cm^2 each; total 20 J/cm^2) provoked the best wound healing at the end of the experiment.[67] Inappropriately high doses may result in delayed wound healing. Use of 50 J/cm^2 decreased wound healing when compared with 20 J/cm^2.[67] The application of laser directly to standardized skin wounds stimulated not only their healing but also the healing of wounds distant from the point of application. According to other publications, wounds where the laser was not applied healed better than those in which the laser was directly applied (best-healing rates were observed in wounds located in an intermediate position when compared with those directly treated with laser and those located more distant).[56] Another study in rats reported that unilateral laser therapy improved bilateral healing of skin wounds when compared with nontreated rats[57] (**Table 2**).

Suggested uses are summarized in **Table 2**. In rabbits, it may also accelerate healing in pododermatitis (case report) (**Fig. 3**) and reduce inflammation and pain in wounds where *Cuterebra* sp larvae were removed (2–4 J/cm^2).[58]

Indications of laser therapy for wounds in avian species are similar to those reported for mammals, although the number of treatments and suggested doses are relatively lower: 1 J/cm^2 for reduction of postoperative pain and speeding healing process in surgical wounds, 2 J/cm^2 for lacerations, 2 to 4 J/cm^2 as an adjunctive therapy for reduction of inflammation and pain at the trauma site, speeding of healing and minimizing scar-tissue formation in self-mutilation cases, and 4 J/cm^2 for deep wounds (**Fig. 4**A, B). Other reported indications include treatment of extensive dermal burn injuries (1 J/cm^2), treatment of pododermatitis (3–4 J/cm^2), and reduction of patagial extension restriction after trauma (4–6 J/cm^2).[75–77] Healing rates and times for pododermatitis after surgical debridement in Magellanic penguins were better in the group treated with laser therapy after instillation of a photosensitizer (aqueous solution of methylene blue) than in the group treated with anti-inflammatories and antibiotics.[78,79]

Indications of laser therapy in reptile wounds include reduction of edema, inflammation, and necrosis in first-intention incisional wounds and enhanced wound healing[80] (**Fig. 5**A, B). In ball pythons, no significant differences in wound healing were observed between incisions treated with 5 J/cm^2 and nontreated ones (control) in the same animal, although lower gross wound scores and more collagen deposition were observed in the laser-treated incisions on day 14.[80] The potential systemic or distance therapeutic effect observed in rats was not considered in this case because all the snakes were treated.[56] In bearded dragons, no histologic differences in healing of full-thickness biopsies were observed after 4 days between treated (single dose of 4 J of 670-nm light) and nontreated animals.[81] A study in iguanas, including a control group, reported that wounds treated with laser at 10 J/cm^2 were significantly smaller

Table 2 Suggested doses of laser therapy	
1–2 J/cm^2	Surgical incisions and lacerations
4–5 J/cm^2	Reduction of edema 4 J/cm^2 accelerates wound healing in some phases of the healing process of full-thickness wounds in rabbits
4–6 J/cm^2	Enhances healing in abscesses treated with antimicrobials
8–10 J/cm^2	Enhances wound repair in rats
8–20 J/cm^2	Enhances air regrowth in mice[58,68–74]

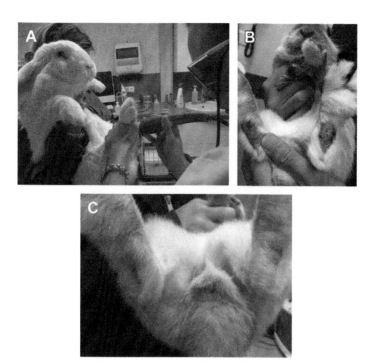

Fig. 3. (*A*) Photobiomodulation therapy in a rabbit with bilateral pododermatitis. (*B*) Macroscopic lesional appearance before photobiomodulation. (*C*) Application of photobiomodulation. Macroscopic lesional appearance after multiple photobiomodulation treatments. (*Courtesy of* M. Huynh, DVM, DipECZM (Avian), Dip. ACZM (Small mammals), Arcueil, France.)

than those treated at 5 J/cm[282] (**Fig. 6**). Faster wound healing after the use of laser therapy alone or in conjunction with other therapies (eg, antibiotics or dressings) has been reported for superficial pododermatitis and thermal wounds (1–2 J/cm^2), deep severe dermal ulcerations in a soft-shelled turtle, deep and contaminated wounds (4 J/cm^2), blister disease (1–6 J/cm^2), abscesses (6 J/cm^2), skin lacerations (5–10 J/cm^2), extensive thermal wounds (8–10 J/cm^2), and rodent bites involving skin and muscle (10 J/cm^2).[82–85]

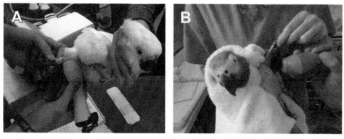

Fig. 4. (*A*) Photobiomodulation therapy in a white cockatoo (*Cacatua alba*). (*B*) Photobiomodulation therapy in an African gray parrot (*Psittacus erithacus*) with axillary dermatitis (*C alba*). (*Courtesy of* M. Huynh, DVM, DipECZM (Avian), Dip. ACZM (Small mammals), Arcueil, France.)

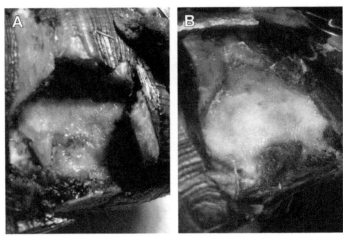

Fig. 5. Macroscopic appearance of a carapacial wound in an Eastern box turtle (*T carolina carolina*) before (*A*) and after (*B*) several photobiomodulation treatments.

Additional information about the use of photobiomodulation in exotic, zoo, and aquatic species has been published.[79,86]

ELECTRICAL STIMULATION THERAPY

EST is the use of exogenous electric waveforms to promote microvascular flow and wound healing. Electrode placement is based on the desired effect and could be reversed during treatment. When the anode is placed on moist sterile gauze over the wound and the cathode is placed on the adjacent skin, the electric current created provokes the migration of negatively charged cells (macrophages and neutrophils)

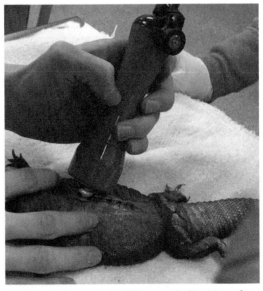

Fig. 6. Photobiomodulation in the ventral midline surgical incision after celomic surgery in a spiny-tailed lizard (*Uromastix* sp).

toward the anode promoting the inflammatory stage of wound healing. Alternatively, placing the cathode over the wound bed and the anode over the adjacent skin provokes the migration of positively charged cells (fibroblasts, keratinocytes, and epidermal cells) toward the cathode[87] (**Box 2**).

Low-intensity EST uses continuous or pulsed electrical current waveforms between 200 µA and 800 µA with low voltage (10–50 V) and long durations (microseconds to milliseconds).[89] The microcurrent dressing Procellera (Vomaris Innovations, Chandler, AZ, USA) uses elemental silver and zinc dot matrix on a sheet to produce a current in the range of 0.6 to 0.7 V and has been associated with antibacterial effects.[60] High-voltage pulsed current therapy uses a monophasic pulsed electric current that consists of double-peaked impulses (<200 microseconds) at very high-peak current amplitude (2–2.5 A), high voltage (75–500 V; typically 150–250 V), and frequencies ranging from 1 to 125 pulses per second.[90] There is no evidence to suggest that 1 polarity is better than the other or that continuous delivery is better than pulsed mode.[89,91]

A comprehensive review of the effects of EST on healing rate and mechanical strength of wounds, and survival rate and viability of skin grafts, donor sites, and musculocutaneous flaps in different small mammal species (eg, rabbits, Guinea pigs, rats, and hamsters) concludes that regardless of the kind of wound, the current, or the polarity applied, EST (especially low-intensity direct current and low-intensity pulsed current) facilitates wound healing and improves the survival of skin and musculocutaneous flaps. It also suggests that the use of EST for a short period may increase collagen deposition but has little or no effect on the formation of cross-linking and collagen realignment in a congruous manner, which may be a phenomenon occurring later and therefore warranting further studies.[89]

THERAPEUTIC ULTRASONOGRAPHY

TU refers to the delivery of ultrasonic waves to the tissues for medical purposes.[91] Among other uses, the administration of ultrasonic waves provokes thermal and nonthermal effects that stimulate soft tissue healing. The interaction of sound waves with densely packed large protein molecules (such as collagen) provokes an elevation of skin temperature that results in an increased extensibility/flexibility of collagen-rich scar tissues and blood flow, which could be beneficial in chronic inflammatory processes. Nonthermal mechanisms for tissue regeneration are mainly based on stable cavitation and acoustic streaming[92] (**Box 3**).

The safe use of TU requires an appropriate selection of frequency, intensity, duty cycle, and duration of the ultrasonic waves delivered.[97] In conventional ultrasound therapy, the hand piece contacts the skin (ultrasound gel may be used to improve transmission) and delivers high-frequency (1.1–3.3 MHz) and intensity (0.1–3.0 W/cm^2) ultrasonic waves in a continuous or pulsed mode, provoking mechanical

---

Box 2
Effects of electrical stimulation therapy

- Promotes directional migration of keratinocytes and macrophages[88]
- Stimulates fibroblasts[88]
- Increases protein and collagen synthesis[88]
- Enhances angiogenesis[88]

> **Box 3**
> **Effects of therapeutic ultrasonography**
>
> - Decreases wound exudate formation, increases collagen deposition, increases vascularity, and allows wound debridement at 0.0225, 0.025, 0.035 MHz by promoting fibrinolysis of the wound surface without damaging the underlying granulation tissue[93]
> - Increases extensibility/flexibility of collagen-rich scar tissues
> - Increases blood flow. Studies in rats reported that TU enhances wound healing by increasing blood perfusion and accelerates healing in normal wounds but not in ischemic ones[94–96]
> - Increases protein synthesis (eg, collagen)[92,93]
> - Activates immune cells to migrate to the site of injury during the inflammatory phase of healing.[92,93]
> - Promotes wound contraction and scar tissue remodeling by altering the collagen fiber pattern[92,93]
> - Enhances transdermal drug delivery[97]
> - Reduces antibiotic resistance of bacterial films[97]
> - Improves treatment of vascular thrombosis[97]

and thermal effects.[87,93] The pulsed mode may be advantageous when mechanical effects are preferred over thermal ones. In low-frequency ultrasound therapy, a mist of sterile saline (instead of the hand piece) transfers ultrasonic energy (<0.04 MHz) to the wound in a continuous mode for 5 to 10 minutes daily.[87]

In relation to skin flaps in a rat model, TU reduced the area of necrosis from 18.3% (nontreated group) to 4.3% (treated), and tissues adjacent to the areas of necrosis presented increased levels of endothelial growth factor in the treated group.[98] Enhanced healing was also observed in a different study about random flaps in rats.[99] In the specific case of ischemic-reperfusion injuries, TU improved flap survival by promoting angiogenesis and inhibiting tissue inflammation.[100] Finally, TU demonstrated beneficial structural effects on full-thickness skin grafts and increased number and density of blood vessels within them.[101] In rabbits, structural benefits in healing of skin grafts have been also described.[102] In mice, a significant increase in CD31$^+$ cells in the epidermis and dermis of TU-treated skin isografts, suggesting an increase in the number of blood vessels, was observed.[103]

The use of TU has some potential risks (mainly related to the thermal effects) and contraindications (hemorrhage, infection, or skin neoplasia).[60,91]

HYPERBARIC OXYGEN THERAPY

Increasing the pressure of oxygen from 1 atm absolute (ATA) to 2 to 2.5 ATA for periods of 90 to 120 minutes twice daily allows the complete saturation of hemoglobin with oxygen and an up to 10-fold increase in dissolved oxygen plasma levels (allowing it to reach deeper tissues).[104,105] Although high oxygen tensions (partial pressures of oxygen, Po_2 > 500 mm Hg) provoke vasoconstriction of arterioles and venules that protect tissues from increased oxidative damage, the increased Po_2 maintains within normal limits the overall tissue oxygenation. In ischemic and postischemic tissues, these vasoconstrictive mechanisms are impaired, which in combination with the vasodilator effect caused by their increased Co_2 concentration result in an increased oxygen delivery that preserves the ATP levels necessary to maintain energy-dependent cellular functions and inhibit swelling and edema formation.[105]

Other potential effects of HBOT include the bactericidal effect of oxygen (eg, in vitro, suppresses 28% *Staphylococcus aureus* methicillin-resistant) and the oxygen-derived free radicals formed in the reperfusion state, the modulation of neutrophil activity, the stimulation of phagocytosis within affected tissues, the promotion of angiogenesis, the stimulation of fibroblast activity, and increased production of growth factors.[105,106]

HBOT improved healing times in full- and partial-thickness wounds in rats, full-thickness wounds in mice (20% increase in wound perfusion when measured with laser Doppler), and second-degree burns in Guinea pigs.[107–109]

Its use in pedicle grafts or skin grafts have been shown to be beneficial in rabbit and rats, especially if the HBOT is started immediately after surgery.[110–120]

Combinations with medicinal leeches have been anecdotally described to improve survival rates for axial skin flaps.[114]

HBOT chambers are available in various sizes, and some models are designed specifically for small animals; however, their elevated costs reduce their availability.

SKIN EXPANDERS

An inflatable or expandable silicone elastomer device of predetermined volume is surgically or endoscopically placed in the subcutaneous tissues of pliable skin adjacent to an existing or proposed defect that cannot be surgically closed owing to a large skin deficit. After an initial healing period of several days, the device is expanded by 10% to 15% of final volume every 48 to 72 hours until the final volume is reached. The constant forces delivered by the expander over the surrounding tissues allow the proliferation of epidermis at the same time subcutaneous fat and dermal thickness decrease. Once the final volume is achieved, a maintenance period appears to improve the quality of the expanded skin. Skin expansion is usually undertaken as part of a delayed reconstructive process.[121] The use of a skin expander has been reported in a rabbit.[122]

XENOGRAFTS

A xenograft is a graft of tissue taken from 1 species and grafted into a different one.

Tilapia collagen nanofibers are inexpensive, have good thermal stability, and could be used as wound dressing. They promote the proliferation of human keratinocytes and stimulate epidermal differentiation. In rats, they improve and speed skin regeneration by promoting cell adhesion, proliferation, and differentiation.[123,124] In deep partial-thickness scald wounds in rabbits, marine collagen peptides prepared from the skin of tilapia enhanced wound healing with adequate tensile strength and antibacterial activity.[125] The use of tilapia skin has been reported in nonscientific literature to manage burn wounds in a mountain lion and 2 bears.

PORCINE-DERIVED BIOMATERIALS

VetBioSISt (Smiths Medical North America, Waukesha, WI, USA), a collagen-rich biological mesh derived from dehydrated and sterilized porcine small intestine submucosa (PSIS), has been used as a scaffold and stimulant for tissue regeneration and remodeling. This product contains fibronectin, decorin, hyaluronic acid, chondroitin sulfate A, and growth factors.[126] The utility of PSIS for wound healing remains controversial. PSIS does not seem to provide any benefit for the treatment of acute full-thickness wounds in dogs, where contraction is a desired part of the wound repair process but may be a dermal substitute to prepare the wound bed for a split-thickness autograft, a cultured epidermal graft, or other reconstructive option in those cases where wound contraction is contraindicated.[127] In rats, equal rates of epithelialization

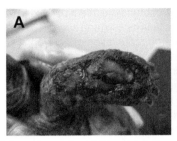
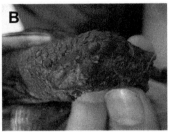

Fig. 7. (*A*) Extensive rodent biting wound on the front leg of a spur-thighed tortoise (*Testudo graeca*). (*B*) Postoperative appearance of the VetBioSISt graft used to cover the defect. (*Courtesy of* M. Huynh, DVM, DipECZM (Avian), Dip. ACZM (Small mammals), Arcueil, France.)

were observed for the group treated with PSIS and the control group; however, wound contraction rate was smaller in the treated group.[128] Permacol (Tissue Science Laboratory, Covington, GA, USA) is a porcine acellular dermal collagen-derived product. In rats, it provided better inflammatory scores, type I/type III collagen ratio, and wound contraction rates than saline moisturized dressings.[129] A different study in rats reported that both PSIS and Permacol were able to support an overlying skin graft, but neither had any beneficial effect on skin graft contraction when compared with skin grafts alone.[130] VetBioSISt has been used for the repair of skin defects in 1 Guinea pig, 1 red-tailed hawk, 2 barn owls, 1 umbrella cockatoo, 1 American crow, a large shell defect and soft tissue damage in a Horsfield's tortoise, severe digit trauma in an American alligator, deep ulceration of the spectacle in a king snake, and a large ventral skin wound in a water snake[131–133] (**Figs. 7** and **8**). In rats, PSIS sponges created with a pore size of 100 to 200 μm showed higher extent of exudate absorption, wound contraction, and faster granulation tissue formation in full-thickness wounds than the synthetic polyurethane wound dressing Tegaderm.[134]

IN VIVO BIOREACTOR

A modular adaptable in vivo bioreactor capable of generating vascularized new skin has been developed and patented (US 2014/0024112 A1). The modular components

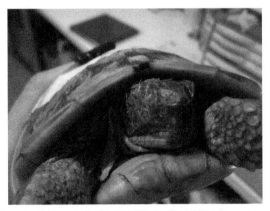

Fig. 8. Postoperative appearance of a VetBioSISt graft used to cover an enucleation wound in a tortoise. (*Courtesy of* M. Huynh, DVM, DipECZM (Avian), Dip. ACZM (Small mammals), Arcueil, France.)

of the bioreactor allow the delivery of growth factors, nutrients, and therapeutics to guide tissue growth (www.surgery.northwestern.edu/divisions/plastic/research/galiano_bsres-lab/models.html).

REFERENCES

1. Knapp-Hoch H, De Matos R. Clinical technique: negative pressure wound therapy-general principles and use in avian species. J Educ Perioper Med 2014;23:56–66.
2. Stanley BJ. Negative pressure wound therapy. Vet Clin Small Anim 2017;47: 1203–20.
3. Scherer SS, Pietramaggiori G, Mathews JC, et al. The mechanism of action of the vacuum-assisted closure device. Plast Reconstr Surg 2008;122:786–97.
4. Malmsjö M, Ingemansson R, Martin R, et al. Negative-pressure wound therapy using gauze of open-cell polyurethane foam: similar early effects on pressure transduction and tissue contraction in an experimental porcine wound model. Wound Repair Regen 2009;17:200–5.
5. Peinemann F, Sauerland S. Negative-pressure wound therapy: systematic review of randomized controlled trials. Dtsch Arztebl Int 2011;108(22):381–9.
6. Howe LM. Current concepts in negative pressure wound therapy. Vet Clin Small Anim 2015;45:565–84.
7. Morykwas MJ, Argenta LC, Shelton-Brown EI, et al. Vacuum-assisted closure: a new method for wound control and treatment: animal studies and basic foundation. Ann Plast Surg 1997;38:553–62.
8. Wackenfors A, Sjogren J, Gustafsson R, et al. Effects of vacuum-assisted closure therapy on inguinal wound edge microvascular blood flow. Wound Repair Regen 2004;12:600–6.
9. Wackenfors A, Gustafsson R, Sjogren J, et al. Blood flow responses in the peristernal thoracic wall during vacuum-assisted closure therapy. Ann Thorac Surg 2005;79:1724–30.
10. Erba P, Ogawa R, Ackermann M, et al. Angiogenesis in wounds treated by microdeformational wound therapy. Ann Surg 2011;253(2):402–9.
11. Pietramaggiori G, Liu P, Scherer SS, et al. Tensile forces stimulate vascular remodeling and epidermal cell proliferation in living skin. Ann Surg 2007;246(5): 896–902.
12. Saxena V, Hwang CW, Huang S, et al. Vacuum-assisted closure: microdeformations of wounds and cell proliferation. Plast Reconstr Surg 2004;114(5):1086–96.
13. Sano H, Ichioka S. Involvement of nitric oxide in the wound bed microcirculatory change during negative pressure wound therapy. Int Wound J 2015;12(4): 397–401.
14. Hunter J, Teot L, Horch R, et al. Evidence-based medicine: vacuum-assisted closure in wound care management. Int Wound J 2007;4:256–69.
15. Cross SE, Thompson MJ, Roberts MS. Distribution of systemically administered ampicillin, benzylpenicillin, and flucloxacillin in excisional wounds in diabetic and normal rats and effects of local topical vasodilator treatment. Antimicrob Agents Chemother 1996;40:1703–10.
16. Borgquist O, Ingemansson R, Malmsjö M. Wound edge microvascular blood flow during negative-pressure wound therapy: examining the effects of pressures from -10 to -175 mmHg. Plast Reconstr Surg 2010;125(2):502–9.
17. Malmsjö M, langemannson R, Lindstedt S, et al. Comparison of bacteria and fungus-binding mesh, foam, and gauze as fillers in negative pressure wound

therapy–pressure transduction, wound edge contraction, microvascular blood flow and fluid retention. Int Wound J 2013;10:597–605.

18. Chen SZ, Li J, Li XY, et al. Effects of vacuum-assisted closure on wound microcirculation: an experimental study. Asian J Surg 2005;28(3):211–7.

19. Malmsjö M, Gustafsson L, Lindstedt S, et al. The effects of variable, intermittent, and continuous negative pressure wound therapy, using foam or gauze, on wound contraction, granulation tissue formation, and ingrowth into the wound filler. Eplasty 2012;12:e5.

20. Borgquist O, Gustafsson L, Ingemansson R, et al. Micro- and micromechanical effects on the wound bed of negative pressure wound therapy using gauze and foam. Ann Plast Surg 2010;64(6):789–93.

21. Borgquist O, Ingemansson R, Malmsjö M. The effect of intermittent and variable negative pressure wound therapy on wound edge microvascular blood flow. Ostomy Wound Manage 2010;56(3):60–7.

22. Braakenburg A, Obdeijn MC, Feitz R, et al. The clinical efficacy and cost effectiveness of the vacuum-assisted closure technique in the management of acute and chronic wounds: a randomized controlled trial. Plast Reconstr Surg 2006; 118(2):390–7.

23. Mouës CM, Vos MC, Van den Bemd GJ, et al. Bacterial load in relation to vacuum assisted closure wound therapy: a prospective randomized trial. Wound Repair Regen 2004;12:11–7.

24. Mouës CM, Heule F, Hovius SE. A review of topical negative pressure therapy in wound healing: sufficient evidence? Am J Surg 2011;201(4):544–56.

25. Khashram M, Huggan P, Ikram R, et al. Effect of TNP on the microbiology of venous leg ulcers: a pilot study. J Wound Care 2009;18:164–7.

26. Morykwas MJ, Simpson J, Punger K, et al. Vacuum-assisted closure: state of basic research and physiologic foundation. Plast Reconstr Surg 2006;117(7 Suppl):121S–6S.

27. Patmo AS, Krijnen P, Tuinebreijer WE, et al. The effect of vacuum-assisted closure on the bacterial load and type of bacteria: a systematic review. Adv Wound Care (New Rochelle) 2014;3(5):383–9.

28. Demaria M, Stanley BJ, Hauptman JG, et al. Effects of negative pressure wound therapy on healing of open wounds in dogs. Vet Surg 2011;40:658–69.

29. Wysocki AB, Staiano-Coico L, Grinnell F. Wound fluid from chronic leg ulcers contains elevated levels of metalloproteinases MMP-2 and MMP-9. J Invest Dermatol 1993;101:64–8.

30. Tarnuzzer RW, Schultz GS. Biochemical analysis of acute and chronic wound environments. Wound Repair Regen 1996;4:321–5.

31. Mast BA, Schultz GS. Interactions of cytokines, growth factors, and proteases in acute and chronic wounds. Wound Repair Regen 1996;4:411–20.

32. Younan G, Ogawa R, Ramirez M. Analysis of nerve and neuropeptide patterns in vacuum-assisted closure-treated diabetic murine wounds. Plast Reconstr Surg 2010;126(1):87–96.

33. Argenta LC, Morykwas MJ. Vacuum-assisted closure: a new method for wound control and treatment: clinical experience. Ann Plast Surg 1997;38(6):563–76.

34. Blackburn JH 2nd, Boemi L, Hall WW, et al. Negative-pressure dressings as a bolster for skin grafts. Ann Plast Surg 1998;40(5):453–7.

35. Schneider AM, Morykwas MJ, Argenta LC. A new and reliable method of securing skin grafts to the difficult recipient bed. Plast Reconstr Surg 1998; 102(4):1195–8.

36. Chang KP, Tsai CC, Lin TM, et al. An alternative dressing for skin graft immobilization: negative pressure dressing. Burns 2001;27(8):839–42.
37. Ben-Amotz R, Lanz OI, Miller JM, et al. The use of vacuum-assisted closure therapy for the treatment of distal extremity wounds in 15 dogs. Vet Surg 2007;36(7): 684–90.
38. Guille AE, Tseng LW, Orsher RJ. Use of vacuum-assisted closure for management of a large skin wound in a cat. J Am Vet Med Assoc 2007;230(11): 1669–73.
39. Nolff MC, Meyer-Lindenberg A. Negative pressure wound therapy augmented full-thickness free skin grafting in the cat: outcome in 10 grafts transferred to six cats. J Feline Med Surg 2015;17(12):1041–8.
40. Stanley BJ, Pitt KA, Weder CD, et al. Effects of negative pressure wound therapy on healing of free full-thickness skin grafts in dogs. Vet Surg 2013;42(5):511–22.
41. Willy C, Agarwal A, Andersen CA, et al. Closed incision negative pressure therapy: international multidisciplinary consensus recommendations. Int Wound J 2017;14(2):385–98.
42. Bayer LR. Negative pressure wound therapy. In: Orgill DP, editor. Interventional treatment of wounds. Cham (Switzerland): Springer; 2018. p. 193–213.
43. Murphey GC, Macias BR, Hargens AR. Depth of penetration of negative pressure wound therapy into underlying tissues. Wound Repair Regen 2009;17(1): 113–7.
44. Jacobs S, Simhaee DA, Marsano A, et al. Efficacy and mechanisms of vacuum-assisted closure (VAC) therapy in promoting wound healing: a rodent model. J Plast Reconstr Aesthet Surg 2009;62(10):1331–8.
45. LaFortune M, Fleming GJ, Wheeler JL, et al. Wound management in a juvenile tiger (*Panthera tigris*) with vacuum-assisted closure (V.A.C.) therapy. J Zoo Wildl Med 2007;38:341–4.
46. Harrison TM, Stanley BJ, Sikarski JG, et al. Surgical amputation of a digit and vacuum-assisted closure (V.A.C.) for management in a case of osteomyelitis and wound care in an eastern black rhinoceros (*Diceros bicornis michaeli*). J Zoo Wildl Med 2011;42:317–21.
47. De Matos R, Krotscheck U, Morrisey J. Management of extensive skin wounds in two raptors using vacuum assisted wound closure. Proceedings 1st Scientific Conf ECZM, April 26-30, 2011. Madrid, Spain. p. 61–2.
48. Lafortune M, Wellehan JFX, Heard DJ, et al. Vacuum-assisted closure (turtle VAC) in management of traumatic shell defects in chelonians. J Herpetol Med Surg 2005;15:4–8.
49. Hedley J, Woods S, Eatwell K. The use of negative pressure wound therapy following subcarapacial abscess excision in a tortoise. J Small Anim Pract 2013;54:610–3.
50. Coke R, Reyes-Fore P. Treatment of a carapace infection in an Aldabra tortoise (*Geochelone gigantea*) with negative pressure wound therapy. J Herp Med Surg 2006;16:102–5.
51. Adkesson MJ, Travis EK, Weber MA, et al. Vacuum-assisted closure for treatment of a deep shell abscess and osteomyelitis in a tortoise. J Am Vet Med Assoc 2007;231:1249–54.
52. Bezjian M, Wellehan JFX, Walsh MT, et al. Management of wounds in a loggerhead sea turtle (*Caretta caretta*) caused by traumatic bycatch injury from the spines of a spotted eagle rat (*Aetobatus narinari*). J Zoo Wildl Med 2014; 45(2):428–32.

53. Pryor B, Millis DL. Therapeutic laser in veterinary medicine. Vet Clin North Am Small Anim Pract 2015;45:45–56.

54. Barolet D, Christiaens F, Hamblin MR. Infrared and skin: friend or foe. J Photochem Photobiol B 2016;155:78–85.

55. Poyton RO, Ball KA. Therapeutic photobiomodulation: nitric oxide and a novel function of mitochondrial cytochrome c oxidase. Discov Med 2011;11(57): 154–9.

56. Rodrigo SM, Cunha A, Pozza DH, et al. Analysis of the systemic effect of red and infrared laser therapy on wound repair. Photomed Laser Surg 2009;27(6): 929–35.

57. Gal P, Vidinsky B, Toporcer T, et al. Histological assessment of the effect of laser irradiation on skin wound healing in rats. Photomed Laser Surg 2006;24(4): 480–8.

58. Mayer J, Ness RD. Laser therapy for exotic small mammals. In: Riegel RJ, Godbold JC, editors. Laser therapy in veterinary medicine. Photobiomodulation. Ames (IA): Wiley Blackwell; 2017. p. 287–97.

59. Silva JCE, Lacava ZGM, Kuckelhaus S, et al. Evaluation of the use of low level laser and photosensitizer drugs in healing. Lasers Surg Med 2004;34:451–7.

60. Thompson E. Debridement techniques and non-negative pressure wound therapy wound management. Vet Clin North Am Small Anim Pract 2017;47: 1181–202.

61. Sun L, Liu P, Quan S. Hemodynamic changes of pregnant rats with preeclampsia after treatment with low-energy laser irradiation of the chest. Nan Fang Yi Ke Da Xue Xue Bao 2010;30(10):2259–62.

62. Myakishev-Rempel M, Stadler I, Brondon P, et al. A preliminary study of the safety of red light phototherapy of tissues harboring cancer. Photomed Laser Surg 2012;30(9):551–8.

63. Santana-Blank L, Rodríguez-Santana E, Santana-Rodríguez KE. Concurrence of emerging developments in photobiomodulation and cancer. Photomed Laser Surg 2012;30(11):615–6.

64. Melo VA, Anjos DC, Albuquerque JR, et al. Effect of low level laser on sutured wound healing in rats. Acta Cir Bras 2011;26(2):129–34.

65. Rezende SB, Ribeiro MS, Nunez SC, et al. Effects of a single near infrared laser treatment on cutaneous wound healing: biometrical and histological study in rats. J Photochem Photobiol B 2007;87:145–53.

66. Al-Watban FAH, Zhang XY, Andres BL. Low-level laser therapy enhances wound healing in diabetic rats: a comparison of different lasers. Photomed Laser Surg 2007;25(2):72–7.

67. Mendez TM, Pinheiro AL, Pacheco MT, et al. Dose and wavelength of laser light have influence on the repair of cutaneous wounds. J Clin Laser Med Surg 2004; 22:19–25.

68. Maiya GA, Kumar P, Rao L. Effect of low intensity helium-neon (He-Ne) laser irradiation on diabetic wound healing dynamics. Photomed Laser Surg 2005;23(2): 187–90.

69. Hodjati H, Rakei S, Johari HG, et al. Low-level laser therapy: an experimental design for wound management: a case-controlled study in rabbit model. J Cutan Aesthet Surg 2014;7(1):14–7.

70. Ezzati A, Mohsenifar Z, Taheri S, et al. Low-level laser therapy with pulsed infrared laser accelerates third-degree burn healing process in rats. J Rehabil Res Dev 2009;46(4):543–54.

71. Ezzati A, Bayat M, Khoshvaghti A. Low-level laser therapy with a pulsed infrared laser accelerates second-degree burn healing process in rat. Photomed Laser Surg 2010;28(5):603–11.
72. Mester E, Szende B, Gärtner P, et al. The effect of laser beams on the growth of hair in mice. Radiobiol Radiother 1968;9(5):621–6.
73. Wikramanayake TC, Rodriguez R, Choudhary S, et al. Effect of the Lexington LaserComb on hair regrowth in the C3H/HeJ mouse model of alopecia areata. Lasers Med Sci 2012;27(2):431–6.
74. Wikramanayake TC, Villasante AC, Mauro LM, et al. Low-level laser treatment accelerated hair regrowth in a rat model of chemotherapy-induce alopecia. Lasers Med Sci 2013;28(3):701–6.
75. Blair J. Bumblefoot: a comparison of clinical presentation and treatment of pododermatitis in rabbits, rodents, and birds. Vet Clin North Am Exot Anim Pract 2013;16(3):715–35.
76. Zehnder A, Wyre N, Kottwitz J, et al. Physical rehabilitation in exotic species. Proceedings AAV Conference. Providence, RI, August 4–9, 2007.
77. Ness RD, Mayer J. Laser therapy for birds. In: Riegel RJ, Godbold JC, editors. Laser therapy in veterinary medicine. Photobiomodulation. Ames (IA): Wiley Blackwell; 2017. p. 298–305.
78. Nascimento CL, Riberiro MS, Sellera FP, et al. Comparative study between photodynamic and antibiotic therapies for treatment of footpad dermatitis (bumblefoot) in Magellanic penguins (*Spheniscus magellanicus*). Photodiagnosis Photodyn Ther 2015;12(1):36–44.
79. Dadone L, Harrison T. Zoological applications of laser therapy. In: Riegel RJ, Godbold JC, editors. Laser therapy in veterinary medicine. Photobiomodulation. Ames (IA): Wiley Blackwell; 2017. p. 320–33.
80. Cole GL, Lux CN, Schumacher JP, et al. Effect of laser treatment on first-intention incisional wound healing in ball pythons (Python regius). Am J Vet Res 2015;76:904–12.
81. Gustavsen KA. Evaluation of low-level laser therapy in a model of cutaneous wound healing in bearded dragons (*Pogona vitticeps*). Proceedings of the annual conference of the AAZV. Salt Lake City, UT, September 28 - October 4, 2013.
82. Mayer J, Ness RD. Laser therapy for reptiles. In: Riegel RJ, Godbold JC, editors. Laser therapy in veterinary medicine. Photobiomodulation. Ames (IA): Wiley Blackwell; 2017. p. 306–11.
83. Kraut S, Fischer D, Heuser W, et al. Laser therapy in a soft-shelled turtle (*Pelodiscus sinensis*) for the treatment of skin and shell ulceration. A case report. Tierarztl Prax Ausg K Kleintiere Heimtiere 2013;41(4):261–6.
84. Pelizzone I, Ianni F, Parmigiani E, et al. Laser therapy for wound healing in chelonians: two case reports. Veterinaria (Cremona) 2014;28(5):33–8.
85. Cushing AC, Knafo E, Abou-Madi N, et al. The use of class IV laser therapy in zoo and wildlife medicine. Proceedings of the Annual Conference of the AAZV, September 28 - October 4, 2013. Salt Lake City, UT. p. 68–9.
86. Stremme DW. Laser therapy for aquatic species. In: Riegel RJ, Godbold JC, editors. Laser therapy in veterinary medicine. Photobiomodulation. Ames (IA): Wiley Blackwell; 2017. p. 312–9.
87. Belanger AY. Therapeutic electrophysical agents: evidence behind practice. 2nd edition. Philadelphia: Lippincott Williams & Wilkins; 2013.
88. Torkaman G. Electrical stimulation of wound healing: a review of animal experimental evidence. Adv Wound Care 2014;3(2):202–18.

89. Kloth LC. Electrical stimulation for wound healing: a review of evidence from in vitro studies, animal experiments, and clinical trials. Int J Low Extrem Wounds 2005;4:23–44.

90. Polak A, Franek A, Taradaj J. High-voltage pulsed current electrical stimulation in wound treatment. Adv Wound Care 2014;3(2):104–17.

91. Davidson JR. Current concepts in wound management and wound healing products. Vet Clin Small Anim 2015;45:537–64.

92. Paliwal S, Mitragotri S. Therapeutic opportunities in biological responses of ultrasound. Ultrasonics 2008;48:271–8.

93. Pavletic MM. Topical wound care products and their use. In: Pavletic MM, editor. Atlas of Small animal wound management and reconstructive surgery. 4th edition. Ames (IA): Wiley Blackwell; 2018. p. 53–94. USA.

94. Djedovic G, Kamelger FS, Jeschke J, et al. Effect of extracorporeal shock wave treatment on deep partial-thickness burn injury in rats: a pilot study. Plast Surg Int 2014;2014:495967.

95. Kuo YR, Wang CT, Wang FS, et al. Extracorporeal shock-wave therapy enhanced wound healing via increasing topical blood perfusion and tissue regeneration in a rat model of STZ induced diabetes. Wound Repair Regen 2009;17(4):522–30.

96. Altomare M, Nascimento A, Romana-Souza B, et al. Ultrasound accelerates healing of normal wounds but not of ischemic ones. Wound Repair Regen 2009;17(6):825–31.

97. Mitragotri S. Healing sound: the use of ultrasound in drug delivery and other therapeutic applications. Nat Rev Drug Discov 2005;4(3):256–60.

98. Meier R, Brunner A, Deibl M, et al. Shock wave therapy reduces necrotic flap zones and induces VEGF expression in animal epigastric skin flap mode. J Reconstr Microsurg 2007;23(4):231–6.

99. Emsen IM. The effect of ultrasound on flap survival: an experimental study in rats. Burns 2007;33:369–71.

100. Reichenberger MA, Heimer S, Schaefer A, et al. Extracorporeal shock wave treatment protects skin flaps against ischemia-reperfusion injury. Injury 2012; 43(3):374–80.

101. Antonic V, Hartmann B, Balks P, et al. Extracorporeal shockwave therapy as supplemental therapy for closure of large full thickness defects—rat full-thickness skin graft model. Wound Medicine 2018;20:1–6.

102. Gonçalves AB, Barbieri CH, Mazzer N, et al. Can therapeutic ultrasound influence the integration of skin grafts? Ultrasound Med Biol 2007;33:1406–12.

103. Stojadinovic A, Elster EA, Anam K, et al. Angiogenic response to extracorporeal shock wave treatment in murine skin isografts. Angiogenesis 2008;11(4): 369–80.

104. Francis A, Baynosa RC. Hyperbaric oxygen therapy for the compromised graft or flap. Adv Wound Care 2017;6(1):23–32.

105. Edwards ML. Hyperbaric oxygen therapy. Part 1: history and principles. J Vet Emerg Crit Care (San Antonio) 2010;20(3):284–97.

106. Bumah VV, Whelan HT, Masson-Meyers DS, et al. The bactericidal effect of 470-nm light and hyperbaric oxygen on methicillin-resistant Staphylococcus aureus (MRSA). Lasers Med Sci 2015;30(3):1153–9.

107. Shulman AG, Krohn HL. Influence of hyperbaric oxygen and multiple skin allografts on the healing of skin wounds. Surgery 1967;62:1051–8.

108. Sheikh AY, Rollins MD, Hopf HW, et al. Hyperoxia improves microvascular perfusion in a murine wound model. Wound Repair Regen 2005;13(3):303–8.

109. Korn HN, Wheeler ES, Miller TA. Effect of hyperbaric oxygen on second degree burn wound healing. Arch Surg 1977;122:732–7.

110. Champion WM, McSherry CK, Goulian D. Effect of hyperbaric oxygen on survival of pedicled skin flaps. J Surg Res 1967;7:583–6.

111. Richards L, Lineaweaver WC, Stile F, et al. Effect of hyperbaric oxygen therapy on the pedicle flap survival in a rat model. Ann Plast Surg 2003;50(1):51–6.

112. Jurell G, Kayser L. The influence of varying pressure and duration of treatment with hyperbaric oxygen on the survival of skin flaps: an experimental study. Scand J Plast Reconstr Surg 1973;7:25–8.

113. Ulkur E, Yuksel F, Acikel C, et al. Effect of hyperbaric oxygen on pedicle flaps with compromised circulation. Microsurg 2002;22:16–20.

114. Lozano DD, Stephenson LL, Zamboni WA. Effect of hyperbaric oxygen and medicinal leeching on survival of axial skin flaps subjected to total venous occlusion. Plast Reconstr Surg 1999;104:1029–32.

115. Arturson GG, Khanna NN. The effects of hyperbaric oxygen, dimethyl sulfoxide and Complamin on survival of experimental skin flaps. Scand J Plast Reconstr Surg 1970;4:8–10.

116. Prada FS, Arrunategui G, Alves MC, et al. Effect of allopurinol, superoxide-dismutase, and hyperbaric oxygen on flap survival. Microsurgery 2002;22:352–60.

117. Zhang T, Gong W, Li Z, et al. Efficacy of hyperbaric oxygen on survival of random pattern skin flap in diabetic rats. Undersea Hyperb Med 2007;34(5):335–9.

118. Nemiroff PM, Merwin GE, Brant T, et al. Effects of hyperbaric oxygen and irradiation on experimental flaps in rats. Otolaryngol Head Neck Surg 1985;93:485–91.

119. Zhang F, Cheng C, Gerlach T, et al. Effect of hyperbaric oxygen on survival of the composite ear graft in rats. Ann Plast Surg 1998;41:530–4.

120. Li EN, Menon NG, Rodriguez ED, et al. The effect of hyperbaric oxygen therapy on composite graft survival. Ann Plast Surg 2004;53:141–5.

121. Stanley BJ. Tension-relieving techniques. In: Tobias KM, Johnston SA, editors. Veterinary surgery small animal. St. Louis (MO): Elsevier Saunders; 2012. p. 3781–810.

122. Cotter M, Stanzione G, Hassan M. Use of tissue expanders to prepare for skin grafts/flaps in rabbits. Proceedings ICE, January, 2000. p. 52–5.

123. Hu Z, Tang P, Zhou C, et al. Marine collagen peptides from the skin of Nile tilapia (*Oreochromis niloticus*): characterization and wound healing evaluation. Mar Drugs 2017;15(4):102–13.

124. Zhou T, Liu X, Sui B, et al. Electrospun tilapia collagen nanofibers accelerating wound healing via inducing keratinocytes proliferation and differentiation. Colloids Surf B Biointerfaces 2016;143:415–22.

125. Zhou T, Sui B, Mo X, et al. Multifunctional and biomimetic fish collagen/bioactive glass nanofibers: fabrication, antibacterial activity and inducing skin regeneration in vitro and in vivo. Int J Nanomedicine 2017;12:3495–507.

126. Hernández-Divers SJ, Hernández-Divers SM. Xenogeneic grafts using porcine small intestinal submucosa in the repair of skin defects in 4 birds. J Avian Med Surg 2003;7(4):224–34.

127. Schallberger SP, Stanley BJ, Haupman JG, et al. Effect of porcine small intestinal submucosa on acute full-thickness wounds in dogs. Vet Surg 2008;37:515–24.

128. Prevel CD, Eppley BL, Summerlin DJ, et al. Small intestinal submucosa: utilization as a wound dressing in full-thickness rodent wounds. Ann Plast Surg 1995; 35:381–8.
129. Kalin M, Kuru S, Kismet K. The effectiveness of porcine dermal collagen (Permacol) on wound healing in the rat model. Indian J Surg 2015;77(2):407–11.
130. MacLeod TM, Sarathchandra P, Williams G, et al. Evaluation of a porcine origin acellular dermal matrix and small intestinal submucosa as dermal replacements in preventing secondary skin graft contraction. Burns 2004;30:431–7.
131. Foerster SH. Innovations in wound care for exotic pets. Proceedings ICE, January, 2000. p. 56–61.
132. Stroud PK, Amalsadvala T, Swain SF. The use of skin flaps and grafts for wound management in raptors. J Avian Med Surg 2003;17:78–85.
133. Divers S. Use of VEtBioSISt skin grafting techniques in reptiles. Proceedings ICE, January, 2000. p. 62–5.
134. Kim MS, Hong KD, Kim SH, et al. Preparation of porcine small intestinal submucosa sponge and their application as a wound dressing in full-thickness skin defect of rat. Int J Biol Macromol 2005;36(1–2):54–60.

Technological Advances in Surgical Equipment in Exotic Pet Medicine

Lucile Chassang, Dr med vet, IPSAV (Zoological Medicine)[a],*,
Camille Bismuth, Dr med vet, DECVS[b]

KEYWORDS

- Exotic pets • Lasers • Radiosurgery • Ultrasound devices • Vessel-sealing devices

KEY POINTS

- Surgery is challenging is exotic pets and several surgical devices can be used to facilitate surgical procedures.
- Vessel-sealing devices and radiosurgery can improve safety and rapidity of various surgeries.
- Lasers and ultrasound devices also proved useful in numerous surgical procedures.

VESSEL-SEALING DEVICES AND RADIOSURGERY
Historical Background and Technological Description

Vessel-sealing devices use electrothermal bipolar electrosurgery energy and pressure to induce denaturing and fusion of collagen and elastin within the vessel and surrounding tissues for vascular occlusion.[1] Electrosurgery refers to generating heat inside tissues using an alternating electric current that passes through the tissue creating a circuit.[2] The LigaSure (Covidien, Inc, Mansfield, MA, USA) is the most commonly used of these devices in veterinary medicine, and the one available at the authors' practice. It uses a generator (**Fig. 1**) attached to a variety of handheld instruments (**Fig. 2**) with jaws designed to deliver bipolar energy into the grasped tissues.[1] Devices for open and laparoscopic procedures are available.[3] This system generator measures the electrical impedance (density) of the tissues, and a precise amount of bipolar radiofrequency energy is generated to ensure an effective seal. An audible tone is

Disclosure: This research did not receive any specific grant from funding agencies in the public, commercial, or not-for-profit sectors. No conflicts of interest to disclose.
[a] Service NAC, CHV Fregis, 43 Avenue Aristide Briand, 94110 Arcueil, France; [b] Service de Chirurgie, CHV Fregis, 43 Avenue Aristide Briand, 94110 Arcueil, France
* Corresponding author. Service NAC, Centre Hospitalier Universitaire Vétérinaire d'Alfort, Ecole Nationale Vétérinaire d'Alfort, 7 avenue du Général de Gaulle, 94700 Maisons-Alfort, France.
E-mail address: chassang.lucile@gmail.com

Vet Clin Exot Anim 22 (2019) 471–487
https://doi.org/10.1016/j.cvex.2019.05.005

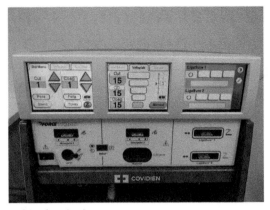

Fig. 1. Generator used in the LigaSure system.

emitted when the cycle is complete, indicating that adequate levels for occlusion have been reached.[1] In contrast, an incomplete seal is documented by an alarm tone giving the surgeon the opportunity to apply the jaws properly and avoid severe bleeding due to an incomplete seal.[4] If used properly, it should ensure a permanent seal with minimal thermal damage (maximum of 2 mm in the surrounding tissue).[1] The device is approved for vessels measuring up to 7 mm diameter and creates a seal that can resist 3 times the normal blood pressure.[4] Large bundles can be grasped and effectively sealed when the instrument is used for tissue dissection.[1] This device has been shown to be more efficient and cause less thermal injury than conventional bipolar electrocautery when used for coagulating rabbit gastric veins and arteries in an experimental study.[5] Other units have also become available in the marketplace, particularly the SurgRx EnSeal device (Ethicon, Cincinnati, OH, USA). Thermal spread is better controlled and tissue damage is theoretically limited to 1 mm by restricting the tissue temperature to 100°C.[1] Unwanted thermal effects are limited by high compression jaw force and application of polymer sensors to the jaw contact surface, enabling a more precise control of the power delivered to the tissue surface.[1,3]

Radiosurgery relies on the same principles, except that the energy is generated by a low-temperature, high-frequency current (4.0 MHz). It enables precise tissue dissection with excellent incisional hemostasis but minimal thermal damage to the surrounding tissues.[2]

Use in Veterinary Surgery

Vessel-sealing device use has been reported for numerous surgical procedures in small animals, but is scarcely mentioned in exotic pet medicine literature. It is

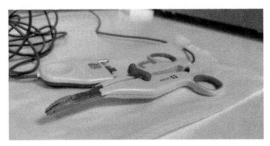

Fig. 2. LigaSure Small Jaw open sealer/divider.

particularly useful for laparoscopic procedures and has been described in another is-sues of this journal.[6]

The authors have been using the LigaSure regularly over the last few years for various surgical procedures (**Table 1**). The current and potential use of this device for surgery in exotic pets is discussed based on the authors' experience and the pub-lished data in exotic pets, laboratory animals, and small animals.

Table 1			
Use of LigaSure in various small mammal surgery			
Organ System	Surgery	Species	Diagnosis
Liver	Hepatic biopsy	Ferret	Chronic pleocellular hepatitis (1), lymphoma (1)
		Guinea pig	Nodular hepatic hyperplasia
		Rabbit	Bacterial hepatitis (yersiniosis)
	Liver lobectomy	Ferret	Hepatocellular carcinoma (1), biliary cystadenocarcinoma (1)
		Rabbit	Liver lobe torsion (3)
Reproductive system	Ovariectomy	Degu	Elective spaying
	Ovariohysterectomy	Hamster	Pyometra
		Rabbit	Uterine adenocarcinoma
Pancreas	Partial pancreatectomy	Ferret	Nodular pancreatic hyperplasia
Spleen	Splenectomy	Ferret	Extramedullary hematopoiesis (1), splenic torsion (1)
		Guinea pig	Splenoma
		Rabbit	Bacterial splenitis (yersiniosis)
	Splenic biopsy	Ferret	Lymphoid hyperplasia and extramedullary hematopoiesis

Splenectomy

The use of the LigaSure for splenectomy in exotic pets have been mentioned by several authors, and seems to contribute to a reduction of the surgical time for sple-nectomy in ferrets.[7] The authors have performed this procedure in several small mam-mals (**Fig. 3**; see **Table 1**). As described in dogs,[8,9] the procedure was fast and easy to perform, and the device provided adequate hemostasis and resistance to blood pres-sure. In dogs, surgical time is significantly shorter with a vessel-sealing device compared with a traditional stapler, and the difference was not affected by the expe-rience of the surgeon in 1 study.[8]

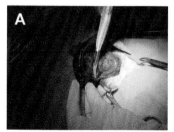
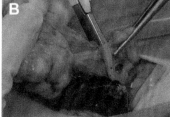

Fig. 3. (*A*) Splenectomy in ferret (*Mustela putorius*) using a vessel-sealing device (LigaSure). (*B*) Splenectomy in a rabbit (*Oryctolagus cuniculus*) using a vessel-sealing device (LigaSure).

Liver Resections and Biopsies

Liver surgery is not uncommon in small mammals, mostly in rabbits with liver lobe torsions and ferrets with hepatic neoplasms or chronic hepatitis. In the authors practice, liver biopsies and most hepatectomies are performed using LigaSure in small animals and small mammals. In the last 5 years, liver lobectomies have been performed in 2 ferrets and 3 rabbits (**Fig. 4**), and the device was used for liver biopsies in a rabbit, a guinea pig, and a ferret (**Fig. 5**; see **Table 1**). Vessel-sealing devices were shown to be efficient and safe for performing liver resection in healthy laboratory rats compared with suture techniques.[10] However, when compared with other techniques (including sutures, surgical staplers, and ultrasonic devices) in dogs, LigaSure showed no significant difference in surgical time or blood loss.[11] The SurgRx EnSeal device showed superiority to LigaSure in inflammatory response and caused lower lateral thermal injury and inflammatory score.[10] Mild hemorrhage has occurred in several cases, requiring a second application of the LigaSure and/or use of other hemostatic methods (bipolar electrosurgery, absorbable hemostat wraps). This may be related to wear of the device (see "Technical Limitation and Perspective").

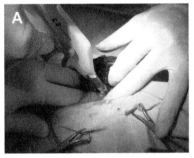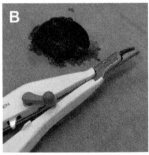

Fig. 4. (*A*) Liver lobectomy in a rabbit (*Oryctolagus cuniculus*) with liver lobe torsion, using a vessel-sealing device (LigaSure). (*B*) Removed liver lobe and vessel-sealing device after a liver lobectomy in rabbit (*O cuniculus*).

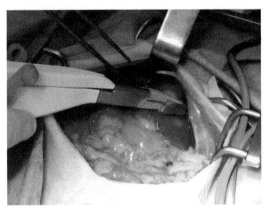

Fig. 5. Liver biopsy using a vessel-sealing device (LigaSure) in a ferret (*Mustela putorius*).

Castration and Spaying

Neutering and spaying, either for elective or therapeutic indications, are common surgical procedures in exotic pets. In small mammals, vessel-sealing devices can be used for castration and ovariectomy or ovariohysterectomy. The authors sporadically used the LigaSure for ovariohysterectomy in rodents (**Fig. 6**) and a rabbit (see **Table 1**). Although it enabled quick and safe hemostasis for ovariohysterectomy in the Syrian hamster (total surgery time from opening of the abdomen to closure of the skin was 7 minutes), it was responsible for excess tissue damage when performing ovariectomy in 1 degu, which died from intestinal entrapment a week later.

Some clinicians seem to be using this technique regularly for ovariohysterectomy or ovariectomy, especially in rabbits.[12,13] It was reported to be time saving and may facilitate surgery in species in which the ovaries are not easily exposed (eg, guinea pigs).[12] Ovariectomy using the LigaSure was shown to be significantly faster (almost 15 minutes shorter) and reduced perioperative complications when compared with ovariohysterectomy with ligatures in pet pigs (*Sus scrofa*).[14] Pain and postoperative partial anorexia was reduced.[14] In birds and reptiles, the use of the LigaSure was reported to facilitate salpingohysterectomies, because it can be used to seal the oviduct in addition to the blood vessels.[7] In dogs, the LigaSure enables a reduction of ovariohysterectomy surgical time of 15 minutes in dogs and 9 minutes in cats.[15] Another study showed similar findings, with a reduction of almost half the time needed for hemostasis using the LigaSure to perform ovarian pedicle hemostasis than with conventional ligatures in dogs.[16] None of the patients had significant complications in the first study, but, in 3/20 dogs from the second study, the electrode of the vessel-sealing device failed and had to be replaced to enable sealing.[15,16] In a rabbit, steatonecrosis and abdominal pain developed 2 months after ovariohysterectomy with this device, requiring surgical removal.[13] However, the authors have encountered several cases of steatitis and steatonecrosis following ovariohysterectomy in pet rabbits with a conventional technique (sutures). An increased risk of postoperative inflammatory response associated with the vessel-sealing device compared with the conventional techniques cannot be stated based on this single report,[13] and further studies would be required.

The LigaSure can also be used for castration in small mammals, reducing significantly surgical time, in open and closed castrations. The entire tissue bundle encompassing the vas deferens, testicular vessels, and cremaster muscle can be sealed at

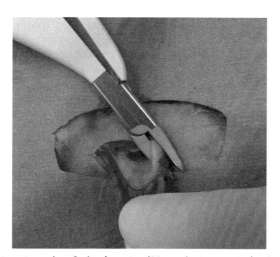

Fig. 6. Ovariohysterectomy in a Syrian hamster (*Mesocricetus auratus*) using a vessel-sealing device (LigaSure).

the same time.[7] In dogs, castration duration was reported to be reduced by 4 minutes when using the LigaSure.[15] It has been shown particularly useful for orchidectomy and scrotal ablation in marsupials, and the technique using the LigaSure has been described in sugar gliders (*Petaurus breviceps*), an opossum (*Didelphis virginianus*), and Bennett's wallabies (*Macropus rufogriseus*).[17,18] In these species, surgery can be challenging because postoperative wound dehiscence, infection, or automutilation are frequent because of overgrooming. The device is used to cauterize and cut the skin and testicular pedicles simultaneously. With this technique, the surgery and anesthesia were very quick, with a mean surgical time of 4 seconds (from the placement of LigaSure to scrotal excision) in sugar gliders and the opossum.[17] Grooming behavior returned to normal within 48 hours, with only mild excessive grooming in the immediate postoperative period. In 1 sugar glider, dehiscence of the incision site occurred due to licking behavior of conspecific animals.[17,18] Castration and scrotectomy in sugar gliders (*P breviceps*) was also described using radiosurgery in the form of an electrosurgical diamond loop electrode pen. Outcomes and benefits of this technique were comparable with the LigaSure technique.[19] Orchidectomy was also performed successfully in 2 asiatic black bears (*Ursus thibetanus*) with a prescrotal closed technique using the LigaSure.[20]

Pancreatectomy

Partial pancreatectomy is a frequent surgical procedure in ferrets with insulinomas, and has been performed with LigaSure in 1 case in the authors' practice. The technique has been reported in dogs[21] and a cat[4] with insulinoma, and seemed safe and time saving. In dogs with insulinoma, the use of the LigaSure allowed for a significantly shorter surgical time compared with the conventional suture-fracture method. Hospitalization was also significantly shorter and no postoperative clinical signs associated with pancreatitis were observed with this technique.[21] Reduced risk of postoperative complications was also demonstrated in pigs undergoing pancreatectomy, with lower postoperative markers for pancreatitis, reduced tissue handling, and shorter surgical time using the LigaSure.[22]

Miscellaneous Soft Tissue Surgeries and Potential Use

Vessel-sealing devices can also be used for any soft tissue surgery requiring hemostasis or dissection, such as removal of soft tissue neoplasms.[7] Their use was reported in rabbits for abdominal mass resection,[23,24] adrenalectomy,[25] and nephrectomy.[24,25] Enucleation in a guinea pig and a seal was also reported, as was removal of soft tissue neoplasms.[7] Although not reported in exotic pets, vessel-sealing device use has been described in various other surgical procedures in small animals, such as lung lobectomies,[1] vasectomy,[26] or tonsillectomy.[27,28]

Rabbits are widely used as experimental models for appendicitis and appendicectomy in humans. However, naturally occurring appendicitis has only been reported recently in a pet rabbit.[29] In this case, appendicectomy was not needed, but it can be required in some cases.[30] The use of LigaSure for appendicectomy have been evaluated in several studies in rabbits and rats, and seemed to be as efficient as conventional techniques in healing of the appendiceal stump.[31] In humans, a significant reduction of the operating time without significant differences in complication rate, use of analgesics, and hospital stay was demonstrated between LigaSure technique and a conventional approach.[32] In rats with and without experimentally induced appendicitis, operating time was also decreased and healing was not impaired.[33,34]

Regarding radiosurgery, it has been mostly used for skin and muscular incision, and has been shown to cause significantly less necrosis and collateral damage than CO_2

laser immediately following incision in ball pythons (*Python regius*).[35] In pigeons (*Columba livia*) and green iguanas (*Iguana iguana*), radiosurgery was also evaluated and caused significantly less thermal injury than CO_2 laser.[36,37]

Technical Limitations

The vessel-sealing device handpieces are designed for a single use. However, repeated use is possible with chemical disinfection or gas sterilization (**Fig. 7**).[7] Depending on the study and the device, multiple use was considered possible, with proper use and maintenance, up to approximately 10 to 25 times without loss of efficiency (eg, sealing and bursting pressure).[8,38,39] Some authors even report using the device over 500 times without loss of function.[7] Wear on the cutting tool and degradation of the insulation on the jaws were the most common problems encountered.[8] Failure of the vascular seal was associated with inadequate tissue apposition on histopathology.[39]

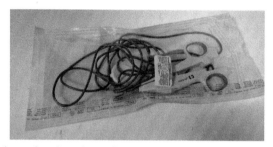

Fig. 7. Resterilized vessel-sealing device (LigaSure Small Jaw).

Adhesions are an important concern after surgery in human and veterinary medicine. It is especially a source of concern in small mammals and severe complications associated with adhesions have been reported in rabbits.[40–42] Several authors hypothesized a beneficial effect of vessel-sealing devices on adhesion occurrence, compared with sutures. However, the LigaSure did not seem to provide any significant reduction in adhesions either in rats[10,43] or in rabbits[31] after abdominal surgery. But, the SurgRx EnSeal was demonstrated superior to suture and Liga-Sure in term of adhesion formation in a model of liver lobe resection in rats.[10]

LASER

Historical Background and Technological Description

The first operational laser was developed by Theodore Maiman in 1960. But the basis necessary for the concept of laser development date from as early as the nineteenth century with the theory of optical resonance.[44] The term laser is an acronym for light amplification by stimulated emission of radiation. Most lasers have a photothermal effect on tissue that can be used to cut, cauterize, coagulate, vaporize, or weld. Heat production can be intense and must be localized precisely to avoid damage to surrounding tissues. Heat production depends on laser-related factors, tissue-related factors, and the surrounding medium.[3] Several types of surgical lasers are available and include argon lasers, carbon dioxide lasers, diode lasers, Nd:YAG lasers, HO:YAG lasers, and Excimer lasers.

CO_2 and diode lasers are probably the most commonly available lasers in veterinary practice (**Fig. 8**). The CO_2 laser produces its effects through instantaneous heating of intracellular water to boiling point, causing cells to explode in its path.[3] Compared with the diode laser, lateral thermal injury is limited and tissue penetration is minimal.[35] Thermal damage depth can range from less than 0.1 to 0.5 mm. It can be used to incise tissues, coagulate vessels under 1 mm in diameter, seal lymphatics, and control intraoperative blood loss and postoperative edema.[35] When using the CO_2 laser, there is no tissue contact: this precludes tactile feedback but prevents tissue drag during incisions.

Use in Exotic Pet Medicine

Carbon dioxide laser

The use of a CO_2 laser in exotic pets have been described by several authors.[45,46] Various soft tissue surgeries were reported as successfully performed in exotic animals.

In small mammals, the use of a CO_2 laser was reported for routine skin incision and cutaneous mass removal such as mammary fibroadenoma in a rat[47] or papillomaviral lesions in a porcupine (Erethizon dorsatum),[48] resection of oral lesions such as reported in a rabbit,[49] limb amputation such as performed in a rabbit,[50] celiotomy, laparotomy, orchidectomy, ovariohysterectomy, subcutaneous abscesses, adrenalectomy, insulinoma removal, and anal sacculectomy in ferrets.[45] Regarding skin incision and mass removal, thermal damage is a source of concern for postoperative healing, and for histologic diagnosis, because charring occurs at the edges of the specimen and may impair assessment of lesion margins.[51,52] However, in 1 study, skin incision made with a pulsed CO_2 laser in healthy rats healed at a rate similar to scalpel incisions.[53] More specifically, the CO_2 laser was evaluated for orchiectomy and scrotal ablation in sugar gliders (P breviceps). Grooming of the surgical site was only observed for 24 hours, and no significant complication was noted, making this technique a valuable alternative to the techniques using a vessel-sealing device or radiosurgery, as described previously. The use of the CO_2 laser also is commonly reported as reducing postoperative edema,[35] and supposedly decreasing postoperative pain. In cats, it is associated with reduced postoperative complications and lower pain scores when performing onychectomies.[54,55]

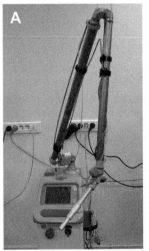
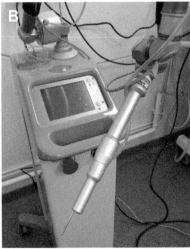

Fig. 8. (A) Handpiece and generator of a CO_2 laser. (B) Close-up view of the handpiece of a CO_2 laser.

In birds, 1 study evaluated the use of a CO_2 laser to remove lipomas in budgerigars (*Melopsittacus undulatus*). It was compared with the use of an ultrasonic aspirator, and no statistically significant difference was observed between the 2 techniques regarding surgical time and blood loss. The technique was considered safe and effective, but the CO_2 laser was less easy to use than the ultrasonic aspirator.[56] Hysterectomy and surgery of infraorbital sinus abscesses were performed in cockatiels with success.[45] The authors used the CO_2 laser to remove bumblefoot lesions in a common duck, with a good postoperative healing (**Fig. 9**). As reported in iguanas, thermal injury was greater with the CO_2 laser than radiosurgery for skin incisions in pigeons (*C livia*).[36]

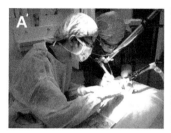
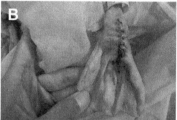

Fig. 9. (*A*) Bumblefoot surgery in a domestic duck (*Anas platyrhynchos*) operated with a CO_2 laser. (*B*) Postoperative aspect after proliferative growth resection.

In reptiles, orchidectomy and ovariohysterectomy using a CO_2 laser were described in the iguana, and also auricular abscess surgery in the turtle.[45] The authors performed CO_2 laser resection of an oral granuloma in an Indian python (*Python molurus*), and this technique enabled bloodless surgery, and wound healing was considered good (**Fig. 10**). It is also commonly used in turtles for removal of papillomas and fibropapillomatosis lesions and is the treatment of choice of fibropapillomatosis in sea turtles according to some authors.[57–59] Its use for skin incision has been studied in ball pythons (*P regius*), and demonstrated an increased necrosis, dehiscence, and granuloma frequency than with scalpel incisions.[35] When compared with radiosurgery, the area of thermal injury was larger when performing skin incisions in green iguanas (*I iguana*).[37] The CO_2 laser also has been used in fish. One case of surgical resection of a fibrosarcoma has been reported,[60] and it has been used in the authors' practice for removal of a cutaneous neoplasm in a goldfish (*Carassius auratus*).

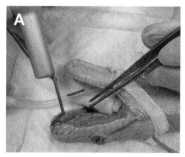
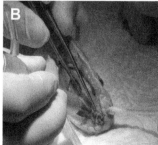

Fig. 10. (*A*) Resection of an oral granuloma in a reticulated python (*Malayopython reticulatus*) with a CO_2 laser. (*B*) Close-up view of the resection of the oral granuloma showing the tissue charring caused by the CO_2 laser.

Diode Laser

The diode laser has been used for various exotic pet surgeries. In small mammals, several authors advocated its use for adrenalectomy in ferrets,[45,46] and its use for elective neutering and spaying was reported.[46] In birds, hysterectomies and orchiectomies, removal of cutaneous granulomas, cloacal papillomas, neoplasms, and abscesses, as well as amputations, have been successfully performed using a diode laser.[45,46] It has been more specifically recommended to perform ablation of the primary feather follicles in birds for flight prevention and has been evaluated in common pintails (*Anas acuta acuta*), a white-faced whistling duck (*Dendrocygna viduata*), and domestic pigeons (*C livia*).[61,62] The diode laser technique was successful in 70% of feathers for the common pintails, but only 33% in the white-faced whistling duck.[61] It was faster, easier to perform, and caused minimal tissue damage compared with cryosurgery in pigeons.[62] In reptiles, diode laser use has been described for numerous celomic surgeries, for example, ovariosalpingectomy, orchiectomy, cystotomy, intestinal surgery, and abscess/neoplasm excision, as well as amputations, oral surgery, or enucleation. The main limitation of this device concerns skin incisions, due to variable pigmentation and keratinization depending on species.[46] According to 1 author, wound healing did not seem delayed, and the laser proved particularly helpful for breaking down adhesions between coelomic viscera, or dissecting abscesses of large granulomas.[46] It has been used successfully in amphibians and fish for celomic surgeries, and for surgical removal of proliferative skin alterations caused by *Dermocystidium* sp in 2 koi ponds.[63]

Technical Limitation and Perspective

Laser energy can be dangerous to eyes and other tissues, and eye protection is suggested for all operating personnel as well as for the patient. Regarding radiofrequency devices, smoke is produced by lasers and may cause safety concerns, so products of tissue vaporization must be safely evacuated from the room environment.[3]

The potential fire hazard is another concern. In 1 experimental study,[64] incidence of fire ignition was 11% in rat cadavers maintained under volatile anesthesia during diode laser surgery. Fire events only occurred when performing cheek skin biopsies, and most of these occurred with open masks (only 1 occurred with tight-fitting masks). The authors concluded that surgical lasers should be avoided for facial surgery of non-intubated anesthetized rodents. This study was performed following 2 cases of severe burns due to fire ignition during laser surgery in the authors' practice in a pet mouse (*Mus musculus*) and a Dzungarian hamster (*Phodopus sungorus*).[65]

ULTRASOUND DISSECTORS AND ASPIRATORS
Historical Background and Technological Description

The concept of ultrasonic surgical devices arose in the 1960s and was primarily developed for ophthalmology (especially cataract surgery).[66] The most commonly used ultrasonic device is the Harmonic system (Ethicon Endo-surgery), which was first introduced in 1998.[67] It coagulates and cuts tissues with delivery of ultrasonic waves at about 55,000 vibrations per second (55.5 kHz). It can seal vessels up to 5 mm in diameter. Compared with vessel-sealing devices, lower temperatures (ranging from 50°C to 100°C) are produced and applied to form an "oscillating saw" effect, enabling to cut tissues and denature proteins to seal vessels.[1] The Harmonic system consists of a generator, a handpiece that houses an ultrasonic transducer, an instrument with an end effector used to cut tissue, a foot pedal, and a hand-switching adaptator.[3] Energy can be delivered by a wide variety of surgical devices, including scalpel, shears, blades, and ball tips. As a vessel-sealing devices, it is widely used in laparoscopic surgery, which is not be discussed here. The second most common device is the cavitron ultrasonic surgical aspirator (or CUSA) (**Fig. 11**), first popularized in 1979.[68] Ultrasonic waves generate energy to fragment and aspirate parenchymal tissue. It is particularly used for liver surgery, as the contact of the oscillating titanium tip causes fragmentation of hepatocytes owing to the high water content, while selectively sparing blood vessels and bile ducts. It does not coagulate, so additional hemostatic techniques are required.[68]

Perspectives and Limitations

The use of these devices has been very rarely mentioned in exotic pets. In a Dzungarian hamster (*P sungorus*), an ultrasonic activated scalpel was used to excise a check pouch following a prolapse. Surgical procedure required only 5 minutes from the induction of anesthesia to the end of surgery.[69] In dogs and cats, ultrasonic scalpels have been used to perform splenectomies,[70] partial pancreatectomies,[71] soft palate resection,[72] partial prostatectomy,[73] and hepatic biopsies.[74] The use of an ultrasonically activated scalpel for hepatic biopsies seemed to be a safe method in dogs,[11,75] causing significantly less hemorrhage and yielding good quality specimens than other methods.[74] However, it caused significantly more collateral damage in dogs.[74] The Harmonic scalpel has been shown to reduce significantly adhesion scores after partial omentectomy in

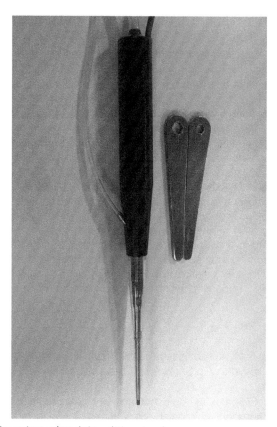

Fig. 11. Ultrasonic aspirator handpiece (Dissectron).

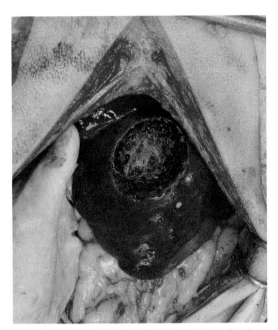

Fig. 12. Resection of an hepatic nodule in the left liver lobe of a dog using an ultrasonic aspirator.

rats, in comparison with standard ligatures and LigaSure.[43] This device may be promising to reduced postoperative complications associated with adhesions.

CUSAs have mostly been evaluated in small animals for neurologic surgeries, such as intervertebral disk fenestration,[76] or brain surgery for mass removal.[77–79] In budgerigars (*M undulatus*), lipomas were removed using the CUSA and this technique was compared with the CO_2 laser. Although no statistically significant difference was observed regarding surgical time or blood loss, the CUSA seemed to cause less tissue trauma, provided superior visualization in the surgical field, and was considered easier to use than the CO_2 laser.[56] In small animals, CUSA use in hepatic surgery is being developed and was initially described for identification and isolation of an intrahepatic portosystemic shunt in a dog.[80] Recently, the use of the CUSA to perform single or multiple hepatectomies in dogs based on the functional anatomic model of the canine liver has been reported.[81] This technique allows preservation of essential vasculature and permits sparing of liver parenchyma, particularly in front of multiple masses (**Fig. 12**). Long-term follow-up and the potential oncological interest of this technique in dogs is currently under evaluation by the same team. This technique could be applied to our exotic pet patients when facing liver tumors.

REFERENCES

1. Peycke LE. Facilitation of soft tissue surgery: surgical staplers and vessel sealing devices. Vet Clin North Am Small Anim Pract 2015;45(3):451–61.

2. MacPhail CM. Biomaterials, suturing, and hemostasis. In: Fossum TW, editor. Small animal surgery. 4th edition. St Louis (MO): Elsevier Health Sciences; 2013. p. 64–83.

3. Sackman JE. Surgical modalities: laser, radiofrequency, ultrasonic and electrosurgery. In: Tobias KM, Johnston SA, editors. Veterinary surgery: small animal, vol. 1, 1st edition. Philadelphia: Elsevier Health Sciences; 2012. p. 183.

4. Knell S, Venzin C. Partial pancreatectomy and splenectomy using a bipolar vessel sealing device in a cat with an anaplastic pancreatic carcinoma. Schweiz Arch Tierheilkd 2012;154(7):298–301.

5. Diamantis T, Kontos M, Arvelakis A, et al. Comparison of monopolar electrocoagulation, bipolar electrocoagulation, Ultracision, and Ligasure. Surg Today 2006; 36(10):908–13.

6. Proença LM. Two-portal access laparoscopic ovariectomy using LigaSure atlas in exotic companion mammals. Vet Clin North Am Exot Anim Pract 2015;18(3): 587–96.

7. Stanford M. Use of a blood vessel sealing instrument in exotic animal surgeries. Exotic DVM 2005;7(2):13–7.

8. Monarski CJ, Jaffe MH, Kass PH. Decreased surgical time with a vessel sealing device versus a surgical stapler in performance of canine splenectomy. J Am Anim Hosp Assoc 2014;50(1):42–5.

9. Rivier P, Monnet E. Use of a vessel sealant device for splenectomy in dogs. Vet Surg 2011;40(1):102–5.

10. Sahin DA, Kusaslan R, Sahin O, et al. Comparison of LigaSure, SurgRx, and suture techniques in intra-abdominal adhesions that occur after liver resection in rats: an experimental study. Int Surg 2007;92(1):20–6.

11. Risselada M, Ellison GW, Bacon NJ, et al. Comparison of 5 surgical techniques for partial liver lobectomy in the dog for intraoperative blood loss and surgical time. Vet Surg 2010;39(7):856–62.

12. Miwa Y, Sladky KK. Small mammals: common surgical procedures of rodents, ferrets, hedgehogs, and sugar gliders. Vet Clin North Am Exot Anim Pract 2016; 19(1):205–44.

13. Linsart A, Buttin R, Matres-Lorenzo L, et al. Steatonecrosis following ovariohysterectomy with a vessel sealing device (LigaSureTM) in a rabbit. Paper presented at: ICARE2017. Venice, Italy, March 25–29, 2017.

14. Biedrzycki A, Brounts SH. A less invasive technique for spaying pet pigs. Vet Surg 2013;42(3):346–52.

15. Faluvegi A, Bedi D, Banhidy J, et al. Neutering of dogs and cats using LigaSure device. Magy Allatorvosok Lapja 2018;140(4):217–21.

16. Schwarzkopf I, Van Goethem B, Vandekerckhove PM, et al. Vessel sealing versus suture ligation for canine ovarian pedicle haemostasis: a randomised clinical trial. Vet Rec 2015;176(5):125.

17. Cusack L, Cutler D, Mayer J. The use of the ligasure device for scrotal ablation in marsupials. J Zoo Wildl Med 2017;48(1):228–31.

18. Anderson K, Kanda I, Brandao J. The use of LigaSure device for scrotal ablation in juvenile male Bennett's wallabies (*Macropus rufogriseus*). Paper presented at: ExoticsCon2018 Atlanta, GA, September 22–27, 2018.

19. Malbrue RA, Arsuaga CB, Collins TA, et al. Scrotal stalk ablation and orchiectomy using electrosurgery in the male sugar glider (*Petaurus breviceps*) and histologic anatomy of the testes and associated scrotal structures. J Exot Pet Med 2018; 27(2):90–4.

20. Jeong D-H, Lee S-Y, Yang J-J, et al. Orchiectomy in the Asiatic black bear (*Ursus thibetanus*). J Vet Clin 2015;32(4):363.

21. Wouters EG, Buishand FO, Kik M, et al. Use of a bipolar vessel-sealing device in resection of canine insulinoma. J Small Anim Pract 2011;52(3):139–45.

22. Hartwig W, Duckheim M, Strobel O, et al. LigaSure for pancreatic sealing during distal pancreatectomy. World J Surg 2010;34(5):1066–70.
23. Whittington J, Meyer A. Diagnostic challenge. J Exot Pet Med 2018;27(4):61–4.
24. Graham J, Mavromatis MV, McCarthy RJ, et al. An unusual case of ascending pyelonephritis in a rabbit (*Oryctolagus cuniculus*). Paper presented at: Association of Exotic Mammal Veterinarians Conference 2015.
25. Rose JB, Vergneau-Grosset C, Steffey MA, et al. Adrenalectomy and nephrectomy in a rabbit (*Oryctolagus cuniculus*) with adrenocortical carcinoma and renal and ureteral transitional cell carcinoma. J Exot Pet Med 2016;25(4):332–41.
26. Kneifel W, Schäfer-Somi S. Vasectomy in a cat using the Ligasure device - case report. Wien Tierarztl Monatsschr 2017;104(5–6):157–63.
27. Cook DA, Moses PA, Mackie JT. Clinical effects of the use of a bipolar vessel sealing device for soft palate resection and tonsillectomy in dogs, with histological assessment of resected tonsillar tissue. Aust Vet J 2015;93(12):445–51.
28. Belch A, Matiasovic M, Rasotto R, et al. Comparison of the use of LigaSure versus a standard technique for tonsillectomy in dogs. Vet Rec 2017;180(8):196.
29. Longo M, Thierry F, Eatwell K, et al. Ultrasound and computed tomography of sacculitis and appendicitis in a rabbit. Vet Radiol Ultrasound 2018;59(5):E56–60.
30. Di Girolamo N. Successful intestinal surgery in rabbits. Paper presented at: ExoticsCon2018. Atlanta, GA.
31. Souza LC, Ortega MR, Achar E, et al. Application of high frequency bipolar electrocoagulation LigaSure in appendix vermiformis of rabbits with or without acute inflammatory process. Acta Cir Bras 2012;27(5):322–9.
32. Sucullu I, Filiz AI, Kurt Y, et al. The effects of LigaSure on the laparoscopic management of acute appendicitis: "LigaSure assisted laparoscopic appendectomy". Surg Laparosc Endosc Percutan Tech 2009;19(4):333–5.
33. Elemen L, Yazir Y, Tugay M, et al. LigaSure compared with ligatures and endoclips in experimental appendectomy: how safe is it? Pediatr Surg Int 2010;26(5):539–45.
34. Yeh CC, Jan CI, Yang HR, et al. Comparison and efficacy of LigaSure and rubber band ligature in closing the inflamed cecal stump in a rat model of acute appendicitis. BioMed Research International 2015;2015:260312.
35. Hodshon RT, Sura PA, Schumacher JP, et al. Comparison of first-intention healing of carbon dioxide laser, 4.0-MHz radiosurgery, and scalpel incisions in ball pythons (*Python regius*). Am J Vet Res 2013;74(3):499–508.
36. Hernandez-Divers S, Stahl SJ, Cooper T, et al. Comparison between CO2 laser and 4.0 MHz radiosurgery for incising skin in white Carneau pigeons (*Columba livia*). J Avian Med Surg 2008;22(2):103–7.
37. Hernandez-Divers SJ, Stahl SJ, Rakich PM, et al. Comparison of CO(2) laser and 4.0 MHz radiosurgery for making incisions in the skin and muscles of green iguanas (*Iguana iguana*). Vet Rec 2009;164(1):13–6.
38. Blake JS, Trumpatori BJ, Mathews KG, et al. Carotid artery bursting pressure and seal time after multiple uses of a vessel sealing device. Vet Surg 2017;46(4):501–6.
39. Kuvaldina A, Hayes G, Sumner J, et al. Influence of multiple reuse and resterilization cycles on the performance of a bipolar vessel sealing device (LigaSure) intended for single use. Vet Surg 2018;47(7):951–7.
40. Duhamelle A, Tessier E, Larrat S. Ureteral stenosis following ovariohysterectomy in a rabbit (*Oryctolagus cuniculus*). J Exot Pet Med 2017;26(2):132–6.
41. Guzman DS-M, Graham JE, Keller K, et al. Colonic obstruction following ovariohysterectomy in rabbits: 3 cases. J Exot Pet Med 2015;24(1):112–9.

42. Lamb S. Large bowel resection and anastomosis in a domestic rabbit following obstruction. J Exot Pet Med 2017;26(3):224–9.
43. Kucuk GO, Ertem M, Kepil N. Histopathological response and adhesion formation after omentectomy with ultrasonic energy, bipolar sealing, and suture ligation. Indian J Surg 2015;77(Suppl 3):799–804.
44. Bartels KE. Lasers in veterinary medicine - where have we been, and where are we going? Vet Clin North Am Small Anim Pract 2002;32(3):495–515.
45. Rupley AE, Parrott-Nenezian T. The use of surgical lasers in exotic and avian practice. Vet Clin North Am Small Anim Pract 2002;32(3):703–21.
46. Hernandez-Divers SJ. Radiosurgery and laser in zoological practice: separating fact from fiction. J Exot Pet Med 2008;17(3):165–74.
47. Kathio IH, Tunio AN. Surgical removal of a fibroadenoma in a domesticated rat (*Rattus norvegicus*): original case study. Parkistan Journal of Agriculture, Agricultural Engineering and Veterinary Sciences 2016;32(1):132–5.
48. Schwartz S, Lockwood SL, Sledge D, et al. Diagnosis and treatment of a novel papillomavirus in a North American porcupine (*Erethizon dorsatum*). Vet Rec Case Rep 2018;6(2). https://doi.org/10.1136/vetreccr-2018-000609.
49. Miwa Y, Nakata M, Takimoto H. A retrospective study of oral tumors in rabbits: 18 cases (2005-2013). Paper presented at: ExoticsCon2016. Portland, Oregon.
50. Wakamatsu I. A case of liposarcoma in a rabbit. J Jpn Vet Med Assoc 2009;62(6): 476–8.
51. Rizzo LB, Ritchey JW, Higbee RG, et al. Histologic comparison of skin biopsy specimens collected by use of carbon dioxide or 810-nm diode lasers from dogs. J Am Vet Med Assoc 2004;225(10):1562–6.
52. Silverman EB, Read RW, Boyle CR, et al. Histologic comparison of canine skin biopsies collected using monopolar electrosurgery, CO_2 laser, radiowave radiosurgery, skin biopsy punch, and scalpel. Vet Surg 2007;36(1):50–6.
53. Sanders DL, Reinisch L. Wound healing and collagen thermal damage in 7.5-μsec pulsed CO_2 laser skin incisions. Lasers Surg Med 2000;26(1):22–32.
54. Clark K, Bailey T, Rist P, et al. Comparison of 3 methods of onychectomy. Can Vet J 2014;55(3):255–62.
55. Wilson DV, Pascoe PJ. Pain and analgesia following onychectomy in cats: a systematic review. Vet Anaesth Analg 2016;43(1):5–17.
56. Wilson H, Rawlings C, Latimer K, et al. Comparison of the cavitron ultrasonic surgical aspirator and CO_2 laser for lipoma resection in budgerigars (*Melopsittacus undulatus*). J Avian Med Surg 2004;18(2):95–100.
57. Page-Karjian A, Norton TM, Krimer P, et al. Factors influencing survivorship of rehabilitating green sea turtles (*Chelonia mydas*) with fibropapillomatosis. J Zoo Wildl Med 2014;45(3):507–19.
58. Glazkova A. Treating sea turtle fibropapillomatosis with CO_2 laser surgery. Veterinary Practice News 2015;34–5.
59. Raiti P. Carbon dioxide (CO_2) laser treatment of cutaneous papillomas in a common snapping turtle, *Chelydra serpentina*. J Zoo Wildl Med 2008;39(2):252–6.
60. Leclerc J-M. Fibrosarcoma in a goldfish treated with CO_2 laser. Vet Pract News 2013;30:12–3.
61. Shaw SN, D'Agostino JJ, Davis MR, et al. Primary feather follicle ablation in common pintails (*Anas acuta acuta*) and a white-faced whistling duck (*Dendrocygna viduata*). J Zoo Wildl Med 2012;43(2):342–6.
62. D'Agostino JJ, Snider T, Hoover J, et al. Use of laser ablation and cryosurgery to prevent primary feather growth in a pigeon (*Columba livia*) model. J Avian Med Surg 2006;20(4):219–24.

63. Pees M, Schmidt V, Pees K. Pilot study on the use of diode laser therapy for treatment of dermatitis in koi carp (*Cyprinus carpio*). Tierarztl Prax Ausg K Kleintiere Heimtiere 2011;39(2):89–96 [in German].

64. Selleri P, Di Girolamo N. A randomized controlled trial of factors influencing fire occurrence during laser surgery of cadaveric rodents under simulated mask anesthesia. J Am Vet Med Assoc 2015;246(6):639–44.

65. Collarile T, Di Girolamo N, Nardini G, et al. Fire ignition during laser surgery in pet rodents. BMC Vet Res 2012;8:177.

66. Williams S, Rader JS. Physical principles of ultrasonic aspiration. In: Rader JS, Rosenshein NB, editors. Ultrasonic surgical techniques for the pelvic surgeon. New York: Springer New York; 1995. p. 1–8.

67. Dutta DK, Dutta I. The harmonic scalpel. J Obstet Gynaecol India 2016;66(3): 209–10.

68. Huang K-W, Lee P-H, Kusano T, et al. Impact of cavitron ultrasonic surgical aspirator (CUSA) and bipolar radiofrequency device (Habib-4X) based hepatectomy for hepatocellular carcinoma on tumour recurrence and disease-free survival. Oncotarget 2017;8(55):93644–54.

69. Sato Y. A case of cheek pouch prolapse in a Djungarian hamster and its excision using an ultrasonic surgical apparatus (SonoSurg, Olympus). Jpn J Vet Anesth Surg 2010;41(2):59–62.

70. Royals SR, Ellison GW, Adin CA, et al. Use of an ultrasonically activated scalpel for splenectomy in 10 dogs with naturally occurring splenic disease. Vet Surg 2005;34(2):174–8.

71. Jiyoung P, Hae-Beom L, Seong Mok J. Partial pancreatectomy using an ultrasonic-activated scalpel in two spaniel dogs with canine insulinoma. J Vet Clin 2017;34(5):359–65.

72. Michelsen J. Use of the harmonic scalpel for soft palate resection in dogs: a series of three cases. Aust Vet J 2011;89(12):511–4.

73. Rawlings CA, Mahaffey MB, Barsanti JA, et al. Use of partial prostatectomy for treatment of prostatic abscesses and cysts in dogs. J Am Vet Med Assoc 1997;211(7):868–71.

74. Vasanjee SC, Bubenik LJ, Hosgood G, et al. Evaluation of hemorrhage, sample size, and collateral damage for five hepatic biopsy methods in dogs. Vet Surg 2006;35(1):86–93.

75. Risselada M, Polyak MM, Ellison GW, et al. Postmortem evaluation of surgery site leakage by use of in situ isolated pulsatile perfusion after partial liver lobectomy in dogs. Am J Vet Res 2010;71(3):262–7.

76. Forterre F, Dickomeit M, Senn D, et al. Microfenestration using the CUSA Excel ultrasonic aspiration system in chondrodystrophic dogs with thoracolumbar disk extrusion: a descriptive cadaveric and clinical study. Vet Surg 2011; 40(1):34–9.

77. Marino DJ, Dewey CW, Loughin CA, et al. Severe hyperthermia, hypernatremia, and early postoperative death after transethmoidal cavitron ultrasonic surgical aspirator (CUSA)-assisted diencephalic mass removal in 4 dogs and 2 cats. Vet Surg 2014;43(7):888–94.

78. Axlund TW, Behrend EN, Sorjonen DC, et al. Canine hypophysectomy using a ventral paramedian approach. Vet Surg 2005;34(3):179–89.

79. Nagaya Y, Kitoh K, Katoh T, et al. Surgical removal of meningioma using an ultrasonic surgical instrument in two dogs. J Jpn Vet Med Assoc 2006;59(3):193–6.

80. Tobias KS, Barbee D, Pluhar GE. Intraoperative use of subtraction angiography and an ultrasonic aspirator to improve identification and isolation of an intrahepatic portosystemic shunt in a dog. J Am Vet Med Assoc 1996;208(6):888–90.
81. Sellier C, Gomes E, Poncet C, et al. Use of a cavitron ultrasonic surgical aspirator for functional anatomic model based hepatectomies in dogs. Paper presented at: ECVS Annual Scientific Meeting. Athens, Greece, July 4–6, 2018.

Technological Advances in Endoscopic Equipment in Exotic Pet Medicine

Izidora Sladakovic, MVS, DACZM[a],*,
Stephen J. Divers, BSc, BVetMed, DZooMed, DECZM (Herpetology, Zoo Health Management), DACZM, FRCVS[b],*

KEYWORDS

- Endoscopy • Endosurgery • Laparoscopy • Laser lithotripsy • SILS
- 3D visualization • 4K resolution

KEY POINTS

- There are many opportunities for improved diagnosis and management of diseases using endoscopic equipment familiar and accessible to most exotic pet practitioners.
- Minimally invasive endoscopy-guided approach to urolith resolution should be considered before pursuing a surgical approach, particularly as laser lithotripsy becomes more readily available.
- Laparoscopic surgery is advancing toward reducing number of ports, and single incision laparoscopic surgeries are becoming increasingly reported in veterinary medicine, including exotic pets.
- Advances in camera technology and visualization continue to pave the way for more efficient and safer endoscopic procedures.
- Wireless and compact endoscopy sets, along with WiFi capabilities, provide an added benefit of being quick, easy, and portable, and their use within a consultation setting enables client interaction and education in real time.

INTRODUCTION

Advances in technology to further improve endoscopic procedures and minimally invasive techniques continue to evolve in the human field. Many of these techniques are crossing over into the veterinary field, including zoologic medicine. From interventional endoscopy, to advances in visualization, improvements in minimally invasive

The authors have nothing to disclose.
[a] Northside Veterinary Specialists, 335 Mona Vale Road, Terrey Hills, New South Wales 2085, Australia; [b] Department of Small Animal Medicine and Surgery, College of Veterinary Medicine, University of Georgia, 2200 College Station Road, Athens, GA 30602, USA
* Corresponding authors.
E-mail addresses: izidora@avesvet.com.au (I.S.); sdivers@uga.edu (S.J.D.)

endosurgical procedures, and advancements in equipment and instrumentation, the broad spectrum of these technological leaps and their possible applications in exotic pets is endless and almost bound by one's imagination. The authors have selected a few technological advances to discuss, which are relevant to exotic pets and are more likely to become widespread in the foreseeable future.

ADVANCES IN DIAGNOSIS AND MANAGEMENT OF DISEASES

Endoscopy has become an integral part of exotic pet medicine. The 2010 Endoscopy and Endosurgery issue of Veterinary Clinics of North America: Exotic Animal Practice continues to be relevant to exotic pets, with ongoing advances in diagnosis and management of diseases using the endoscopic equipment familiar to most exotic pet practitioners, particularly the versatile 2.7-mm system. There has been an increase in literature on the use of endoscopy for diagnosis of conditions not previously reported in exotic pets and improvements in their management, including interventional techniques. The use of the 2.7-mm system was recently described and validated for gastroscopy and acquisition of gastric biopsies in pigeons (*Columba livia*).[1] The use of the 1.9-mm integrated endoscope and 3-Fr biopsy forceps has been validated by the authors for acquisition of liver and kidney biopsies in budgerigars (*Melopsittacus undulatus*) (Sladakovic et al, unpublished data, 2017). In scenarios where larger tissue samples are required, optical biopsy forceps can be used instead of the standard biopsy forceps (**Fig. 1**); this has been described in free-ranging river sturgeon (*Scaphirhynchus*) for toxicologic analysis.[2] A recent report describes the use of the 2.7-mm

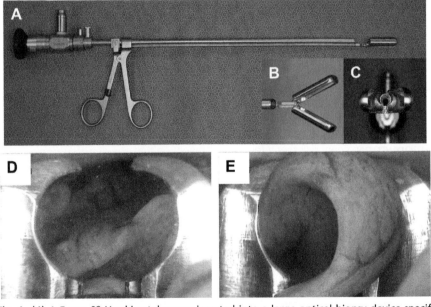

Fig. 1. (*A*) A 5 mm 0° Hopkins telescope inserted into a large optical biopsy device specifically designed to collect up to 1 gram of tissue for toxicologic analyses. Close up view of the open biopsy jaws side-on (*B*) and head-on (*C*) illustrating the position of the terminal lens. (*D*) The biopsy forceps are open thereby allowing visualization in the coelom of this sturgeon. (*E*) Once the forceps have been advanced onto a suitable tissue site, the jaws are closed to harvest a large sample, and the entire unit is removed from the animal.

system for cystoscopy and biopsy of urinary bladder masses in 2 rabbits (*Oryctolagus cuniculus*), leading to a first report of polypoid cystitis in this species.[3] The use of endoscopy was described for removal of a vaginal calculus in a rabbit, concurrently identifying the presence of uterine ostia, a possible predisposing factor.[4] Ear diseases are common in exotic mammals, particularly rabbits and guinea pigs (*Cavia porcellus*). Surgical intervention of middle ear disease is frequently advocated as medical management often ineffective at clearing the infection. A recent case report describes the use of otoscopy and myringotomy for successful management of otitis media and otitis interna in a guinea pig.[5] Management of tracheal strictures in an Eclectus parrot (*Eclectus roratus*) using a combination of endoscopy-guided resection and placement of a nitinol wire stent has also been described.[6] Human pediatric laparoscopic instruments, available in 2 and 3 mm, has allowed the development of endosurgical techniques in exotic pets, including endosurgical removal of *Aspergillus* granulomas in birds, avoiding the need for invasive surgical approaches or prolonged medical therapy (**Fig. 2**).[7]

ADVANCES IN UROLITH MANAGEMENT

Cystoliths and urethroliths are common, and cystotomy has traditionally been the treatment of choice, as most of the uroliths are not amenable to medical dissolution. Because of the high incidence of recurrence and invasiveness of surgical management, there is a need for a minimally invasive approach. ACVIM Consensus Statement recommends a nonsurgical approach in dogs and cats where feasible, with the aim of reducing patient discomfort, particularly if there is recurrence and need for repeat surgery. This is particularly encouraged in cases of urethral stones, where urethrotomies are associated with a high risk of adverse effects, such as strictures.[8] Smaller uroliths can be removed endoscopically using a transurethral approach if they are small enough to pass through the urethra or fragmented using grasping forceps before removal. These techniques have been described in female guinea pigs.[9]

Endoscopy-guided or intracorporeal laser lithotripsy is widely used in human medicine for management of ureteral, bladder, and urethral stones and is considered the standard of care for these conditions. The most commonly used laser is holmium:yttrium-aluminum-garnet (Ho:YAG). The laser works by generating photothermal energy, which is absorbed by the stones, causing fragmentation. The energy is absorbed by water and can safely be used 0.5 to 1 mm away from mucosal surfaces. The energy is delivered via a laser fiber that is passed through an endoscopy sheath. The fiber must be in direct contact with the stone, which is enabled by endoscopic visualization. In dogs, laser lithotripsy has been shown to be safe and effective for removal of uroliths and urethroliths and is a minimally invasive alternative to cystotomy.[10,11] There are a couple of published reports on its use in exotic pets. In a female guinea pig, Ho:YAG laser was used for management of a urethrolith. The procedure was performed under visualization of a 10.5-Fr rigid endoscope. Stone fragmentation and complete removal was achieved, and the guinea pig was recovered uneventfully.[12] Similarly, laser lithotripsy was used for successful management of a urolith in a red-eared slider (*Trachemys scripta elegans*). In the same report, a urolith measuring approximately 10 cm in a marginated tortoise (*Testudo marginata*) could not be fragmented and removed, presumably due to the large size.[13] There are additional reports on the use of laser lithotripsy for management of uroliths in tortoises.[14] The availability of an 8.5-Fr flexible video ureteroscope (Flexible Video-Uretero-Renoscope [FLEX-XC], Karl Storz) may overcome some of the size limitations faced in exotic pets and

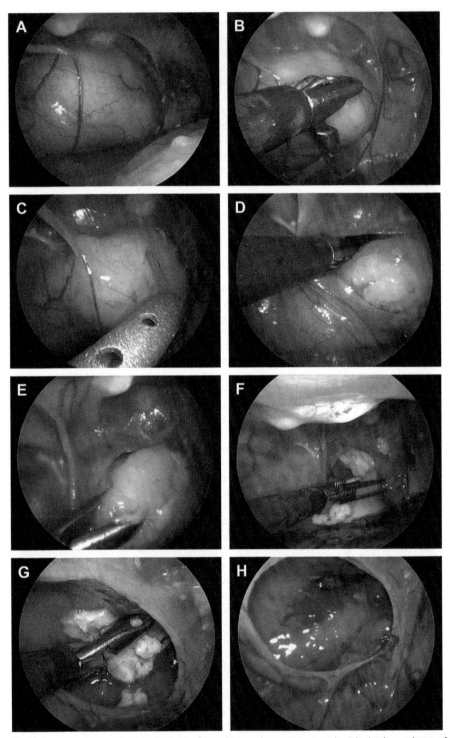

Fig. 2. Endosurgical removal of a large fungal granuloma associated with the heart base of a gyr-prairie falcon. (*A*) View of the large granuloma from within the left cranial thoracic air

enable this technique to be used in males and very small animals. One of the main limitations of laser lithotripsy is the cost and availability of the equipment.

ADVANCES IN ENDOSURGICAL TECHNIQUES AND INSTRUMENTATION
Single-Incision Laparoscopic Surgery

Laparoscopy technique in exotic pet practice was described previously in a recent article of this journal.[15] Laparoscopic surgery is increasingly becoming less invasive, with novel techniques being explored and developed in the human field, including single incision laparoscopic surgery (SILS), and natural orifice approaches, including natural orifice transluminal endoscopic surgery. In comparison to multiport laparoscopic surgeries, there are reports in human medicine that single-port techniques are associated with less pain and shorter hospitalization periods. There is less tissue damage associated with multiple ports and trocar placements. Single-port laparoscopic surgeries have made their way into the veterinary field, and numerous procedures, including ovariectomies, adrenalectomies, splenectomies, and intestinal surgeries, have been performed with favorable results.[16–20] A study comparing single and multiple port access for elective ovariectomy in dogs found that the single-port approach resulted in reduced surgical time and less complications.[16] However, this study had limitations with regard to study design, namely multiple surgeons with different skill level involved. One of the disadvantages of single-port surgeries is the reduced working space and limited ability for triangulation; however, this is being overcome by development of angled endoscopes and articulating instrumentation. A recent report described single-port laparoscopic-assisted ovariohysterectomy in rabbits using the foam SILS port.[21] The procedure was successfully performed, with no intraoperative or postoperative complications encountered. Whether straight or articulating instruments were used was not described; however, the photographs indicate that straight laparoscopic instruments were used. Ovariectomy and salpingectomy in captive cheetahs (*Acinonyx jubatus*) have also been described, using the SILS foam port and straight instruments.[22]

Anesthesia

Anesthetic management during laparoscopic surgery is a greater challenge in small exotic pets, compared with domesticated dogs and cats. Cardiorespiratory compromise created by CO_2 insufflation is an important consideration. Comparison between 4, 8, and 12 mm Hg intraabdominal pressures in rabbits was recently investigated. There was a significant difference in working space between 4 and 8 mm Hg, but there was no difference in working space between 8 and 12 mm Hg. Because 8 mm Hg results in less cardiorespiratory changes, this pressure may be suitable for laparoscopic surgeries.[23]

◀─────────────────────────────────

sac completely obscuring the heart. (*B*) Initial breach of the granuloma capsule using 3-mm debriding/biopsy forceps. (*C*) Use of a 3-mm suction probe to remove any fluid from within the capsule. (*D*) Use of a 3-mm babcock forceps (closed) to help separate the caseous debris from the capsule. (*E*) Initial granuloma removal using 3-mm babcock forceps. (*F*) Continued removal of debris using less traumatic, 3-mm fenestrated forceps. (*G*) Final removal of any remaining fragments using 3-mm debriding/biopsy forceps. (*H*) View of the completely debrided granuloma before endosurgical application of amphotericin B via an endoscopic injection needle. The bird made a complete recovery.

ADVANCES IN VISUALIZATION

Advanced camera capabilities, including high-resolution, contrast-enhanced, 3-dimensional (3D) visualization, and use of fluorescence imaging are emerging as important contributors to intraoperative surgical management and decision-making in the human field.

Image Enhancement

Using the standard white light, there are certain limitations to the nonspecific brightness and contrast functions, which can affect image quality and visualization. Structures that are further away from the camera are darker. Simply increasing brightness causes the structures that are closer to the camera to be overexposed, creating a glare. Likewise, electronic contrast enhancement is nonspecific. These limitations have been overcome by creation of visual enhancement modalities (Storz Professional Image Enhancement System [Spies], Karl Storz). This technology performs digital reprocessing, generating a new image using 1 of 5 different modalities. A preliminary study found that CLARA and CLARA + CHROMA modalities provided a higher-quality image compared with white light.[24] CLARA modality alters brightness to create better visualization of darker areas, providing a completely illuminated image. CHROMA modality enhances color contrast of difficult to see areas. Although there are no published studies yet in exotic pets evaluating the differences between modalities, the authors have used these in education and research settings (**Fig. 3**).

Three-Dimensional and 4K Resolution

Lack of depth perception is an important limitation in endosurgery, affecting accuracy and procedures times. To overcome this, 3D visualization systems were created. A video telescopic operating microscope (Karl Storz) has recently evolved to a 3D system, allowing this technology to be used for extracorporeal surgeries in exotic pets (**Fig. 4**). Comparing 2D and 3D technologies, there is improved accuracy and speed, with less errors, and quicker acquisition of endosurgical skills using 3D.[25,26] However, 3D technology is not without shortcomings. Apart from the cost and the need for 3D glasses, there are also operator side effects to consider, such as dizziness, fatigue, nausea, and headaches.[26] 4K resolution provides images of 4 times higher resolution than high definition. It provides images of superb detail and greater depth perception. Compared with 3D systems, it is associated with less visual adverse effects.[26]

Fluorescence Imaging

Fluorescence imaging has applications for both diagnostic and surgical endoscopy. Diagnosis and identification of inflammatory and neoplastic conditions using fluorescein imaging is already widespread in the human field. Fluorophores administered intravenously or topically, and using a confocal microscope, have been investigated in dogs for evaluation of gastric mucosa. Confocal endomicroscopy enabled real-time diagnosis of gastrointestinal diseases and in some cases identified abnormalities that were missed on routine histopathology.[27] Indocyanine green (ICG) fluorescence imaging has been used for oncologic surgery and identification of tumor margins and intraoperative identification of vessels, lymphatics, and ducts. In veterinary medicine, the use of ICG fluorescence imaging has been used for thoracic duct identification during thoracoscopy in dogs.[28] There are no reports of this imaging modality in exotic pets at the current time; however, there is a scope to explore this technology

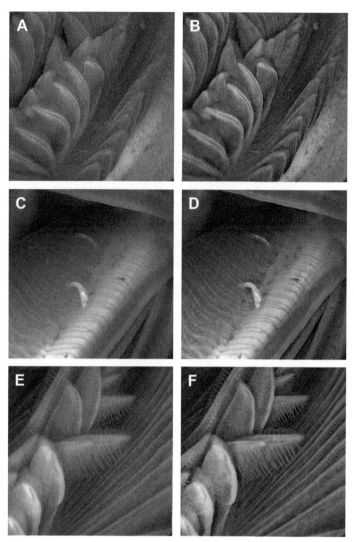

Fig. 3. Endoscopic images of gills in catfish. Image (*A*) was obtained using a high-definition camera; in comparison image (*B*) was obtained using the CHROMA modality. Image (*C*) was obtained using a high-definition camera; in comparison image (*D*) was obtained using the CHROMA modality. Image (*E*) was obtained using a high-definition camera; in comparison image (*F*) was obtained using the CHROMA modality.

in cases where targeted biopsies are required, particularly where the size of the patient limits multiple biopsy collection.

Adjustable Angle Telescope

Traditionally, the telescope selected for an endoscopic procedure is set, most commonly to 0° or 30°. A telescope with adjustable viewing angle, from 0° to 120° is now available, allowing improved visualization of a significantly larger intracorporeal space. This may be particularly useful in chelonians where the presence of a shell limits the manoeuvrability of the scope and in endosurgical procedures (**Fig. 5**).

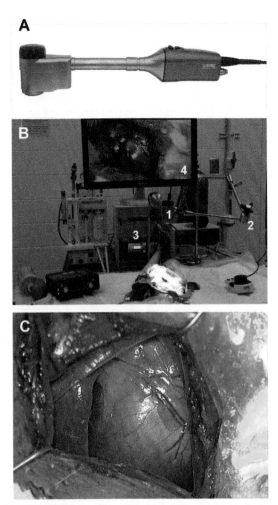

Fig. 4. (*A*) The VITOM 3D TH200 (Karl Storz) houses 2 camera units that provide a 3D image onto a high-definition screen. The device is used in open surgery and positioned above the patient to provide microsurgical capability with 3D depth perception. (*B*) The VITOM 3D (1) is positioned above the patient using a mechanical holding arm (2) attached to the surgery table. The images are processed using an Image-1 camera system (3) and displayed onto the HD monitor. Note that the image on the screen appears blurry compared with the record image (*C*). This is because the monitor displays 2 interposing images; however, a surgeon wearing 3D glasses perceives a crystal clear 3D image with depth perception. ([*A*] © Karl Storz SE & Co. KG, Germany.)

Portable and Compact Endoscopy Units

Wireless portable endoscopy units allow real-time endoscopy during a consultation and examination of the patient in client's presence (Firefly Global). This has the added advantage of providing opportunities for client education, which is integral in exotic pet medicine (Firefly Global). Attachments for smartphones are also available, allowing added flexibility of using the features of modern smartphones (SMART SCOPE, Karl Storz) described in Minh Huynh's article "Smartphone-based Device in the Exotic Pet Medicine" in this same issue.

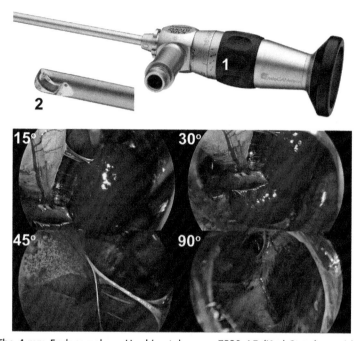

Fig. 5. The 4-mm Endocameleon Hopkins telescope 7230 AE (Karl Storz) provides the expected clarity of a rod-lens telescope but with the added advantage of variable viewing angle from 15° to 90°. The current selector is pointing to 45° (1). The terminal lens rotates within a protected housing (2), and illumination is provided by 6 windows to provide coverage over the entire field of view. The endoscopic images are taken with the telescope pointing at the cranial division of the left kidney in a pigeon (15°) and selecting the different angle deflections from 30° to 90° without moving the telescope. (© Karl Storz SE & Co. KG, Germany.)

ACKNOWLEDGMENTS

We thank Karl Storz Veterinary Endoscopy for continuing to support the educational and research endoscopy programs at the University of Georgia.

REFERENCES

1. Sladakovic I, Ellis AE, Divers SJ. Evaluation of gastroscopy and biopsy of the proventriculus and ventriculus in pigeons (*Columba livia*). Am J Vet Res 2017; 78(1):42–9.

2. Divers SJ, Boone SS, Berliner A, et al. Nonlethal acquisition of large liver samples from free-ranging river sturgeon (*Scaphirhynchus*) using single-entry endoscopic biopsy forceps. J Wildl Dis 2013;49(2):321–31.

3. Girolamo ND, Bongiovanni L, Ferro S, et al. Cystoscopic diagnosis of polypoid cystitis in two pet rabbits. J Am Vet Med Assoc 2017;251(1):84–9.

4. Tarbert DK, de Matos R. Endoscopic removal of a vaginal calculus in a domestic rabbit (*Oryctolagus cuniculus*). J Exot Pet Med 2016;25(3):253–60.

5. Pignon C, Volait L, Donnelly T. Endoscopic myringotomy to treat middle ear infection in a guinea pig. Proc AEMV and ARAV Conf. September 23–28, 2017, Dallas, Texas.

6. Mejia-Fava J, Holmes SP, Radlinsky M, et al. Use of a nitinol wire stent for management of severe tracheal stenosis in an eclectus parrot (*Eclectus roratus*). J Avian Med Surg 2015;29(3):238–49.

7. Sladakovic I, Divers S. Endosurgical treatment of severe air sac aspergillosis in a blue-fronted Amazon (Amazona aestiva) and a gyrfalcon x prairie falcon (Falco rusticolus x mexicanus). Proc 3rd ICARE Conf. March 25-28, 2017, Venice, Italy. p. 688.

8. Lulich JP, Berent AC, Adams LG, et al. ACVIM Small animal consensus recommendations on the treatment and prevention of uroliths in dogs and cats. J Vet Intern Med 2016;30(5):1564–74.

9. Wenger S, Hatt JM. Transurethral cystoscopy and endoscopic urolith removal in female guinea pigs (*Cavia porcellus*). Vet Clin North Am Exot Anim Pract 2015; 18(3):359–67.

10. Bevan JM, Lulich JP, Albasan H, et al. Comparison of laser lithotripsy and cystotomy for the management of dogs with urolithiasis. J Am Vet Med Assoc 2009; 234(10):1286–94.

11. Lulich JP, Osborne CA, Albasan H, et al. Efficacy and safety of laser lithotripsy in fragmentation of urocystoliths and urethroliths for removal in dogs. J Am Vet Med Assoc 2009;234(10):1279–85.

12. Coutant T, Dunn M, Langlois I, et al. Cystoscopic-guided lithotripsy for the removal of a urethral stone in a guinea pig. J Exot Pet Med 2019;28:111–4.

13. Nardini G, Bielli M, Nicoli S, et al. Endoscopic laser lithotripsy in chelonians: two cases. Veterinaria 2014;28(6):33–7 [abstract in English].

14. Westropp JL. Holmium: YAG Laser lithotripsy. Proc 33rd World Small Animal Veterinary Association. August 20–24, 2008, Dublin, Ireland.

15. Sladakovic IS, Divers SJ. Exotic mammal laparoscopy. Vet Clin North Am Exot Anim Pract 2016;19(1):269–86.

16. Gonzalez-Gasch E, Monnet E. Comparison of single port access versus multiple port access systems in elective laparoscopy: 98 dogs (2005-2014). Vet Surg 2015;44(7):895–9.

17. Ko J, Jeong J, Lee S, et al. Feasibility of single-port retroperitoneoscopic adrenalectomy in dogs. Vet Surg 2018;47(S1):O75–83.

18. Mayhew PD, Sutton JS, Singh A, et al. Complications and short-term outcomes associated with single-port laparoscopic splenectomy in dogs. Vet Surg 2018; 47(S1):O67–74.

19. Case JB, Ellison G. Single incision laparoscopic-assisted intestinal surgery (SILAIS) in 7 dogs and 1 cat. Vet Surg 2013;42(5):629–34.

20. Runge JJ, Mayhew PD. Evaluation of single port access gastropexy and ovariectomy using articulating instruments and angled telescopes in dogs. Vet Surg 2013;42(7):807–13.

21. Coleman KA, Monnet E, Johnston MS. Single port laparoscopic-assisted ovariohysterectomy in 3 rabbits. J Exot Pet Med 2018;27(1):21–4.

22. Hartman MJ, Monnet E, Kirberger RM, et al. Single-incision laparoscopic sterilization of the cheetah (*Acinonyx jubatus*). Vet Surg 2015;44(S1):76–82.

23. Kabakchiev C, Beaufrere H, zur Linden A, et al. Effect of intra-abdominal pressure on working space and cardiorespiratory parameters in the domestic rabbit (Oryctolagus cuniculus). Proc Veterinary Endoscopy Society Annual Meeting. May 21–23, 2018, Lisbon, Portugal.

24. Emiliani E, Talso M, Baghdadi M, et al. Evaluation of the Spies™ modalities image quality. Int Braz J Urol 2017;43(3):476–80.
25. Alaraimi B, El Bakbak W, Sarker S, et al. A randomized prospective study comparing acquisition of laparoscopic skills in three-dimensional (3D) vs. two-dimensional (2D) laparoscopy. World J Surg 2014;38(11):2746–52.
26. Abdelrahman M, Belramman A, Salem R, et al. Acquiring basic and advanced laparoscopic skills in novices using two-dimensional (2D), three-dimensional (3D) and ultra-high definition (4K) vision systems: a randomized control study. Int J Surg 2018;53:333–8.
27. Sharman MJ, Bacci B, Whittem T, et al. In vivo histologically equivalent evaluation of gastric mucosal topologic morphology in dogs by using confocal endomicroscopy. J Vet Intern Med 2014;28(3):799–808.
28. Steffey MA, Mayhew PD. Use of direct near-infrared fluorescent lymphography for thoracoscopic thoracic duct identification in 15 dogs with chylothorax. Vet Surg 2018;47(2):267–76.

Advances in Therapeutics and Delayed Drug Release

Thomas Coutant, Dr med vet, IPSAV (Zoological Medicine)[a],*,
Delphine Laniesse, Dr med vet, DVSc, IPSAV (Zoological Medicine), DECZM-Avian[b],
John M. Sykes IV, DVM, DACZM[c]

KEYWORDS

- Osmotic pump • Nanoparticle • Hydrogel • Sustained-released • Nanomedicine
- Exotic pet medicine • Therapeutics

KEY POINTS

- Reducing frequency of drug administration is crucial to limit stress and injuries secondary to frequent handling in exotic pets.
- Sustained-released drug delivery systems can increase duration of action.
- Three promising technologies are currently being investigated with some possible applications: osmotic pumps, nanoparticles, and hydrogels.
- Osmotic pumps are commercially available, whereas nanoparticles and hydrogels need to be specifically ordered in compounding pharmacies.
- They are implantable device or injectable formulations, which cannot be removed easily by the treated animal.

INTRODUCTION

Medical therapy in exotic pet medicine relies widely on daily or even more frequent oral, parenteral, or topical drug administration, which can be stressful and even harmful in some cases, either for the patient or for the handler.[1] Long-acting formulations are of great interest in exotic practice if they can allow significant reduction in drug administration frequency, thereby decreasing the need to handle medicated animals by the practitioner or the owner.

Furthermore, the level of care of exotic patients is sometimes suboptimal because of the absence of practical therapeutic options. This is the case with pain management in birds using butorphanol requiring intramuscular injections about every 2 hours for

Disclosure: This research did not receive any specific grant from funding agencies in the public, commercial, or not-for-profit sectors. No conflicts of interest to disclose.
[a] Service NAC, CHV Fregis, 43 Avenue Aristide Briand, Arcueil 94110, France; [b] Eläinsairaala Evidensia Tammisto Vantaa, Tammiston Kauppatie 29, Vantaa 01510, Finland; [c] Wildlife Conservation Society, Zoological Health Program, 2300 Southern Boulevard, Bronx, NY 10460, USA
* Corresponding author.
E-mail address: thomas_c_93@hotmail.fr

Vet Clin Exot Anim 22 (2019) 501–520
https://doi.org/10.1016/j.cvex.2019.05.006
vetexotic.theclinics.com

analgesic efficacy. This administration frequency may not be compatible with a clinical setting, leading to inadequate pain management in avian patients.[2–4] A similar problem is encountered in a zoologic setting when dealing with animals that must be under general anesthesia to be manipulated for safety reasons.

Increasing duration of drug action is therefore an absolute necessity in these cases because external constant-rate infusion is not always a valid option for obvious practical reasons.[5] This review thus focuses on recent advances in sustained-released drug delivery systems: osmotic pumps, nanoparticles, and hydrogels.

Osmotic Pumps

Osmotic pumps are pharmaceutical devices that use one of the most fundamental biological properties of life: osmosis. It results in an original way of drug administration offering stable controlled continuous rate delivery over a prolonged period of time.[6,7] The relative small size of the device, added to the fact that fluids can be found in every body area of a living organism, enables drug delivery systemically or at multiple potential site-specific locations.[8]

The theory
Osmosis principles Osmosis is a physical concept explaining the force generating a flow between 2 solutions of different solute concentrations when separated by a semi-permeable membrane, only allowing passage of the solvent and blocking the passage of any other molecules (**Fig. 1**A).[6] Equilibrium is reached when the hydrostatic pressure difference between the 2 solutions balances the osmotic pressure difference, resulting in the absence of solvent flow between the compartments (**Fig. 1**B).[6] According to the Van't Hoff equation, the concentration of the solution and its temperature are the 2 main parameters increasing the osmotic pressure.[6,8]

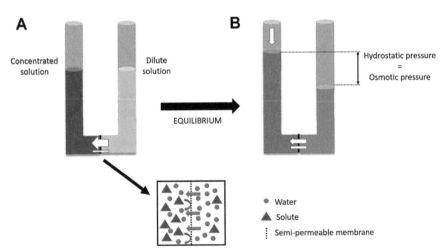

Fig. 1. Principle of osmosis. (*A*) Two solutions of equal volume and different concentration in a given solute are separated by a semi-permeable membrane, which allows for passage of water but not solute molecules. There is a resulting water flow through the membrane from the solution with the lowest concentration to the solution and with the highest concentration following the direction of the osmotic pressure. (*B*) Because the volume of the solution with the highest concentration increases, the hydrostatic pressure rises against the osmotic pressure. When the 2 pressures are equal, equilibrium is reached.

Constitution and general properties of osmotic pumps The key property of the osmotic pumps is that drug delivery is solely dependent on the osmotic force generated
by the osmotic pressure of the osmogen (the solution creating the osmotic pressure
which can be the drug itself).[6,8] Consequently, the drug delivery rate only depends on
the 2 parameters previously mentioned as part of the Van't Hoff equation. The temperature (**Fig. 2**) usually shows little variation between 2 individuals of the same species and
thus can be considered as fixed. The second parameter, which is the concentration
of the solution, can also be maximized and made almost independent of the osmolarity
of the body fluids by supersaturating the device with the osmogen. The consequence of
the control on these parameters is a robust constant drug release rate, which is highly
comparable in vivo and in vitro if the same temperature is applied (**Fig. 3**).[6,8]

Osmotic pumps basically comprise 2 principal elements in their simplest form (single-compartment system **Fig. 4A**):

- A drug core, playing the role of the osmogen
- A semi-permeable membrane coating the drug core

To these 2 fundamental constituents, several more can be added that make the device more sophisticated.[8]

One important characteristic of the semi-permeable membrane in the fabrication of
an osmotic pump is its permeability, which depends on the nature of the polymers
used; indeed, this influences the rate at which the solvent will enter the system. The
semi-permeable membrane is also perforated by 1 or more ports allowing the drug

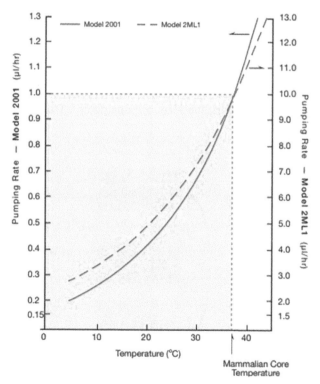

Fig. 2. The pumping rate of 2 Alzet osmotic pumps varying in direct proportion to temperature (tested from 4°C to over 40°C in 0.9% saline). (DURECT Corporation, Cupertino, CA).

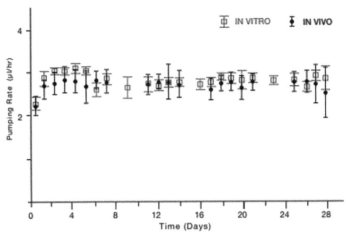

Fig. 3. Pumping rate of an Alzet osmotic pump over time in vitro and in vivo in Sprague-Dawley rats after subcutaneous implantation (n = 105). (DURECT Corporation, Cupertino, CA).

to be released and preventing the formation of an equilibrium between the osmotic and hydrostatic pressure.[6] The size of these ports should be of adequate diameter because too large a port will allow drug diffusion independently of the pump mechanism, and too small a port will generate high hydrostatic pressure blocking the exit of the drug, which can lead to unpredictable drug delivery. In some osmotic devices, the delivery port can be formed in situ after pump implantation using a pore-forming agent that dissolves in contact with aqueous body fluids.[8]

Applications in veterinary exotic pet medicine
Osmotic pumps used in veterinary practice There is at this time only 2 osmotic pump models that have been described as being used in veterinary medicine, and both are 2-compartment osmotic devices: the Alzet osmotic pumps (DURECT Corporation,

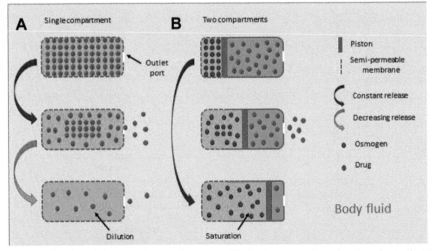

Fig. 4. Mechanism of 2 types of osmotic pumps. (A) single-compartment system (note that in this case the osmogen is the drug itself) and (B) 2-compartment system.

Cupertino, CA, USA)[1,4,7,9–11] and the Ivomec SR Bolus pump (Merck & Co, Inc, Rahway, NJ, USA).[6,12,13] In 2-compartment systems, the drug and the osmogen are separated with an expandable nonpermeable membrane (**Fig. 4**B), and only the osmogen compartment is in contact with the semi-permeable membrane. Body fluids can enter the osmogen compartment, increasing its hydrostatic pressure and displacing the inter-compartment membrane, resulting in drug release through the port.[6] The drug delivery is therefore completely independent from the drug osmotic pressure; therefore, any kind of drug solution or suspension can be used in these systems.

The Alzet osmotic pumps are by far the most commonly used models of osmotic pumps in veterinary medicine and especially in exotic pet practice. These miniature osmotic pumps can be implanted in animals as small as mice, and their cylindrical shape makes them suitable for almost every anatomic site.[1,4,11,14] They are composed of a core reservoir containing the drug surrounded by an impermeable thermoplastic hydrocarbon elastomer. The osmotic agent is placed between the core and a semi-permeable membrane, which forms the outer surface of the pump.[4,6,7] They are commercially provided empty of drug, and have to be filled before use, after which a cannula acting as a flow modulator is inserted in the device (**Fig. 5**), and the drug can be released slowly through this cannula at a constant rate. Three different reservoir storage capacities are currently available (100 µL, 200 µL, and 2 mL) allowing delivery constant continuous rates ranging from 0.11 to 10 µL/h for up to 6 weeks.[6] If drug delivery in a site-specific location is needed, there is the possibility to connect a catheter to the flow modulator.[15–18]

The Ivomec SR Bolus pump is a more specific device because it has been design to sediment into the rumen of cattle and deliver ivermectin as a mean of antiparasitic continuous treatment for up to 135 days.[12,13] It is based on push-melt technology, in which the drug is embedded in a thermoresponsive wax which melts at body temperature and is pushed out by a piston moved by increased hydrostatic pressure in the osmogen compartment.[6]

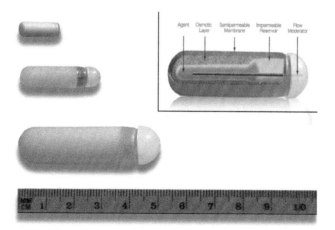

Fig. 5. Examples of available models of Alzet osmotic pumps with a detailed view of their inner composition. (DURECT Corporation, Cupertino, CA).

How to use these osmotic pumps Several models of Alzet osmotic pumps are available and can be chosen according to the size of the animal in which the pump will be implanted, the route of administration, the desired drug dose, delivery rate, and duration as recommended by the manufacturer.[19] A calculator is available on the manufacturer's Web site to correct the default delivery rate of each pump model taking into account the temperature and osmolality of the targeted animal species.[1,4,11,19] For a given calculated delivery rate, the quantity of drug delivered across time can further be adjusted by adapting the concentration of the drug loaded in the device.[1] The value of this concentration is given by the formula: IR × BW/PR (IR, wanted infusion rate; BW, body weight of the treated animal; and PR, the pump delivery rate calculated previously by giving temperature and osmolality parameters). The infusion rate can be determined by multiplying the desired plasmatic concentration of the drug by the clearance of this drug. This implies that the pharmacokinetics parameters for the drug are known in the species of interest.[4]

The loading of the drug compartment is usually done using micrometric scales for optimal quantity precision.[1,7,20] If the device is to work at the time of implantation, pumps need to be primed for at least 6 hours (preferably overnight) in warm sterile saline (0.9% NaCl) before implantation.[10,20] If not primed, there is usually a delay in the drug delivery of a few hours; this can be compensated by, first, a traditional injection of the drug, which can act as a loading dose, a technique commonly using more classical constant rate infusion (Dr John Sykes, personal communication, 2018).

In the case of the Ivomec SR Bolus, the device is ready to use, so no previous manipulations or calculations have to be performed.

How to administer osmotic pumps One of the main drawbacks of the Alzet osmotic pumps (and of osmotic pumps in general) is the necessity for a light surgical procedure under general anesthesia to implant the device. It is also recommended to surgically remove the implant at the end of the treatment period to avoid the persistence of a foreign body with unknown consequences in terms of potential for infection and inflammation. However, new devices made of biodegradable materials are under development for future application.[6]

The subcutaneous route is the most common route of osmotic pump administration and several techniques have been described depending on the targeted animal species. In a clinical setting, it requires general anesthesia of the patient with local analgesia on the site of implantation. Regardless of the site, a 1- to 2-cm skin incision is made and a pocket big enough to hold the pump is created by blunt dissection of the subcutaneous tissue. The pump is usually placed with the exiting port away from the incision, which is then closed using conventional surgical techniques. The subcutaneous sites already described include the dorsal midline between scapula in felids, canines, and rodents,[7,10,21] the lateral part of the body in snakes,[9] the left inguinal region in common peafowls and Japanese quails (Coturnix coturnix japonica),[4,22] and the dorsal cervical area in hens (Gallus domesticus).[23]

Intraperitoneal implantation has also been described in snakes and passerine birds but are not recommended in clinical practice owing to the serious risk of complication (peritonitis, coelomic perforation, and tracheal obstruction).[1,11]

The Ivomec SR Bolus is designed for oral administration using a standard bailing gun.[12,13]

Cost and commercialization of these osmotic pumps One more advantage of osmotic pumps is their relative low cost of between 30 and 60 USD for 1 Alzet osmotic pump depending on the features of the pump (reservoir capacity and delivery rate). To this has to be added the cost of the drug loaded in the device.

Uses of osmotic pumps in exotic pet medicine

In birds One study reported the pharmacokinetic of butorphanol using an Alzet osmotic pump in common peafowls (*Pavo cristatus*) without adverse effects (**Fig. 6**).[4] The plasma concentration suspected to be above therapeutic threshold was reached. These investigators also reported the use of this system in a merlin (*Falco columbarius*) and in a pink pigeon (*Nesoenas mayeri*) with evident sedation. Pharmacokinetic studies in other species, pharmacodynamic studies, and evaluation of potential adverse effects are warranted before use in the clinical setting. It is worth noting that this device could also be used in small birds because intraperitoneal and subcutaneous implantation of Alzet osmotic pumps have already been described in laboratory settings.[11,22]

In reptiles Use of osmotic pumps for antimicrobial therapy in snakes has also been studied in an attempt to avoid daily injections, which are necessary with conventional therapies (particularly useful in venomous snake species that cannot be manipulated on a daily basis).[9] Pharmacokinetics of amikacin delivered intraperitoneally by osmotic pump to corn snakes (*Elaphe guttata guttata*) have been reported to result in predictable and constant plasma concentrations, but a pharmacodynamic study has not been performed, and potential renal side effects were not evaluated in that study.[1] One case of migration of the pump in the trachea secondary to accidental implantation in an air sac was reported in 1 case in a snake. This led the investigators to recommend avoiding intraperitoneal implantation of osmotic pumps in these animals in favor of subcutaneous implantation (**Fig. 7**). There is 1 case report of successful treatment of osteomyelitis caused by *Salmonella* sp in a Taylor's cantil (*Agkistrodon bilineatus taylori*) using a subcutaneous Alzet osmotic pump delivering amikacin. The implant was changed every 4 weeks for 10 months without observed side effects.[9] There is also a study on 20 Mojave rattlesnakes (*Crotalus scutulatus*) with spinal osteomyelitis due to *Salmonella arizonae*, in which osmotic pumps were used to deliver amikacin subcutaneously without success.[24] In the same study, some snakes were treated with

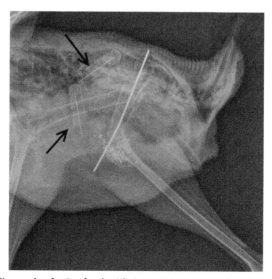

Fig. 6. Lateral radiograph of a Peafowl with 2 osmotic pumps subcutaneously implanted in the inguinal fold (*arrows*) for delivering butorphanol after orthopedic surgery. (*Courtesy of* Meredith Clancy).

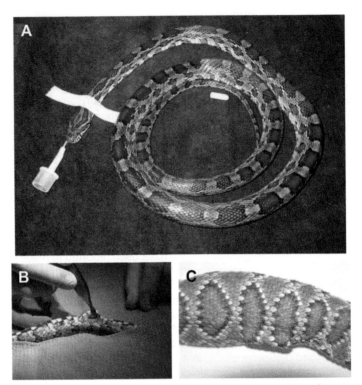

Fig. 7. Steps for the implantation of a subcutaneous osmotic pump in snakes. Anesthetized corn snake (*Pantherophis guttatus*) being prepared for osmotic pump placement (note the relative size of the pump to this animal's body length) (*A*), subcutaneous incision made for placement of an osmotic pump in a corn snake (*B*), and (*C*) Mojave rattlesnake showing the outline of a subcutaneously placed osmotic pump.

florfenicol using osmotic pumps subcutaneously, which resulted in the death of 5 of the 6 treated snakes with severe local necrosis at the site of the pump implantation. Therefore, osmotic pumps to deliver subcutaneous florfenicol in snakes should be avoided. In another study, osmotic pumps were used to deliver voriconazole in 2 Eastern massasauga rattlesnakes (*Sistrurus catenatus*) and 1 timber rattlesnake (*Crotalus horridus*) diagnosed with snake fungal disease (*Ophidiomyces ophiodiicola*).[25] Therapeutic plasmatic concentrations were only achieved in the timber rattlesnake, which was successfully released, whereas the other 2 snakes died secondary to the fungal infection. Finally, the use of intracoelomic osmotic pumps was reported in iguanas (*Iguana iguana*) in a study of reproductive behavior.[26] No complication due to the pump placement was reported in that study.

In small mammals There is currently no report of use of osmotic pumps in a clinical setting in exotic small mammals, although numerous studies exist using these devices in a laboratory research setting.[14,21,27–29] One study reported the pharmacokinetics of fentanyl using an osmotic pump in cats, arguing its potential application in nondomestic felids maintained in zoologic collections.[7] A similar extrapolation could possibly be made for the use of the Ivomec SR Bolus in animals ranging from cattle to wild bovines in zoos for parasitic prevention.[12,13]

It is interesting to note that osmotic pumps have been implanted in mammals as small as Golden Syrian hamsters (*Mesocricetus auratus*) in a laboratory setting.[30]

There are also some anecdotal reports using osmotic pumps for local antibiotherapy in mammals in a zoologic setting. A gelada (*Theropithecus gelada*) with carpal dislocation and infection secondary to a bite wound was successfully treated with an osmotic pump delivering amikacin directly at the infection site.[31] A pudu (*Pudu puda*) and a wallaby (*Macropus rufogriseus*) were also successfully treated for jaw abscess with in situ antibiotic delivery with an osmotic pump; however, a similar treatment failed in a blue monkey (*Cercopithecus mitis*) with osteomyelitis (Dr John Sykes, personal communication, 2018).

In fish Intraperitoneal placement of osmotic pumps has also been reported in fish for research purposes[32,33]; however, there is no clinical application published at this date.

Use of Nanomedicine in Therapeutics

Principles of nanomedicine
What is nanomedicine? In therapeutics, the term "nanomedicine" refers to the use of nanometric particles to enhance the delivery of a drug, thereby increasing its bioavailability, persistence, pharmacokinetics, and reducing its potential toxicity.[34,35] This can be achieved by incorporation of the drug of interest to these nanoparticles via encapsulation within the particles or attachment to the particle's surface.[34]

The mechanism of action of nanoparticles is based on an effect called the "enhanced permeability and retention" (EPR) effect. This involves the capacity of nanoparticles to extravasate at sites of increased vascular permeability (which are usually the targeted sites, such as tumors, and inflamed or infected areas), and to be retained in less-permeable vascular systems.[35] In the specific case of tumors, they are retained within the tumor because of high intratumoral fluid pressure and collapsing lymphatic vessels causing low lymphatic drainage.[36] This EPR effect causes protection of the drug incorporated in/on the nanoparticles, allowing it to reach directly the targeted tissues. With this targeting system, a reduced dose of the drug can be used, thus decreasing its cost and, more importantly, its systemic toxicity, by reducing the dose in nontargeted tissues. It must be noted that nanoparticles also have their own metabolic pathways of elimination and potential toxicity. Because nanoparticles are usually too large for renal glomerular filtration,[36] opsonization by phagocytic cells is the primary route of nanoparticle clearance. Finally reaching its targeted site, the drug can be released by several mechanisms, such as disintegration of the nanoparticle, release from its surface, fusion of the nanoparticle with the targeted cell with intracellular release, or triggered release of the drug by an external factor such as heat, magnetic field, or pH.[34,35]

Mechanism of liposomal medicine in therapeutics Liposomes are the most commonly used therapeutic nanoparticles used in veterinary medicine. They are nanometric spherical vesicles composed of an internal aqueous core surrounded by 1 or more phospholipid bilayers (**Fig. 8A**). The hydrophilic head groups are directed toward the aqueous core and the external environment, and the hydrophobic tail groups are directed toward each other, forming the membrane core. Consequently, they allow transportation of hydrophilic (in their aqueous core) and hydrophobic (in their lipidic membrane) drugs.[34–36] Because they are highly susceptible to gastrointestinal degradation they are mostly administered parenterally or in specific sites.[35]

Composed solely of biodegradable constituents they have poor potential for systemic toxicity; however, hypersensitivity reactions have been observed after administration resulting in life-threatening anaphylactic shock. These reactions are relatively

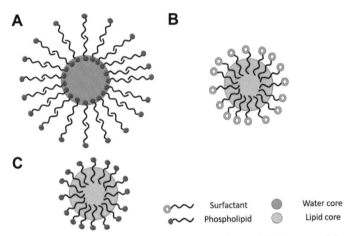

Fig. 8. Lipid-based nanoparticles used in veterinary medicine: (*A*) liposome, (*B*) nanoemulsion particle, and (*C*) micelle.

rare and can be avoided by slow infusion of the liposomal drug and with preventive administration of anti-histaminic and anti-inflammatory treatments.[34,35]

Other types of nanomedicine substances As previously mentioned, liposomes are just one of the numerous types of nanometric particles that have been developed or are under development for drug delivery. Among these types of nanoparticles, the following have been used in veterinary medicine[34,35,37]:

- Nanoemulsions consisting in a dispersion of oil and water in nanodroplets containing the drug stabilized by a surfactant (**Fig. 8**B)
- Micelles loaded with hydrophobic drug in their core stabilized by a hydrophilic shell (composed of phospholipids, polymers, or amino acids) (**Fig. 8**C)
- Polymeric nanoparticles containing the drug either dissolved, entrapped in it, or adsorbed to its surface. Chitosan, a biodegradable and nontoxic carbohydrate polymer is the most represented

Developing uses and applications of nanomedicine in exotic pet medicine
Drug delivery using nanomedicine was mainly developed in 3 major fields of veterinary medicine: chemotherapy, vaccination, and analgesia. More anecdotal use was also described in anti-infectious therapy, ophthalmology, and nutrition. To serve these different purposes, nanoparticle drug delivery systems were developed with multiple possible administration routes, including traditional parenteral, ocular, inhalation, intra-articular, epidural, and topical routes.[35]

   Current studies in exotic species have focused on use of liposome-encapsulated opioid drugs to develop long-acting analgesic formulations.[34,38,39] Several studies investigated the use of liposome-encapsulated butorphanol tartrate (LEBT) in birds and liposome-encapsulated bupivacaine for topical wound administration in rats to increase the short duration of action of the free drug. A pharmacokinetic study evaluating subcutaneous administration of LEBT in Hispaniolan parrots (*Amazona ventralis*) reported butorphanol plasma concentrations above the suspected therapeutic threshold for up to 5 days.[3] Two other experimental studies also showed LEBT anti-nociceptive effect using an arthritis model in Hispaniolan parrots and green-cheeked conures (*Pyrrhura molinae*).[40,41] This formulation is not commercially available at the moment and needs to be prepared by a pharmacist, which complicates its use in a clinical setting. Regarding local analgesia, liposome-encapsulated bupivacaine showed an antinociceptive effect for up to 8 times longer than bupivacaine alone in a wound model in rats. This could represent a promising addition to multimodal analgesic protocols to treat local pain.[42] A commercially available liposome-encapsulated bupivacaine (Exparel) has also been tested for nerve blocks in rabbits with promising results in term of efficacy and safety, and it showed a slow release with a longer duration of action, but a lower plasma concentration, at a given time.[43] No further use in a clinical setting of these 2 analgesic delivery modalities have been reported yet.

Other uses of nanoparticles in veterinary medicine Interest in liposomal-based therapy has also been shown in other fields of medicine. Formulations adapted for use with drugs with poor water solubility have been studied in anti-infectious therapy, with the ability to target specifically the infected tissues, with the goal to decrease potential systemic toxicity.[44,45] In a recent study, an oral nanoparticle formulation of amoxicillin was tested in broiler chickens, resulting in a higher bioavailability and longer half-life than traditional free amoxicillin.[46] Intravenous liposomal voriconazole formulations are currently being developed with good results, and this could be of particular interest, for example, in the treatment of aspergillosis in birds[44]; however, pharmacokinetics, efficacy, and safety studies have yet to be performed before considering the use of such a formulation in a clinical setting. Liposomal-based therapy has also been used in research for topical treatment of glaucoma in a rabbit model, with success using latanoprost and thymoquinone.[47]

In Situ Forming Implants Using Hydrogels

Mechanism and characteristics of hydrogels

General properties of hydrogels Hydrogels are polymeric drug delivery systems characterized by their gel form providing numerous therapeutic advantages, such as increased efficacy of the drug, decreased toxicity, and side effects, as well as improved pharmacokinetics (sustained-release properties for decreased drug administration frequency).[48]

There are several mechanisms that can trigger the gelation of the formulation, but most often it requires the use of a solvent that maintains the formulation in a low viscosity liquid form before administration, hence facilitating the administration and reducing the pain associated with the injection.[48–50] Once injected into the body, the solvent dissolves in body fluids and is dispersed, thereby modifying the physicochemical properties surrounding the formulation. Following these changes, and possible changes in pH, ionic strength, or temperature, the product then becomes a gel.[49] These gels have variable degrees of hydrophobicity and they entrap the drug to which it is mixed, protecting it from the body environment. They then release the drug over long period of time, from several hours to several months.[49,51] Thermoreversible gelation systems are currently the most popular of the studied polymeric systems because they use water as a solvent, avoiding the injection of potentially toxic chemical solvents in the animal's organism.[49,52]

Mechanism of an in situ thermosensitive forming gel: the example of poloxamer Thermogelling is a reversible process, which is characterized by a solution-gel transition temperature ($T_{sol-gel}$). As long as the polymer is maintained below this temperature it presents under the form of a solution showing low viscosity.[51,53] When the environmental temperature increases, the copolymer molecules aggregate into micelles, and, when $T_{sol-gel}$ is reached, micellar packing occurs, forming a highly viscous and partially rigid gel, which dissolves slowly; these particularities make this gel a highly effective system for sustained release of hydrophilic and hydrophobic drugs (**Fig. 9**).[48,51,52,54] $T_{sol-gel}$ as well as the gel strength have been shown to increase as the polymer concentration decreases. Other important characteristics of these compounds in practice are their viscosity at ambient temperature for ease of administration, as well as the gelation time, which needs to be short to avoid the drug being dissolved in the body before the gel is formed.[55] Poloxamer 407, available under several trademarks such as Pluronic F127 or Synperonic F127, is by far the most popular of these thermoreversible gels because of its biocompatibility, its high solubility, and good drug release capacity. $T_{sol-gel}$ is 28°C ± 2°C (SD) for a 20% P407 formulation, so it is in liquid form at ambient temperature, ideal for compounding and administration, and in a gel form at body temperature, generally over 37°C.[2,49,51,55–57] However, at 20% the gel strength is quite poor, so higher concentrations are recommended for use in sustained-release formulations.[58] At a concentration of 30%, $T_{sol-gel}$ is 24°C ± 0.3°C (SD), so it is still liquid at ambient temperature, and the gel strength is improved.[57] It is important to note that the physical characteristics of poloxamer can be altered by the drug or additives (eg, salts and other polymers) it is mixed with; for example, sodium chloride decreases $T_{sol-gel}$ and increases gel strength, whereas diclofenac, ethanol, and hydrochloric acid increase $T_{sol-gel}$ and decrease gel strength.[48,51,59]

Poloxamer also has other interesting properties:
- Surfactant characteristics resulting of its amphiphilic structure: solubilization of poorly water-soluble drugs, making it particularly useful in topical application, as well as giving it a potential microbial inhibition capacity[51,60]
- Sustained-release properties: entrapment of hydrophilic and hydrophobic drugs[2,61]
- Stabilization properties: it can protect proteins and other macromolecules from biological and immune degradation[62]
- Healing potential: it can increase contact time between the drug and its site of action[63]
- Stimulating power on immune response, cell proliferation, fat metabolism, and tissue microcirculation[64]

The release of the drug generally depends on the Fickian diffusion of the drug through the gel on the one hand and on the dissolution of the gel itself in the body

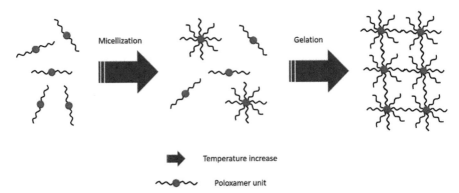

Micellization

Gelation

Temperature increase

Poloxamer unit

Fig. 9. Transition of a thermosensitive polymer from solution to gel as the temperature increases.

environment on the other hand.[49,51] The rapid dissolution of the gel is the main disadvantage of Poloxamer 407, preventing it from lasting longer than a few days.[48] However, adjunct use of other polymers such as Poloxamer 188 can help reduce this dissolution speed in a biological environment and extend the duration of the drug release.[48]

One of the major advantages of poloxamer over other types of hydrogel is its apparent lack of systemic and local toxicity regardless its route of administration.[52,56,65] The major reported side effect of poloxamer so far is dyslipidemia. Increase in plasma cholesterol and triglyceride concentration for at least 4 days have been reported following intraperitoneal and intramuscular injection of poloxamer in rats.[66,67] Another study in rabbits described more precisely these effects, showing that a high dose of intravenous poloxamer injection resulted in decreased plasma high-density lipoprotein levels and increased plasma very low-density lipoprotein levels, with no significant change in low-density lipoprotein plasma levels.[62] It was also reported that poloxamer caused mild decrease in renal glomerular filtration rate in rats without observed clinical significance.[2] Poloxamer toxicity or side effects have not yet been reported in other animal taxons, such as in birds or reptiles.[60] Finally, poloxamer is easy to prepare and inexpensive, which makes it interesting in a clinical setting (around 300 USD/kg).[58]

Applications of hydrogels in exotic pet medicine
Poloxamer and more generally hydrogels have only been anecdotally studied and used in exotic pet medicine.

In birds One study described the pharmacokinetics of a sustained-released butorphanol formulation using poloxamer (12.5 mg/kg of butorphanol in Poloxamer 407 25%) in Hispaniolan Amazon parrots.[2] This study reported butorphanol plasma concentration above suspected therapeutic threshold for more than 3 hours but less than 8 hours without any adverse effects. This could indicate a possibility to significantly decrease the frequency of injections when compared with classic butorphanol solution in this species (every 2 hours). However, pharmacodynamic studies would be required to confirm this hypothesis. In broiler chickens, a long-acting doxycycline formulation containing poloxamer for intramuscular administration (20 mg/kg of doxycycline in Poloxamer 407 15%) was reported to achieve sufficient plasma concentration against *Mycoplasma* spp using a dose interval of 1 week.[68] A sustained-release hydrogel formulation containing sodium salicylate was also tested in broiler chickens via subcutaneous administration (150 mg/kg of sodium salicylate in alginate gel) resulting in plasma concentration above minimum effective concentration for analgesia in human for 24 hours.[69] A voriconazole-poloxamer formulation was studied in brown pelicans, double-crested cormorants, and ring-billed gulls, but no substantial benefit of the poloxamer was identified in this study (preliminary results of the study only).[70] A case report described the successful use of topical formulation of chloramphenicol, doxycycline, and muropicin in poloxamer to treat a persistent methicillin-resistant axillary dermatitis in an African gray parrot (*Psittacus erithacus*).[60]

In rabbits Pharmacokinetics of a sustained-released moxifloxacine poloxamer formulation showed plasma concentrations theoretically effective against most bacterial strains for almost 3 days via subcutaneous injection in rabbits.[71] Sustained release of piroxicam after intramuscular injection of atenolol after sublingual administration was also demonstrated in rabbits.[55,72] Slow release of quinine after intrarectal administration was also shown, but this does not have any clinical application in exotic pet medicine and was studied exclusively for use in the treatment of malaria in humans.[73]

Poloxamer P407 was compared with a labeled eye lubricant (Ocrygel) for use on the eye of rabbits to study prevention of corneal ulcers during anesthesia. Poloxamer was statistically more efficient in preventing corneal lesions, with only 15% lesions identified, compared with the Ocrygel with 32.5% lesions.[74]

In rats A poloxamer-lidocaine formulation injected in the sciatic nerve of rats was used for long-duration local block (240 minutes compared with 150 minutes with lidocaine alone).[56] In another study, the plasmatic half-life of morphine was found to stay 5 times longer above suspected therapeutic threshold when formulated in poloxamer following subcutaneous injection in rats, with no adverse effect.[5] Furthermore, a chlorhexidine-poloxamer gel showed increased healing rate of infected skin wounds in rats.[64] Other drugs were shown to have sustained-release pharmacokinetic profiles when mixed with poloxamer in rats, but with poor clinical applicability (hirudin, urease, fertility-promoting intrauterine infusion liquid vancomycin, insulin, interleukin)[52,54,65,75–78]; however, controlled-release of ibuprofen in poloxamer could not be demonstrated in rats, although poloxamer did enhance the bioavailability of the drug.[79]

In reptiles In situ injection of Poloxamer 407 gel containing ceftazidime and piperacillin was recently used in a case report to successfully treat an epipterygoid bone abscess in a Savannah Monitor (*Varanus exanthematicus*).[80] This case completely resolved with no noted adverse effect in a period of 2 years. The evolution of the lesion was followed by tomodensitometry, giving good information about the healing process.

In fish Sustained-release of estradiol in poloxamer was demonstrated in juvenile goldfish compared with estradiol administered in an oil base.[81]

Table 1		
Advantages and drawbacks of each sustain-released technology described in this review article		
Technology	**Advantages**	**Drawbacks**
Osmotic pumps	• Can be extracted in case of drug overdose or toxicity • Is not altered by its biological environment • Release the drug at a constant rate • Low cost • Commercially available • Release rate and operation time can be chosen	• Necessitate 2 light surgical procedures under anesthesia to be implanted and explanted • Can sometimes migrate in unwanted location (especially if implanted accidently in air sacs during intracoelomic implantation)
Nanoparticles	• Can target very specific location depending on the technology used • Only necessitate an injection	• Not commercially available • Potentially expensive • Very few studied application in exotic pet practice • Potential toxicity, mainly anaphylactic choc
Hydrogels	• Can be administered as a solution • Low cost • Low toxicity and good tissue tolerability • Several studies already available in exotic pet medicine	• Need to be ordered in a compounding pharmacy • Dissolves rapidly in body environment not allowing very long-acting formulations

In zoo/wildlife species An enrofloxacine-poloxamer gel injected subconjunctivally every week showed similar efficacy to more traditional daily oral doxycycline therapy in treating corneal ulcers in Californian sea lions (*Zalophus californianus*), thus reducing the frequency of handling, which is always valuable when dealing with wild animals intended to be released.[82] A case report described the successful use of an intralesional ceftazidime-poloxamer formulation for treatment of a facial abscess in a Golden Lion Tamarin (*Leontopithecus rosalia*).[61]

SUMMARY

Osmotic pumps, nanoparticles, and hydrogels are all interesting sustained-released drug delivery systems, responsible for possible longer therapeutic action of the drug it contains and therefore reduced frequency of administration. This feature is of particular interest in exotic pet practice, especially in species that are difficult to handle or for which repetitive handling is highly stressful and possibly affecting their recovery. Even though these 3 different systems fulfill very similar objectives in drug delivery, their advantages and drawbacks are quite different, as summarized in **Table 1**. It is also interesting to note that formulations incorporating both nanoparticles and hydrogels are currently under study with very promising results to extend further their delayed delivery potential.[51,83] Finally, even though these therapeutic delivery systems show great promise for numerous applications in exotic pet medicine, there is still a need for more research studying efficacy, safety, and potential indications using these technologies.

ACKNOWLEDGMENTS

The authors would like to thank the DURECT Corporation which produce the Alzet osmotic pump system for their kind authorization to use some of their figures in the present paper, as well as Dr John Sykes and Dr Meredith Clancy for sharing their experiences in the use of these devices in exotic animal and for authorizing the use of their personal pictures (see **Figs. 6** and **7**).

REFERENCES

1. Sykes JM, Ramsay EC, Schumacher J, et al. Evaluation of an implanted osmotic pump for delivery of amikacin to corn snake (*Elaphe guttata guttata*). J Zoo Wildl Med 2006;37(3):373–80.

2. Laniesse D, Guzman DS-M, Knych HK, et al. Pharmacokinetics of butorphanol tartrate in a long-acting poloxamer 407 gel formulation administered to Hispaniolan Amazon parrots (*Amazona ventralis*). Am J Vet Res 2017;78(6):688–94.

3. Sladky KK, Krugner-Higby L, Meek-Walker E, et al. Serum concentrations and analgesic effects of liposome-encapsulated and standard butorphanol tartrate in parrots. Am J Vet Res 2006;67(5):775–81.

4. Clancy MM, KuKanich B, Sykes IVJM. Pharmacokinetics of butorphanol delivered with an osmotic pump during a seven-day period in common peafowl (*Pavo cristatus*). Am J Vet Res 2015;76(12):1070–6.

5. Sulimai NH, Ko JC, Jones-Hall YL, et al. Evaluation of 25% poloxamer as a slow release carrier for morphine in a rat model. Front Vet Sci 2018;5. https://doi.org/10.3389/fvets.2018.00019.

6. Herrlich S, Spieth S, Messner S, et al. Osmotic micropumps for drug delivery. Adv Drug Deliv Rev 2012;64(14):1617–27.

7. Sykes JM, Cox S, Ramsay EC. Evaluation of an osmotic pump for fentanyl administration in cats as a model for nondomestic felids. Am J Vet Res 2009;70(8): 950–5.

8. Keraliya RA, Patel C, Patel P, et al. Osmotic drug delivery system as a part of modified release dosage form. ISRN Pharma 2012;2012:1–9.

9. Clancy MM, Newton AL, Sykes JM. Management of osteomyelitis caused by *Salmonella enterica* subsp. *houtenae* in a Taylor's cantil (*Agkistrodon bilineatus taylori*) using amykacin delivered via osmotic pump. J Zoo Wildl Med 2016;47(2): 691–4.

10. Gilberto DB, Motzel SL, Bone AN, et al. Use of three infusion pumps for postoperative administration of buprenorphine or morphine in dogs. J Am Vet Med Assoc 2002;220(11):1655–60.

11. Horton BM, Long JA, Holberton RL. Intraperitoneal delivery of exogenous corticosterone via osmotic pump in a passerine bird. Gen Comp Endocrinol 2007; 152(1):8–13.

12. Miller JA, Davey RB, Oehler DD, et al. The Ivomec SR bolus for control of *Boophilus annulatus* (*Acari: Ixodidae*) on cattle in South Texas. J Econ Entomol 2001; 94(6):1622–7.

13. Miller JA, Davey RB, Oehler DD, et al. Efficacy of the Ivomec SR bolus for control of horn flies (*Diptera: Muscidae*) on cattle in South Texas. Vet Entomol 2003;96(5): 1608–11.

14. Doucette TA, Ryan CL, Tasker RA. Use of osmotic minipumps for sustained drug delivery in rat pups: effects on physical and neurobehavioural development. Physiol Behav 2000;71(1–2):207–12.

15. Strait KR, Orkin JL, Anderson DC, et al. Chronic, constant-rate, gastric drug infusion in nontethered rhesus macaques (*Macaca mulatta*). J Am Assoc Lab Anim Sci 2010;49(2):8.

16. Baron J, Huang Z, Oerter KE, et al. Dexamethasone acts locally to inhibit longitudinal bone growth in rabbits. Am J Physiol Endocrinol Metab 1992;263(3): E489–92.

17. Antoniazzi AQ, Webb BT, Romero JJ, et al. Endocrine delivery of interferon tau protects the corpus luteum from prostaglandin F2 alpha-induced luteolysis in ewes. Biol Reprod 2013;88(6):144.

18. Prieskorn DM, Miller JM. Technical report: chronic and acute intracochlear infusion in rodents. Hear Res 2000;140(1–2):212–5.

19. Pump selection. Alzet osmotic pumps. Available at: http://www.alzet.com/products/guide_to_use/pump_selection.html. Accessed August 23, 2018.

20. Filling & Priming ALZET Pumps. Alzet osmotic pumps. Available at: http://www.alzet.com/products/guide_to_use/filling.html. Accessed August 23, 2018.

21. Smith LJ, Shih A, Miletic G, et al. Continual systemic infusion of lidocaine provides analgesia in an animal model of neuropathic pain. Pain 2002;97(3):267–73.

22. Girling J, Bennett E, Cockrem J. Administration of pregnant mare serum gonadotropin to Japanese quail (*Coturnix coturnix japonica*): dose response over seven days and comparison of delivery by daily injection or osmotic pump. N Z Vet J 2002;50(3):115–21.

23. Petitte JN, Etches RJ. daily infusion of corticosterone and reproductive function in the domestic hen (*Gallus domesticus*). Gen Comp Endocrinol 1991;83:397–405.

24. Sykes J, Folland D, Bemis D, et al. Osmotic pump delivery of florfenicol or amikacin in Mojave rattlesnakes (*Crotalus scutulatus*) with *Salmonella arizonae* osteomyelitis. In: Proceedings AAZV/ARAV. Los Angeles, October 2008.

25. Lindemann DM, Allender MC, Rzadkowska M, et al. Pharmacokinetics, efficacy and safety of voriconazole and itraconazole in healthy cottonmouths (*Agkistrodon piscivorus*) and massasauga rattlesnakes (*Sistrurus catenatus*) with snake fungal disease. J Zoo Wildl Med 2017;48(3):757–66.

26. Phillips JA, Alexander N, Karesh WB, et al. Stimulating male sexual behavior with repetitive pulses of GnRH in female green iguanas, *Iguana iguana*. J Exp Zool 1985;234(3):481–4.

27. Abe C, Tashiro T, Tanaka K, et al. A novel type of implantable and programmable infusion pump for small laboratory animals. J Pharmacol Toxicol Methods 2009; 59(1):7–12.

28. Long JF, Nagode LA, Steinmeyer CL, et al. Comparative effects of calcitriol and parathyroid hormone on serum aluminium in vitamin D-depleted rabbits fed an aluminium-supplemented diet. Res Commun Chem Pathol Pharmacol 1994; 83(1):3–14.

29. Moussy Y, Hersh L, Dungel P. Distribution of [3H]Dexamethasone in rat subcutaneous tissue after delivery from osmotic pumps. Biotechnol Prog 2006;22(3): 819–24.

30. Sonis ST, Costa JW, Evitts SM, et al. Effect of epidermal growth factor on ulcerative mucositis in hamsters that receive cancer chemotherapy. Oral Surg Oral Med Oral Pathol 1992;74(6):749–55.

31. Sykes J, Georoff T, Rodriquez C. Combination of systemic and local treatment of an infected bite wound using an osmotic pump in a Gelada (*Theropithecus gelada*). In: Proceeding 38th Annual Workshop Association of Primate Veterinarians, Atlanta, October 2010.

32. Marte CL, Sherwood NM, Crim LW, et al. Induced spawning of maturing milkfish (*Chanos chanos* Forsskal) with Gonadotropin-Releasing-Hormone (GnRH) analogues admistered in various ways. Aquaculture 1987;60:303–10.

33. Andersen DE, Reid SD, Moon TW, et al. Metabolic effects associated with chronically elevated cortisol in rainbow trout (*Oncorhynchus mykiss*). Can J Fish Aquat Sci 1991;48(9):1811–7.

34. Sadozai H, Saeidi D. Recent developments in liposome-based veterinary therapeutics. ISRN Vet Sci 2013;2013:1–8.

35. Underwood C, van Eps AW. Nanomedicine and veterinary science: the reality and the practicality. Vet J 2012;193(1):12–23.

36. Børresen B, Hansen AE, Kjaer A, et al. Liposome-encapsulated chemotherapy: current evidence for its use in companion animals: BØRRESEN et al. Vet Comp Oncol 2018;16(1):E1–15.

37. Wang C, Wang MQ, Ye SS, et al. Effects of copper-loaded chitosan nanoparticles on growth and immunity in broilers. Poult Sci 2011;90(10):2223–8.

38. Krugner-Higby L, Smith L, Schmidt B, et al. Experimental pharmacodynamics and analgesic efficacy of liposome-encapsulated hydromorphone in dogs. J Am Anim Hosp Assoc 2011;47(3):185–95.

39. Johnson RJ, Kerr CL, Enouri SS, et al. Pharmacokinetics of liposomal encapsulated buprenorphine suspension following subcutaneous administration to cats. J Vet Pharmacol Ther 2017;40(3):256–69.

40. Paul-Murphy JR, Sladky KK, Krugner-Higby LA, et al. Analgesic effects of carprofen and liposome-encapsulated butorphanol tartrate in Hispaniolan parrots (*Amazona ventralis*) with experimentally induced arthritis. Am J Vet Res 2009;70(10): 1201–10.

41. Paul-Murphy JR, Krugner-Higby LA, Tourdot RL, et al. Evaluation of liposome-encapsulated butorphanol tartrate for alleviation of experimentally induced

arthritic pain in green-cheeked conures (*Pyrrhura molinae*). Am J Vet Res 2009; 70(10):1211–9.

42. Grant GJ, Lax J, Susser L, et al. Wound infiltration with liposomal bupivacaine prolongs analgesia in rats. Acta Anaesthesiol Scand 1997;41(2):204–7.

43. Richard BM, Newton P, Ott LR, et al. The safety of EXPAREL ® (Bupivacaine Liposome Injectable Suspension) administered by peripheral nerve block in rabbits and dogs. J Drug Deliv 2012;2012:1–10.

44. Veloso DFMC, Benedetti NIGM, Ávila RI, et al. Intravenous delivery of a liposomal formulation of voriconazole improves drug pharmacokinetics, tissue distribution, and enhances antifungal activity. Drug Deliv 2018;25(1):1585–94.

45. Castro RS, de Amorim IFG, Pereira RA, et al. Hepatic fibropoiesis in dogs naturally infected with Leishmania (Leishmania) infantum treated with liposome-encapsulated meglumine antimoniate and allopurinol. Vet Parasitol 2018; 250:22–9.

46. Güncüm E, Bakırel T, Anlaş C, et al. Novel amoxicillin nanoparticles formulated as sustained release delivery system for poultry use. J Vet Pharmacol Ther 2018; 41(4):588–98.

47. Fahmy HM, Saad EAE-MS, Sabra NM, et al. Treatment merits of latanoprost/thymoquinone – encapsulated liposome for glaucomatus rabbits. Int J Pharm 2018; 548(1):597–608.

48. Bermudez JM, Grau R. Thermosensitive poloxamer-based injectables as controlled drug release platforms for veterinary use: development and in-vitro evaluation. Int Res J Pharm Pharmacol 2011;1(6):109–18.

49. Matschke C. Sustained-release injectables formed in situ and their potential use for veterinary products. J Control Release 2002;85(1–3):1–15.

50. Yu Z-G, Geng Z-X, Liu T-F, et al. *In vitro* and *in vivo* evaluation of an *in situ* forming gel system for sustained delivery of Florfenicol. J Vet Pharmacol Ther 2015;38(3): 271–7.

51. Dumortier G, Grossiord JL, Agnely F, et al. A review of poloxamer 407 pharmaceutical and pharmacological characteristics. Pharm Res 2006;23(12):2709–28.

52. Liu Y, Lu W-L, Wang J-C, et al. Controlled delivery of recombinant hirudin based on thermo-sensitive Pluronic® F127 hydrogel for subcutaneous administration: In vitro and in vivo characterization. J Control Release 2007;117(3):387–95.

53. Katakam M, Ravis WR, Golden DL, et al. Controlled release of human growth hormone following subcutaneous administration in dogs. Int J Pharm 1997; 152(1):53–8.

54. Veyries ML, Couarraze G, Geiger S, et al. Controlled release of vancomycin from Poloxamer 407 gels. Int J Pharm 1999;192(2):183–93.

55. Xuan J-J, Balakrishnan P, Oh DH, et al. Rheological characterization and in vivo evaluation of thermosensitive poloxamer-based hydrogel for intramuscular injection of piroxicam. Int J Pharm 2010;395(1–2):317–23.

56. Paavola A, Yliruusi J, Kajimoto Y, et al. Controlled release of lidocaine from injectable gels and efficacy in rat sciatic nerve block. Pharm Res 1995;12(12): 1997–2002.

57. Baloglu E, Karavana SY, Senyigit ZA, et al. Rheological and mechanical properties of poloxamer mixtures as a mucoadhesive gel base. Pharm Dev Technol 2011;16(6):627–36.

58. Laniesse D, Smith DA, Knych HK, et al. In vitro characterization of a formulation of butorphanol tartrate in a poloxamer 407 base intended for use as a parenterally administered slow-release analgesic agent. Am J Vet Res 2017;78(6):677–87.

59. Barichello J. Absorption of insulin from Pluronic F-127 gels following subcutaneous administration in rats. Int J Pharm 1999;184(2):189–98.

60. Pilny AA. Use of a compounded poloxamer 407 antibiotic topical therapy as part of the successful management of chronic ulcerative dermatitis in a Congo African grey parrot (*Psittacus erithacus*). J Avian Med Surg 2018;32(1):45–9.

61. McBride M, Cullion C. Successful treatment of a chronic facial abscess using a prolonged release antibiotic copolymer in a golden lion tamarin (*Leontopithecus rosalia*). J Zoo Wildl Med 2010;41(2):316–9.

62. Naik H, Kolur A, Maled D, et al. Effect of Poloxamer 407 on serum VLDL, LDL and HDL levels of rabbits. Natl J Physiol Pharm Pharmacol 2014;4(3):221.

63. Kant V, Gopal A, Kumar D, et al. Topical pluronic F-127 gel application enhances cutaneous wound healing in rats. Acta Histochem 2014;116(1):5–13.

64. Babickaite L, Grigonis A, Ramanauskiene K, et al. Therapeutic activity of chlorhexidine-poloxamer antiseptic gel on wound healing in rats: a preclinical study. Pol J Vet Sci 2018. https://doi.org/10.24425/119036.

65. Wang P-L, Johnston TP. Sustained-release interleukin-2 following intramuscular injection in rats. Int J Pharm 1995;113(1):73–81.

66. Blankenship-Paris TL, Dutton JW, Goulding DR, et al. Evaluation of buprenorphine hydrochloride Pluronic® gel formulation in male C57BL/6NCrl mice. Lab Anim 2016;45(10):370–9.

67. Wout ZGM, Pec EA, Maggiore JA, et al. Poloxamer 407-mediated changes in plasma cholesterol and triglycerides following intraperitoneal injection to rats. J Parenter Sci Technol 1992;46(6):192–200.

68. Gutiérrez L, Vargas-Estrada D, Rosario C, et al. Serum and tissue concentrations of doxycycline in broilers after the sub-cutaneous injection of a long-acting formulation. Br Poult Sci 2012;53(3):366–73.

69. Booty SJ, Harding DRK, Whitby CP, et al. Sustained-release injectable hydrogel formulations for administration of sodium salicylate in broiler chickens. J Avian Med Surg 2018;32(4):294.

70. Flammer K, Davidson GS, Massey W, et al. Plasma concentrations of voriconazole delivered in Poloxamer 407 in select aquatic bird species. In: Conference Proceedings. 2018.

71. Carceles CM, Serrano JM, Marin P, et al. Pharmacokinetics of Moxifloxacin in rabbits after intravenous, subcutaneous and a long-acting poloxamer 407 gel formulation administration. J Vet Med A Physiol Pathol Clin Med 2006;53(6):300–4.

72. Monti D, Burgalassi S, Rossato MS, et al. Poloxamer 407 microspheres for orotransmucosal drug delivery. Part II: In vitro/in vivo evaluation. Int J Pharm 2010; 400(1–2):32–6.

73. Fawaz F, Koffi A, Guyot M, et al. Comparative in vitro–in vivo study of two quinine rectal gel formulations. Int J Pharm 2004;280(1–2):151–62.

74. Pignon C, Volait L, Desprez I, et al. Use of thermoreversible gel for the prevention of perioperative corneal ulcers in rabbits. In: Conference Proceedings. ExoticsCon, Atlanta, September 2018.

75. Barichello J. Enhanced rectal absorption of insulin-loaded Pluronic® F-127 gels containing unsaturated fatty acids. Int J Pharm 1999;183(2):125–32.

76. Lu C, Liu M, Fu H, et al. Novel thermosensitive in situ gel based on poloxamer for uterus delivery. Eur J Pharm Sci 2015;77:24–8.

77. Pec EA, Wout ZG, Johnston TP. Biological activity of urease formulated in poloxamer 407 after intraperitoneal injection in the rat. J Pharm Sci 1992;81(7):626–30.

78. Pillai O. Transdermal delivery of insulin from poloxamer gel: ex vivo and in vivo skin permeation studies in rat using iontophoresis and chemical enhancers. J Control Release 2003;89(1):127–40.

79. Newa M, Bhandari KH, Oh DH, et al. Enhanced dissolution of ibuprofen using solid dispersion with poloxamer 407. Arch Pharm Res 2008;31(11):1497–507.

80. Barboza T, Beaufrère H, Chalmers H. Epipterygoid bone salmonella abcess in a Savannah monitor (*Varanus exanthematicus*). J Herpetol Med Surg 2018;28(1–2): 29–33.

81. Cespi M, Bonacucina G, Pucciarelli S, et al. Evaluation of thermosensitive poloxamer 407 gel systems for the sustained release of estradiol in a fish model. Eur J Pharm Biopharm 2014;88(3):954–61.

82. Simeone CA, Colitz CMH, Colegrove KM, et al. Subconjunctival antimicrobial poloxamer gel for treatment of corneal ulceration in stranded California sea lions (*Zalophus californianus*). Vet Ophthalmol 2017;20(5):441–9.

83. Lee J, Kwon HJ, Ji H, et al. Marbofloxacin-encapsulated microparticles provide sustained drug release for treatment of veterinary diseases. Mater Sci Eng C Mater Biol Appl 2016;60:511–7.

Permanent Implantable Medical Devices in Exotic Pet Medicine

Minh Huynh, DVM, DECZM (Avian), DACZM

KEYWORDS

- Stent • Subcutaneous ureteral bypass • Low profile cystotomy tube • Pacemaker

KEY POINTS

- Esophageal stents are mainly palliative.
- Tracheal stents may have several indications, but there is a need to use custom-made devices or alternatively coronary stents.
- Ureteral stents and subcutaneous ureteral bypass are promising techniques to manage ureteral obstruction or malformation in small animal medicine.
- Low-profile gastrotomy tubes can be used as cystotomy tubes in ferrets.
- Pacemakers can be used in ferrets and rabbits, but there are major challenges with the generator placement owing to its size.

INTRODUCTION

Medical devices are defined as implantable if they are intended to remain in the body after the procedure.[1] In the case of anatomic alteration, the technological device may replace or palliate the function of the organ. This trend is observed in human society, whereby 5% to 6% of people in industrialized countries benefit from implantable medical devices.[1] In veterinary medicine, use of such devices is marginal but may find some indications, including in exotic pet medicine. For example, esophageal stricture, tracheal stricture or ureteral obstruction in exotic patients may benefit from such technology. Another example is the pacemaker, which can modify the cardiac electric activity. The use of those devices in exotic pet medicine is even more challenging due to size restriction and the limited data available. The use of bone plating is developed in a different article from this issue (see Sabater M. Advances in exotic animal osteosynthesis).

BIOCOMPATIBILITY

Implant materials can be classified by the type of material and the biologic response they elicit as biotolerant, bioinert, and bioactive materials.[2,3] For example,

Disclosure Statement: None.
Centre Hospitalier Vétérinaire Frégis, 43 Avenue Aristide Briand, Arcueil 94110, France
E-mail address: nacologie@gmail.com

polymers are classified as biotolerant, whereas titanium and titanium alloys are defined as bioinert. However, titanium allows the formation of new bone on its surface and ion exchange with the tissues, leading to formation of a chemical bonding along the interface, bonding osteogenesis.[4] Biocompatibility is evaluated for its potential systemic toxicity, its corrosion and corrosion resistance, its strength, and its surface.[2–4] Because non sterile implant can become potentially lethal, implantable medical devices must allow sterilization before use. The 2 main factors that influence the biocompatibility are the host response induced by the material and the material's degradation in the body environment (**Table 1**).

ESOPHAGEAL STENT
Historical Background

Esophageal stenting is used in humans for the treatment of malignant dysphagia, refractory benign strictures, benign perforations, postoperative anastomotic leaks, and benign fistulae.[5] Recurrent esophageal stricture is one of the most common indications, a situation whereby the stricture cannot be remediated to a diameter of 14 mm over 5 dilatation sessions at 2-week intervals or when a satisfactory luminal diameter cannot be maintained for 4 weeks once the target diameter of 14 mm has been achieved.[6]

Technological Description

Initial plastic tubes were progressively replaced by self-expandable metal stents in human medicine.[5] Four types of stents are available: fully covered metal stents, removable partially covered metal stents, removable covered plastic stents, and biodegradable stents.[5,7] Metallic stents are considered more cost-effective and safer.[5] Recurrence may occur after removal of stents after weeks to months.[5]

Table 1 Classification of biomaterials		
Classification	**Material**	**Response**
Biotolerant materials	Gold Cobalt chromium alloys Stainless steel Zirconium Niobium Tantalum Polyethylene Polyamide Polymethylmethacrylate Polytetrafluoroethylene Polyurethane	Formation of thin connective tissue capsule, but the capsule does not adhere to the implant surface
Bioinert materials	Titanium, titanium alloy, aluminum oxide, zirconium oxide	Allow close approximation of bone on their surface, leading to contact osteogenesis. These materials allow formation of stable oxide layer on its surface
Bioactive materials	Bioglass, synthetic calcium phosphate	Formation of bony tissue around the implant material and strongly integrates with the implant surface
Bioreabsorbable materials	Polyglycolic polymers	Replace by autologous tissue

Data from Refs.[2–4]

Most metallic stents are made of nitinol with or without polyurethane or silicone coating. Other materials include a polyester-silicone combination and stainless steel.[7] Biodegradable stents are made of polydioxanone absorbable surgical suture.[7] Nitinol is a metal alloy of nickel and titanium. The main advantage of nitinol is the superelasticity of the material. It is highly biocompatible. When shape memory alloys are in their martensitic form, they easily form a new shape. However, when the alloy is heated, it reverts to austenite and recovers its previous shape with great force (a process known as shape memory).[8]

The stent is usually placed with an endoscope with or without fluoroscopic guidance. The placement should extend 2 to 4 cm beyond each end of the stricture.[7]

Biodegradable stents may present the advantage of decreasing the need for reinterventions for stent removal. However, unusual complications, such as collapse of the stent in the esophagus, preventing further endoscopic examination, have been reported in humans.[7]

Use in Small Animal Medicine

In dogs, biodegradable stents, self-expanding metallic stents, and a self-expanding plastic stent have been used for the treatment of refractory benign esophageal strictures.[9] A high complication rate has been described, and long-term success is limited. Seven out of 9 dogs experienced major complications necessitating intervention, and half of the cohort was euthanized.[9] It has also been used in 2 cats affected with esophageal stricture.[10,11] One cat survived for a year before it deteriorated and was euthanized.[11] The other cat was able to eat, and the biodegradable stent was absorbed.[10]

Use in Exotic Pet Medicine

In exotic pet medicine, esophageal stricture or neoplasia has been rarely described apart from in ferrets. Ferrets may be prone to esophagitis or foreign body ingestion.[12] One case of esophageal stenting has been described.[12] The ferret had a history of gastric foreign body removal. Esophageal stricture was shown with positive contrast radiography. Balloon dilation was performed initially, but the ferret stricture reoccurred. A nitinol-covered self-expanding metallic stent was placed in the esophagus under fluoroscopic guidance. However, recurrence at the stenting site was seen 6 weeks after implantation and was treated again with balloon dilation and topical triamcinolone. One final balloon dilation occurred 4.5 months later. The ferret survived 5 years after treatment, eating soft food for the first 2 years before progressing to eating solid food. It is unclear if the stent helped to resolve the condition because only 1 dilatation session occurred before stent placement, and several sessions occurred after placement.

Technical Limitation

Luminal diameter is certainly the limiting factor for endoscopic placement. The smallest outer diameter available is 16 mm, with a 5.8-mm introducer diameter.[7] The manufacturer who designed the only ferret case published provides a custom-made diameter biodegradable esophageal stent, which can be up to 4 mm in diameter (Infiniti Medical, Menlo Park, CA, USA).[12]

Perspective

Esophageal disease is rare in exotic pet medicine apart from in ferrets. Esophageal hypertrophy has been described in a rabbit.[13] Benign esophageal tumors have been described in birds and reptiles.[14,15]

AIRWAY STENT
Historical Background

Airway stenting is indicated in patients with extrinsic or intrinsic tracheobronchial stenosis, persistent obstruction despite endobronchial dilation, and loss of tracheal integrity owing to malignant invasion.[16] It can be used as a palliative long-term treatment.[16] It is considered safe and effective. However, complications are reported, such as fibrosis of the tracheal wall, in-stent restenosis, tracheal obstruction, and stent migration.[8]

Technological Description

There are 3 types of stents: silicone stents, polydioxanone biodegradable stents, and self-expandable metallic stents.[17] Metallic stent comes as fully covered, partially covered, or uncovered stents.[17] They are usually made of cobalt alloy filament (Wallstent; Boston Scientific, Marlborough, MA, USA) or nitinol (Ultraflex; Boston Scientific)[18] (**Fig. 1**). Silicone stents can be customized and cut as needed.[17] They are also easily removable.[17] Silicon-based endoprostheses have a higher risk of migration because of their lower radial force.[8] Metallic stents promote reepithelialization and mucous transport, but they also predispose to granuloma formation.[17] The main advantage of the metallic stents is their ability for distorsion, which makes them more adapted to tortuous airway.[17]

Use in Small Animal Medicine

Tracheal stents are used most commonly in dogs with a diagnosis of tracheomalacia.[19] Use of nitinol stents has been reported in dogs, cats, and horses.[19–21] Survival time in dogs may vary from 1 to 48 months.[19] Median survival time according to recent studies was 502 days.[22] Material failure with stent fracture is commonly reported in dogs, occurring in nearly half of the cases.[19,22] Nitinol stent tend to shorten over time compared to post-deployment measurements.[23] Because most dogs succumbed to the tracheal disease, it is more of a palliative treatment than a curative treatment.[19]

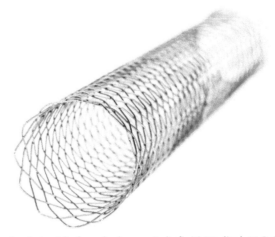

Fig. 1. Nitinol tracheal stent before deployment. (Infiniti Medical, LLC. Redwood City CA, USA.)

Stents come in predetermined sizes from 8-mm diameter to 24-mm diameter (Wallstent and Ultraflex; Boston Scientific; Vet Stent-Trachea; Infiniti Medical). The smallest size is 5-mm diameter × 20 mm (Wallstent; Boston Scientific). Alternatively, it is possible to use a stent designed for coronary use. Coronary stents allow a smaller diameter, with 2.25 mm to 4 mm (Resolute Integrity; Medtronic, Minneapolis, MN, USA). Coronary stents are made of a cobalt alloy coated with a polymer loaded with zotarolimus.

Use in Exotic Pet Medicine

Tracheal stenosis is a relatively common complication of tracheal intubation in avian and small mammal anesthesia.[24] Foreign body inhalation was also suspected as a cause of tracheitis and stenosis in a secretarybird.[25] Spontaneous tracheal collapse has been described in a duck.[26]

An experimental model of rabbit tracheal stenosis was described where the lesion was induced by prolonged endotracheal intubation or by brushing the tracheal mucosa with a nylon brush.[27,28] Tracheal stenosis following intubation was also described in 3 rabbits undergoing ovariohysterectomy.[29,30] Tracheal damage seems relatively common in rabbits following intubation, suggesting some species predisposition.[31]

Tracheal stenting has been experienced in a pet rabbit.[32] The luminal diameter of the trachea was 0.9 mm on the site of the stenosis, whereas the rabbit had a tracheal diameter of 3.6 mm in its cervical portion. The stent used was a metallic coronary stent made of metal with a primer coat and a coating that consisted of a blend of zotarolimus and polymer (Resolute Infinity; Medtronic, Boulogne-Billancourt, France). A bronchoscope could not be technically inserted in the trachea to deploy the stent. The investigator used an esophageal tube to insert the device and controlled deployment with a radiograph (**Fig. 2**). The rabbit died 2 weeks later, but cause of death remain unclear and not related to the stent placement.[32] The rabbit served as an experimental model for tracheal stenosis and tracheal stent insertion.[33–37] New Zealand rabbits, with a relatively wide tracheal lumen diameter (5.5 mm), are usually used. The stent (Wallstent; Boston Scientific; and Zilver Flex; Cook Medical, Bloomington, IN, USA) allows an inner diameter of 6.5 mm and an expanded outer diameter of 8 mm (which is the width of outer diameter of the trachea). The Wallstent seems to promote an important response of the tracheal tissue compared with the Zilver Flex stent.[8] Biodegradable polydioxanone stents were used in the rabbit model of tracheal stenosis.[35] The rabbits were inserted with a 5 × 15-mm stent, which allowed survival for at least a month.[35]

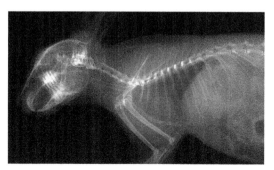

Fig. 2. Rabbit with a coronary stent used as a tracheal stent. (*Courtesy of* Christophe Bulliot with permission from *Le Point vétérinaire*.)

Usually tracheal stenosis in birds is treated medically or surgically with tracheal resection and anastomosis.[24] There is 1 case report using a tracheal stent in an Eclectus parrot with extensive tracheal stenosis, which was considered nonresectable owing to the length of the affected area.[38] Tracheal stenting was performed with a custom-made nitinol wire stent (Vet Stent-Trachea; Infiniti Medical) because the size of the device was the main limitation. The size of the stent was 4 mm × 36 mm. It was designed to be 10% oversized, self-expanding, and equivalent to the maximum diameter of healthy-appearing areas of trachea cranial and caudal to the strictured area. The bird survived for 3 years with the stent with medical management consisting mainly of nebulization of acetylcysteine, dexamethasone, amikacin, and terbinafine. The bird still had some episodes of intermittent dyspnea and stridor during those 3 years.

Anecdotally, a specific airway stenting technique has been used for a permanent rhinostomy in a prairie dog with pseudo-odontoma respiratory obstruction.[39] An earlobe retractor was positioned through the nasal bone preventing reepithelialization and maintaining airway patency.

Technical Limitation

Because of the very tortuous nature of the trachea in rabbits and avian species, metallic or biodegradable stents are more adapted. Size limitation is the main factor. The only case of tracheal stenting in a pet parrot used a custom-made nitinol wire stent. Use of the coronary stent may be advantageous in terms of luminal diameter as long as the length of the stenosis is limited (the maximal length is 40 mm). The coronary implants are small sized, available, and include a coating that inhibits reepithelialization.

Perspective

Endotracheal intubation is recommended for airway management in avian and rabbit species.[40] It is likely that in rabbits especially, when blind techniques are used, tracheal damage may be encountered more often in practice as intubation becomes part of a routine anesthetic procedure. In avian medicine, airway stenting may be an interesting option in the management of tracheal stricture, especially in long-necked birds when surgery is not amenable.

URETERAL STENT
Historical Background

In humans, use of a ureteral stenting device, nephrostomy tube, and subcutaneous nephrovesical bypass is mainly palliative. Indications include pelvic tumor compression, ureteral malignant invasion, and retroperitoneal fibrosis.[41] It is relatively efficient for intrinsic pathologic conditions but relieves only half of the obstructions owing to extrinsic compression.[41]

Ureteral stents by retrograde insertion are the first line of treatment in humans but are also associated with a high rate of failure occurring in nearly half of the patients.[41] It is typically placed by cystoscopy. Recommendations about replacement time vary but may be up to every 3 months.[42]

Technological Description

Ureteral stents can be made of polymeric compounds or metal and can be biodegradable.[43] Morbidity can be very high in humans (80% of cases).[41] Ureteral stents used in veterinary medicine are usually made of polyurethane tubes[44,45] (**Fig. 3**). Ureteral stent diameters exist in 2 (0.67 mm) to 6-F size (2 mm) catheters (Vet Stent-Ureter; Infiniti

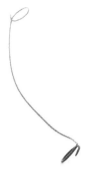

Fig. 3. Double pigtail ureteral stent system. (Infiniti Medical, LLC. Redwood City CA, USA.)

Medical). Some stents are made of a heat adaptive polymer called thermostar. The stent is stiff at room temperature and softens at body temperature. A 6-F-diameter metallic stent made of nickel-cobalt-chromium-molybdenum alloy has been developed in human medicine to prevent reincrustation in contrast to the polymer-based stent (Resonance; Cook Medical).[42]

Use in Small Animal Medicine

Most common indications are reported for benign obstructions with calculi in cats and dogs.[43] It is considered as a gold standard for ureteral obstructions in dogs according to ACVIM guidelines.[46] Ureteral surgery is usually associated with high major complication rates (36%–31%) and high perioperative mortalities (16%–18%) in feline patients.[47] Ureteral stent and ureteral bypass have been developed to overcome complications associated with conventional surgery.[43] In 2011, a first series of 6 cats had stent placement.[48] In 2013, a study comparing ureteral stent and subcutaneous ureteral bypass was published.[49]

Percutaneous placement of ureteral stents can be attempted in dogs but is not generally recommended in cats.[43] The regular procedure includes a celiotomy with antegrade or retrograde placement. A 22-G over-the-needle catheter is inserted in the greater curvature of the kidney. The needle is removed, and the catheter is left in the renal pelvis. Placement is checked under fluoroscopy. A guidewire is inserted in the catheter and passed down the ureter into the bladder. A cystotomy is performed, and the wire is grasped. The ureteral dilator is passed normograde over the guidewire. The dilator is then removed, and the ureteral stent is passed over the guidewire. The cranial pigtail is positioned within the renal pelvis, and the guidewire is removed from the bladder to allow the stent to form a pigtail in the bladder.

Most cats have marked improvement in azotemia after the procedure.[50] Short-term complications occurred in less than 10% of the cases, and long-term complications occurred in 33% of cats.[51] In dogs, retrograde ureteral stenting is usually preferred by cystoscopic and fluoroscopic guidance.[43] Complications included stent encrustation, stent migration, and tissue proliferation at the ureterovesical junction.[52]

Ureteral stents are associated with more urinary tract infections in cats undergoing ureteral surgery.[45] However, ureteral stents are more likely to resolve azotemia in cats.[53]

Complications described include dysuria, hematuria, and stranguria.[45,51] Dysuria was noted in 37% of cats.[51] Stent migration, fracture, encrustation, and obstruction of lower urinary tract signs refractory to medical management are described.[45,51,54]

Use in Exotic Pet Medicine

Ureteral stenting has been described in 3 pet rabbits **(Fig. 4)**.[55,56] Retrograde and anterograde placement have been described. Anorexia and urinary incontinence

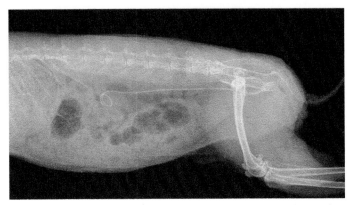

Fig. 4. Ureteral stent placement in a rabbit. (*Courtesy of* Isabelle Langlois and Université de Montréal.)

were observed postoperatively. Two cases had encrustation complications, and 2 cases experienced soft tissue proliferation. One of the cases had a stent replacement with a newer-generation stent 18 months after the first placement because of encrustation. It died 10 months after placement of the second stent. One other case died 3 months after placement of the stent. One of the rabbits developed new calculi and contralateral nephromegaly. The author suggests a role of *Encephalitozoon cuniculi* infection as a comorbid factor.[55]

Technical Limitation

Ureteral stents come in standard size and may not be useable in all sized rabbits. Encrustation seems very common and expected owing to the very specific calciuresis physiology in rabbits. Medical and dietary management must be optimized to avoid stent failure.

Perspective

Drug-eluting stents and novel surface coating strategies may prove beneficial in the future.[57] Use of noncalculogenic metallic stents may be more developed.[42] An experimental coating made of rhenium-doped fullerene-like molybdenum disulfide nanoparticles was found to be encrustation-repellant on silicone catheters, adding some interesting perspective to the device.[58]

SUBCUTANEOUS URETERAL BYPASS
Historical Background

The nephrovesical subcutaneous stent has been developed in humans as an alternative to a permanent nephrostomy tube.[59] It was used mainly in advanced oncologic cases with metastatic prostate or invasive bladder cancer when ureteral stenting failed. It has been shown to provide a better quality of life than with the nephrostomy tube.[60]

Technological Description

The Subcutaneous Ureteral Bypass (SUB; Norfolk Vet Products, Skokie, IL, USA) is a permanent silicon nephrostomy tube and a cystotomy tube, which are placed permanently and connected via a low-profile shunting port. Both tubes are ended with a 6.5-F locking loop catheter and a silicon cuff to prevent dislodgement. The shunting port can be flushed using a flush kit (SUB Flush Kit; Norfolk Vet Products, Skokie, IL, USA).

Use in Small Animal Medicine

In cats, regardless of stent or SUB placement, all cases had successful decompression of the renal pelvis.[49]

The placement of the SUB system is performed after a ventral midline celiotomy. An 18-gauge over-the-needle catheter is inserted into the caudal pole of the kidney equidistant ventrally and dorsally and directed to the renal pelvis. Similar to ureteral stent placement, nephropyelography is performed. A 0.035-in guidewire is then placed into the 18-gauge catheter and coiled in the renal pelvis. The 18-gauge catheter is removed over the guidewire. A 6.5-F pigtail locking-loop nephrostomy tube is placed over the 1190 Palm and Culp guidewire into the renal pelvis and secured to the renal capsule with tissue glue. A 6.5-F cystostomy tube is then inserted into the bladder and secured to the bladder with sutures. The tube ends of both the nephrostomy and the cystostomy tubes are tunneled through the body wall and attached to a titanium shunting port that is secured to the body wall.

SUB does not require ureterotomy and does not affect the ureterovesical junction. One other advantage is that it may be flushed after implantation. One study suggests that the SUB device in cats is associated with lower complication rates and longer survival times than the ureteral stent.[61] Ureteral stents are more indicated in dog patients because it can be performed endoscopically with a high success rate.

Use in Exotic Pet Medicine

One case of SUB was described in a 5-year-old rabbit presented for azotemia and ureteral obstruction caused by urolithiasis.[62] The procedure was unremarkable, and tolerance of the device was good (**Fig. 5**). Renal decompression was achieved. The shunting port was flushed 15 days later. Three months after surgery, the rabbit deteriorated with a ureteral obstruction of the contralateral kidney. The shunting port was also obstructed. The rabbit was euthanized. The investigator of this clinical case report indicates that the device should probably be flushed more frequently compared with small carnivores.[62]

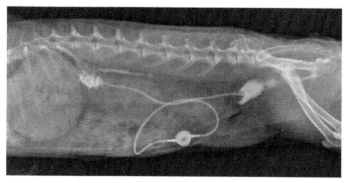

Fig. 5. Postoperative radiograph of a SUB system placement in a rabbit. (*Courtesy of Clementine Haas.*)

Another case of subcutaneous ureteral bypass was used in a ferret with ureterovesical junction stenosis.[63] A 6.5-F pigtail locking loop nephrostomy tube was placed into the renal pelvis under ultrasonographic guidance, and a 7-F cystostomy tube was inserted at the apex of the urinary bladder. The nephrostomy catheter kinked during the first week, and some urinary leakage from the bladder was diagnosed, issues that were resolved surgically.[63] Renal decompression was achieved.[63] Urinary tract infection was diagnosed 3 weeks after implantation, which did not resolve after antibiotic treatment.[63] The SUB device was removed 3 months after the surgery because of reobstruction.[63]

Technical Limitation

The smallest device consists of a 6.5-F catheter (2.2 mm diameter and 20 cm long). It is designed to be used in feline patients. The main limiting factor is the size of the renal pelvis. There are some specific recommendations using the SUB device when the renal pelvis is smaller than 5 to 8 mm. It is reported to be easier and safer to insert the nephrostomy catheter down the ureter rather than coiling in the renal pelvis. The locking string at the loop is cut and removed to use it as a ureterostomy catheter.

Perspective

SUB devices are easy to place and may be advantageous because the device can be easily flushed as needed, lowering the risk of encrustation. In situ injection of antibiotics in the case of urinary tract infection can be also convenient.

LOW-PROFILE CYSTOTOMY TUBE
Use in Small Animal Medicine

Cystotomy tubes are traditionally long and difficult to manage in veterinary medicine. In 2003, 2 articles reported the use of a low-profile gastrotomy tube as a cystotomy tube in 4 dogs and 1 cat[64,65] (**Fig. 6**). The main advantage of the device is that the opening of the tube is very close to the skin, which decreases the likelihood of removal.

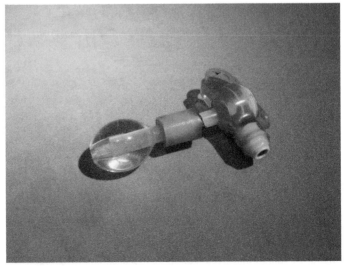

Fig. 6. Low profile gastrotomy tube used as cystotomy tube. (*Courtesy of* Minh Huynh.)

Use in Exotic Pet Medicine

There are 2 reports of the use of a low-profile cystotomy tube in ferrets.[66,67] Both ferrets had severe distension of the bladder and likely had bladder atony. Cystotomy tubes were placed and achieved long-term urinary diversion (**Fig. 7**). One ferret had a tube for at least 4 months. The other ferret had the tube for 1 year and died subsequently of infectious myocarditis related to septicemia and chronic urinary tract infection. Other complications include inadvertent removal of the tube 1 week after placement and recurrent urinary tract infection.[67] Urine cultures are recommended monthly.

Technical Limitation

In one of the cases, the cystotomy tube needed readjustment because of the length of the tube, which provoked minor leakage around the ostium site.

Perspective

Permanent cystotomy tubes may be interesting as palliative treatment for permanent disability of the lower urinary tract.

PACEMAKER
Historical Background

The first pacemakers were developed in 1958 in human medicine.[68] The pacemaker was designed to assume the functions of the natural cardiac pacemaker. The device has evolved progressively, allowing implantation through a peripheral vein rather than a thoracotomy procedure.

Technological Description

Currently, the electric elements and a battery are packaged by a laser welding of titanium, which has a strong mechanical hardness, extreme resistance to corrosion, biocompatibility, and durability.

A pulse generator and pacing lead are required for cardiac pacing. The pulse generator analyzes the cardiac rhythm and provides an appropriately timed pacing stimulus to return it to a more satisfactory heart rate.

Generators are denominated by pacemaker nomenclature: The first letter denotes the site where the heart is paced; the second letter identifies the sensing function; and the third letter identifies the response after sensing. The "I" designation means

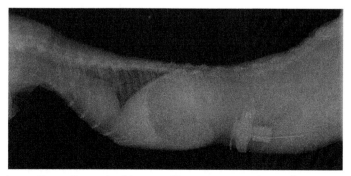

Fig. 7. Postoperative radiograph of Low-profile gastrotomy tube used as a cystotomy tube in a ferret. (*Courtesy of* Minh Huynh.)

that the pacing function is inhibited in response to spontaneous ventricular depolarization. The fourth letter of the pacemaker nomenclature refers to the programmability of the pacemaker, with an "R" designation indicating that there is a rate-responsive feature that adjusts the rate accordingly (**Table 2**).[69]

Use in Small Animal Medicine

In dogs, the first pacemaker was implanted in 1968.[70] Main indications include symptomatic bradyarrhythmia, especially third-degree atrioventricular block and sick sinus syndrome.[71–73] Other causes include second-degree atrioventricular block and atrial standstill.[71–73] Most pacemakers in veterinary medicine are VVIR or VVI.[68]

There are multiple leads, bipolar or unipolar, with passive or active fixation. Unipolar leads are rarely used nowadays.[68]

Temporary pacing is necessary during anesthesia before implantation of the permanent pacemaker. Transvenous pacing is performed via the saphenous or femoral vein. For transthoracic pacing, the electrodes are placed on the clipped right and left hemithorax over the precordial impulse.

TRANSVENOUS PACING

The procedure consists of placing a lead via the right jugular vein, cranial vena cava, and right atrium, through the tricuspid (right atrioventricular) valve into the right ventricle. The lead is advanced into the right ventricle under fluoroscopic guidance. Once in place, the lead is connected to the pulse generator, and the heart will be paced as necessary. The pulse generator is placed into a subcutaneous pocket created by blunt dissection.

Generally, heart rates are kept as low as possible.[68] Sensitivity of the lead is very important. It is important to note that in any paced animal, the jugular vein is no longer available for intravenous access.

EPICARDIAL PACING

In cats, epicardial pacing is the method of choice because of the small size and risk of vena cava syndrome.[71] A coeliotomy is performed to access and incise the diaphragm. A pericardiotomy is performed to access the left ventricular free wall. A lead eyelet is sutured. The pericardiectomy is left open, and a loop of free lead is

Table 2
International Generic Pacemaker Code by Bernstein and others (1987)

I	II	III	IV	V
Chamber paced	Chamber sensed	Response to sensing	Programmable functions	Antitachycardia functions
0 = none	0 = none	0 = none	0 = none	0 = none
A: Atrium	A: Atrium	T: Triggers pacing	P: Rate or output	P: Pacing
V: Ventricle	V: Ventricle	I: Inhibits pacing	M: Multiprogrammable	S: Shock
D: Dual	D: Dual	D: Dual	C: Communicating (telemetric control)	D: Dual
			R: Rate adaptive	

From Bernstein A., Camm J., Fletcher D., et all. The NASPE*/BPEG** Generic Pacemaker Code for Antibradyarrhythmia and Adaptive-Rate Pacing and Antitachyarrhythmia Devices. Official Journal of the World Society of Arrhythmias 1987; with permission.

left in the thoracic cavity. The lead is attached to the generator, which was placed in a muscular pocket in the left body wall created by incising and undermining the transversus muscle.

When transvenous pacing cannot be performed, various surgical approaches have been described for placement of permanent epicardial pacemaker, including thoracotomy, abdominal incision, and epicardial lead implantation via a transdiaphragmatic approach.

Use in Exotic Pet Medicine

Two cases were reported in a ferret and a rabbit (**Fig. 8**).[74,75] In the ferret of this report, the pacemaker implanted was VVIR and was adjusted so that the heart rate could increase to a rate of 180 beats per minute in response to muscle stimulation.[74] Epicardial unipolar pacing was elected for the ferret case because of the size of the animal and the limited vascular access. The pacing electrode (IS-1 Unipolar Epicardial Pacing Lead; Medtronics, Minneapolis, MN, USA) of the permanent pacemaker (Model 5380 Identity; St. Jude Medical, St. Paul, MN, USA) was sutured on 1 side to the outer surface of the myocardium on the left ventricular apex. The pulse generator of the permanent pacemaker was placed freely into the ventral abdominal cavity. Ventricular premature depolarization and ventricular tachycardia were noted and needed adjustment of the refractory period. Cardiac arrhythmia could still be detected on auscultation 3 months after implantation. Pleural effusion and progressive congestive heart failure developed eventually. The ferret died 4 months and 3 weeks after implantation. Fibrosis at the site of the pacing lead attachment may have contributed to the loss of ventricular capture, rising threshold, and need for higher voltage.

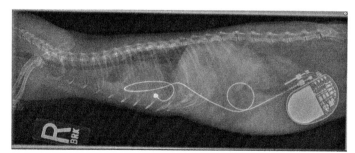

Fig. 8. Post-operative radiograph of an epicardial pacemaker in a ferret. (*Courtesy of* Jessica Comolli and University of Georgia.)

A 7-year-old female rabbit was presented for 2:1 high-grade second-degree atrioventricular block and paroxysmal third-degree atrioventricular block.[75] A transvenous pacing was elected through the right jugular vein. A single bipolar, steroid-eluting, passive-fixation lead wire (52-cm Capsure LET 332995V; Medtronics) was guided into the apical region of the right ventricle. The lead wire was secured locally, and then the lead wire was placed through a tunnel created in the subcutaneous tissue, leading to a second incision at the dorsal midscapular region, where the generator (VVI; Zephyr SR Model 5620, St. Jude Medical) was placed within the subcutaneous tissue. The base rate was set to 160 bpm. Although the generator was sutured to the scapular periosteum, it eventually slid ventrally in the cervical region. The rabbit experienced the complication of abscess around the pacemaker lead, where it exited the jugular vein about 7 months after implantation. The abscess kept recurring over the life of the rabbit despite appropriate antibiotic choice and regular debridement.

Exophthalmia associated with caval syndrome was also noticed 1 year and 3 months later. The lead eventually perforated through the abscess, and the rabbit chewed the device without altering it, 3 years and 5 months after implantation. At this point, the battery of the device was also depleted, and the pacemaker was not replaced. The rabbit died 3 years and 7 months after implantation.

Technical Limitation

The size of the patient makes transvenous placement difficult, making the epicardial approach probably more suitable. Attachment of the generator is complex because it is preferable to avoid placing it in the abdominal cavity in herbivorous species.

Perspective

Dual-chamber pacing has been shown with improved dynamics and quality of life compared with right ventricular pacing.[76]

ACKNOWLEDGMENTS

The author would like to thank Sari Kanfer and Isabelle Langlois for contributing to this issue with their clinical cases. The author would like to thank Mikel Sabater, Kevin Le Boedec and Cecile Damoiseaux for their advice and review of this article.

REFERENCES

1. Joung Y-H. Development of implantable medical devices: from an engineering perspective. Int Neurourol J 2013;17(3):98–106.
2. Saini M, Singh Y, Arora P, et al. Implant biomaterials: a comprehensive review. World J Clin Cases 2015;3(1):52–7.
3. Koppolu P, Macha D, Lingam L, et al. Osseointegration in implants: a review 2016.
4. Manivasagam G, Singh AK, Rajamanickam A, et al. Ti based biomaterials, the ultimate choice for orthopaedic implants–a review. Vol 542009.
5. van Halsema EE, van Hooft JE. Clinical outcomes of self-expandable stent placement for benign esophageal diseases: a pooled analysis of the literature. World J Gastrointest Endosc 2015;7(2):135–53.
6. Kochman ML, McClave SA, Boyce HW. The refractory and the recurrent esophageal stricture: a definition. Gastrointest Endosc 2005;62(3):474–5.
7. Hindy P, Hong J, Lam-Tsai Y, et al. A comprehensive review of esophageal stents. Gastroenterol Hepatol 2012;8(8):526–34.
8. Chaure J, Serrano C, Fernandez-Parra R, et al. On studying the interaction between different stent models and rabbit tracheal tissue: numerical, endoscopic and histological comparison. Ann Biomed Eng 2016;44(2):368–81.
9. Lam N, Weisse C, Berent A, et al. Esophageal stenting for treatment of refractory benign esophageal strictures in dogs. J Vet Intern Med 2013;27(5):1064–70.
10. Battersby I, Doyle R. Use of a biodegradable self-expanding stent in the management of a benign oesophageal stricture in a cat. J Small Anim Pract 2010;51(1):49–52.
11. Glanemann B, Hildebrandt N, Schneider MA, et al. Recurrent single oesophageal stricture treated with a self-expanding stent in a cat. J Feline Med Surg 2008;10(5):505–9.
12. Webb J, Graham J, Fordham M, et al. Diagnosis and treatment of esophageal foreign body or stricture in three ferrets (Mustela putorius furo). J Am Vet Med Assoc 2017;251(4):451–7.

13. Parkinson L, Kuzma C, Wuenschmann A, et al. Esophageal smooth muscle hypertrophy causing regurgitation in a rabbit. J Vet Med Sci 2017;79(11):1848–52.

14. Schmidt RE, Reavill DR, Phalen DN. Gastrointestinal system and pancreas. In: Schmidt RE, Reavill DR, Phalen DN, editors. Pathology of pet and aviary bird. (IA): John Wiley & Sons; 2015. p. 55–94.

15. Gál J, Jakab C, Szabó Z, et al. Haemangioma in the oesophagus of a red-eared slider (Trachemys scripta elegans). Acta Vet Hung 2009;57(4):477–84.

16. Tjahjono R, Chin RY, Flynn P. Tracheobronchial stents in palliative care: a case series and literature review. BMJ Support Palliat Care 2018;8(3):335–9.

17. Flannery A, Daneshvar C, Dutau H, et al. The art of rigid bronchoscopy and airway stenting. Clin Chest Med 2018;39(1):149–67.

18. Sun F, Uson J, Ezquerra J, et al. Endotracheal stenting therapy in dogs with tracheal collapse. Vet J 2008;175(2):186–93.

19. Sura PA, Krahwinkel DJ. Self-expanding nitinol stents for the treatment of tracheal collapse in dogs: 12 cases (2001–2004). J Am Vet Med Assoc 2008;232(2): 228–36.

20. Culp WT, Weisse C, Cole SG, et al. Intraluminal tracheal stenting for treatment of tracheal narrowing in three cats. Vet Surg 2007;36(2):107–13.

21. Couetil LL, Gallatin LL, Blevins W, et al. Treatment of tracheal collapse with an intraluminal stent in a miniature horse. J Am Vet Med Assoc 2004;225(11):1727–32, 1701-1722.

22. Rosenheck S, Davis G, Sammarco CD, et al. Effect of variations in stent placement on outcome of endoluminal stenting for canine tracheal collapse. J Am Anim Hosp Assoc 2017;53(3):150–8.

23. Durant AM, Sura P, Rohrbach B, et al. Use of nitinol stents for end-stage tracheal collapse in dogs. Vet Surg 2012;41(7):807–17.

24. Sykes JMT, Neiffer D, Terrell S, et al. Review of 23 cases of postintubation tracheal obstructions in birds. J Zoo Wildl Med 2013;44(3):700–13.

25. Ludwig C, Lueders I, Schmidt V, et al. Tracheal resection in a secretary bird (Sagittarius serpentarius) with granulomatous, foreign-body induced tracheitis. J Avian Med Surg 2017;31(4):308–13.

26. Henry-Guyot E, Langlois I, Lanthier I, et al. Tracheal collapse in a Pekin duck (Anas platyrhynchos domestica). J Avian Med Surg 2016;30(4):364–7.

27. Lee HS, Kim SW, Oak C, et al. Rabbit model of tracheal stenosis induced by prolonged endotracheal intubation using a segmented tube. Int J Pediatr Otorhinolaryngol 2015;79(12):2384–8.

28. Steehler MK, Hesham HN, Wycherly BJ, et al. Induction of tracheal stenosis in a rabbit model—endoscopic versus open technique. Laryngoscope 2011;121(3): 509–14.

29. Grint NJ, Sayers IR, Cecchi R, et al. Postanaesthetic tracheal strictures in three rabbits. Lab Anim 2006;40(3):301–8.

30. Mancinelli E, Eatwell K. Tracheal stricture after laparoscopic ovariectomy in two rabbits. Paper presented at: International Conference on Avian, Herpetological and Exotic Mammal Medicine. Wiesbaden, 2013.

31. Phaneuf LR, Barker S, Groleau MA, et al. Tracheal injury after endotracheal intubation and anesthesia in rabbits. J Am Assoc Lab Anim Sci 2006;45(6):67–72.

32. Bulliot C, Romain S, Rattez E, et al. A case of tracheal stenosis and its surgical treatment with a coronary stent in a rabbit (Oryctolagus cuniculus). Paper presented at: Internation Conference on Avian, Reptile and Exotic Mammal. Venice, It, 2017.

33. Chao YK, Liu KS, Wang YC, et al. Biodegradable cisplatin-eluting tracheal stent for malignant airway obstruction: in vivo and in vitro studies. Chest 2013;144(1): 193–9.

34. Faria CM, Rodrigues OR, Minamoto H, et al. A new model of self-expanding tracheal stent made in brazil : an experimental study in rabbits. J Bras Pneumol 2012;38(2):214–7.

35. Kawahara I, Ono S, Maeda K. Biodegradable polydioxanone stent as a new treatment strategy for tracheal stenosis in a rabbit model. J Pediatr Surg 2016;51(12): 1967–71.

36. Novotny L, Crha M, Rauser P, et al. Novel biodegradable polydioxanone stents in a rabbit airway model. J Thorac Cardiovasc Surg 2012;143(2):437–44.

37. Serrano C, Lostale F, Rodriguez-Panadero F, et al. Tracheal self-expandable metallic stents: a comparative study of three different stents in a rabbit model. Arch Bronconeumol 2016;52(3):123–30.

38. Mejia-Fava J, Holmes SP, Radlinsky M, et al. Use of a Nitinol wire stent for management of severe tracheal stenosis in an Eclectus Parrot (Eclectus roratus). J Avian Med Surg 2015;29(3):238–49.

39. Bulliot C, Mentré V. Original rhinostomy technique for the treatment of pseudoodontoma in a prairie dog (Cynomys ludovicianus). J Exot Pet Med 2013;22(1): 76–81.

40. Varga M. Airway management in the rabbit. J Exot Pet Med 2017;26(1):29–35.

41. Chung SY, Stein RJ, Landsittel D, et al. 15-year experience with the management of extrinsic ureteral obstruction with indwelling ureteral stents. J Urol 2004;172(2): 592–5.

42. Rao MV, Polcari AJ, Turk TM. Updates on the use of ureteral stents: focus on the Resonance(®) stent. Med Devices (Auckl) 2010;4:11–5.

43. Palm CA, Culp WT. Nephroureteral obstructions: the use of stents and ureteral bypass systems for renal decompression. Vet Clin North Am Small Anim Pract 2016;46(6):1183–92.

44. Pavia PR, Berent AC, Weisse CW, et al. Outcome of ureteral stent placement for treatment of benign ureteral obstruction in dogs: 44 cases (2010-2013). J Am Vet Med Assoc 2018;252(6):721–31.

45. Wormser C, Clarke DL, Aronson LR. Outcomes of ureteral surgery and ureteral stenting in cats: 117 cases (2006-2014). J Am Vet Med Assoc 2016;248(5): 518–25.

46. Lulich JP, Berent AC, Adams LG, et al. ACVIM small animal consensus recommendations on the treatment and prevention of uroliths in dogs and cats. J Vet Intern Med 2016;30(5):1564–74.

47. Kyles AE, Hardie EM, Wooden BG, et al. Management and outcome of cats with ureteral calculi: 153 cases (1984-2002). J Am Vet Med Assoc 2005;226(6): 937–44.

48. Zaid MS, Berent AC, Weisse C, et al. Feline ureteral strictures: 10 Cases (2007-2009). J Vet Intern Med 2011;25(2):222–9.

49. Horowitz C, Berent A, Weisse C, et al. Predictors of outcome for cats with ureteral obstructions after interventional management using ureteral stents or a subcutaneous ureteral bypass device. J Feline Med Surg 2013;15(12):1052–62.

50. Manassero M, Decambron A, Viateau V, et al. Indwelling double pigtail ureteral stent combined or not with surgery for feline ureterolithiasis: complications and outcome in 15 cases. J Feline Med Surg 2014;16(8):623–30.

51. Berent AC, Weisse CW, Todd K, et al. Technical and clinical outcomes of ureteral stenting in cats with benign ureteral obstruction: 69 cases (2006-2010). J Am Vet Med Assoc 2014;244(5):559–76.

52. Kuntz JA, Berent AC, Weisse CW, et al. Double pigtail ureteral stenting and renal pelvic lavage for renal-sparing treatment of obstructive pyonephrosis in dogs: 13 cases (2008-2012). J Am Vet Med Assoc 2015;246(2):216–25.

53. Culp WT, Palm CA, Hsueh C, et al. Outcome in cats with benign ureteral obstructions treated by means of ureteral stenting versus ureterotomy. J Am Vet Med Assoc 2016;249(11):1292–300.

54. Kulendra NJ, Syme H, Benigni L, et al. Feline double pigtail ureteric stents for management of ureteric obstruction: short- and long-term follow-up of 26 cats. J Feline Med Surg 2014;16(12):985–91.

55. Rembeaux H, Langlois I, Burdick S, et al. Ureteral stenting for management of ureterolithiasis in three domestic rabbits (Oryctolagus cuniculus). Paper presented at: Exoticscon. Atlanta, 2018.

56. Langlois I. Ureteral stenting for management of ureterolithiasis in a domestic rabbit (Oryctolagus cuniculus). Paper presented at: AEMV. Orlando, 2014.

57. Yang L, Whiteside S, Cadieux PA, et al. Ureteral stent technology: drug-eluting stents and stent coatings. Asian J Urol 2015;2(4):194–201.

58. Ron R, Zbaida D, Kafka IZ, et al. Attenuation of encrustation by self-assembled inorganic fullerene-like nanoparticles. Nanoscale 2014;6(10):5251–9.

59. Nissenkorn I, Gdor Y. Nephrovesical subcutaneous stent: an alternative to permanent nephrostomy. J Urol 2000;163(2):528–30.

60. Wang Y, Wang G, Hou P, et al. Subcutaneous nephrovesical bypass: treatment for ureteral obstruction in advanced metastatic disease. Oncol Lett 2015;9(1): 387–90.

61. Deroy C, Rossetti D, Ragetly G, et al. Comparison between double-pigtail ureteral stents and ureteral bypass devices for treatment of ureterolithiasis in cats. J Am Vet Med Assoc 2017;251(4):429–37.

62. Haas C, Lapiere M, Kinon L, et al. Subcutaneous ureteral bypass (SUBTM) for the treatment of ureteral obstruction in a rabbit. Paper presented at: Yaboumba congress. Paris, 2018.

63. Vilalta L, Dominguez E, Altuzarra R, et al. Imaging diagnosis-radiography and ultrasonography of bilateral congenital ureterovesical junction stenosis causing hydronephrosis and hydroureter in a Ferret (Mustela Putorius Furo). Vet Radiol Ultrasound 2017;58(3):E31–6.

64. Stiffler KS, McCrackin Stevenson MA, Cornell KK, et al. Clinical use of low-profile cystostomy tubes in four dogs and a cat. J Am Vet Med Assoc 2003;223(3): 325–9, 309-310.

65. Salinardi BJ, Marks SL, Davidson JR, et al. The use of a low-profile cystostomy tube to relieve urethral obstruction in a dog. J Am Anim Hosp Assoc 2003; 39(4):403–5.

66. Smith M, Mankin KT, Hoppes S. Clinical use of a low profile cystotomy tube in a ferret. Paper presented at: Association of Exotic Mammal Veterinarians Conference. Indianapolis, 2013.

67. Huynh M, Desenclos MC, Devaux L, et al. Long-term use of a low profile Cystotomy tube in a Ferret. Paper presented at: Exoticscon. Portland, 2016.

68. James R. Use of pacemakers in dogs. Practice 2007;29(9):503–11.

69. Bernstein AD, Camm AJ, Fletcher RD, et al. The NASPE/BPEG generic pacemaker code for antibradyarrhythmia and adaptive-rate pacing and antitachyarrhythmia devices. Pacing Clin Electrophysiol 1987;10(4 Pt 1):794–9.

70. Buchanan JW. First pacemaker in a dog: a historical note. J Vet Intern Med 2003; 17(5):713–4.
71. Visser LC, Keene BW, Mathews KG, et al. Outcomes and complications associated with epicardial pacemakers in 28 dogs and 5 cats. Vet Surg 2013;42(5): 544–50.
72. Swanson LE, Huibregtse BA, Scansen BA. A retrospective review of 146 active and passive fixation bradycardia lead implantations in 74 dogs undergoing pacemaker implantation in a research setting of short term duration. BMC Vet Res 2018;14(1):112.
73. Johnson MS, Martin MW, Henley W. Results of pacemaker implantation in 104 dogs. J Small Anim Pract 2007;48(1):4–11.
74. Sanchez-Migallon Guzman D, Mayer J, Melidone R, et al. Pacemaker implantation in a ferret (Mustela putorius furo) with third-degree atrioventricular block. Vet Clin North Am Exot Anim Pract 2006;9(3):677–87.
75. Kanfer S. Transvenous pacemaker implantation for complete heart block in a Rabbit (Oryctolagus cuniculi). Paper presented at: Association of Exotic Mammal Veterinarian Conference. Indianapolis, 2013.
76. Genovese DW, Estrada AH, Maisenbacher HW, et al. Procedure times, complication rates, and survival times associated with single-chamber versus dual-chamber pacemaker implantation in dogs with clinical signs of bradyarrhythmia: 54 cases (2004-2009). J Am Vet Med Assoc 2013;242(2):230–6.

Advances in Retrieval and Dissemination of Medical Information

Nicola Di Girolamo, DVM, MS, PhD, DECZM(Herpetology)[a,b,]*

KEYWORDS

- Knowledge dissemination • Knowledge retrieval • PubMed • Google scholar
- Instagram • Facebook • YouTube

KEY POINTS

- In recent years there has been a dramatic change in how information can be disseminated in health care, including exotic pet medicine.
- The exotic animal veterinarian needs know how to retrieve scientific information from the web, including strength and weaknesses of PubMed, Ovid Medline, and Google Scholar.
- Effective use of social media was listed as one of the 10 priorities to improve visibility and dissemination of research findings.
- Platforms such as YouTube, Instagram, Facebook, Snapchat, and their specific use needs to be understood to make them a tool for dissemination of scientific knowledge.
- Oversimplification is a risk of social media use in health care, and should be a concern for the veterinary community.

INTRODUCTION

In recent years, there has been a dramatic change in how information can be disseminated in the scientific world. This factor is especially true for health care in general, and exotic pet practice hardly make an exception. From the constant growth of online repositories that archives scholarly articles such as PubMed, to the creation of hashtags specifics for health care that can be followed by millions of persons, we need to understand that communication is changing and we can either embrace the change or succumb ignoring it.

The author has no commercial or financial conflicts of interest to declare. This study was not supported by a grant.
[a] Center for Veterinary Health Sciences, Oklahoma State University, 2065 W Farm Road, Stillwater, OK 74078, USA; [b] Tai Wai Small Animal and Exotic Hospital, 69-75 Chik Shun Street, Tai Wai, Sha Tin, New Territories, Hong Kong
* Center for Veterinary Health Sciences, Oklahoma State University, 2065 W Farm Road, Stillwater, OK 74078.
E-mail address: nicoladiggi@gmail.com

RETRIEVAL OF PEER-REVIEWED INFORMATION
Databases

Medline and PubMed
MEDLINE is the first journal citation database available to the public. It was launched by the National Library of Medicine in 1971 as an online extension of the Medical Literature Analysis and Retrieval System, a computerized biomedical bibliographic retrieval system existent from 1964. Medline currently includes more than 5000 scientific biomedical and life sciences journals, providing more than 25 million references to articles dating back to 1946.

PubMed, available from 1996, is a world-renowned interface used to search Medline, as well as additional biomedical content including the following types of citations[1]:

- In-process citations and "ahead of print" citations
- Citations of articles from journals that are not included in MEDLINE, certain general science and general chemistry journals
- Citations that precede the date that a journal was selected for MEDLINE indexing (when provided electronically by the publisher) and pre-1966 citations that have not yet been updated with current Medical Subject Headings and converted to MEDLINE status.
- Citations to author articles of articles published by National Institutes of Health-funded researchers.

Regardless of these additional sources, MEDLINE remains the largest subset of PubMed articles, representing 88.9% of all citations in PubMed.[2] Other than PubMed, there are other ways to access MEDLINE, the more popular being Ovid Medline. In general, Ovid Medline is considered to be less user friendly, but to permit a more focused search. When formally compared, PubMed was found to have greater sensitivity than Ovid-MEDLINE with comparable precision.[3] In addition to the comprehensive journal selection process, what sets MEDLINE apart from the rest of PubMed is the added value of using a specific vocabulary based on keywords, called Medical Subject Headings, to index citations.

PubMed search strategy Although the PubMed interface was developed to be easy to use, using basic search strings often retrieve nonspecific results. It has been proved that health care professionals often search PubMed in an ineffective manner, either by using limited search terms, narrowing the search inappropriately, or confusing Boolean operators.[4] For a more efficient search process, the Advanced Search Builder interface can be used. This interface allows a targeted search in specific fields, with the convenience of being able to select the intended search field from a list. It also provides a history of your previous searches, which is useful to develop a complex search query by combining several previous searches using Boolean operators. The Boolean operators currently available are AND, OR, and NOT and can be used to refine searches by combining search terms or previous searches. It is key to understand that, when using multiple Boolean operators in PubMed, they are processed left to right. To change the order in which terms are processed, a set of parentheses can be used to process the terms into parentheses as a unit (**Fig. 1**).[5] The use of the Boolean operator NOT is generally discouraged to have a more comprehensive result (less specific, more sensitive). A useful technique for a quick, scoping search focusing on veterinary journals, is the application a specialty filter for veterinary science. This filter is available on the Filters sidebar, or can be added in the search builder as "veterinary [sb]"; for example, "hyperparathyroidism AND veterinary [sb]". However,

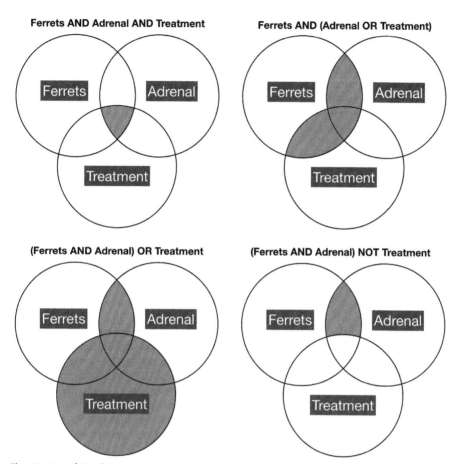

Fig. 1. Use of Boolean operators and parenthesis on platforms such as PubMed may be initially confusing for the user. Notice the 4 completely different results retrieved from searches including the same keywords. The use of AND includes articles that have both keywords. The use of OR includes articles that have either one or the other keyword. The use of NOR excludes the articles with one keyword (usually NOT is discouraged). The parentheses are key to make a search effective, for example, enclosing synonyms in parenthesis with OR between them.

investigators should be aware that the sensitivity and specificity of subject filters on Pubmed is less than ideal[6] and that relevant information could be missed if a preliminary search is not implemented with scrutiny of all the sources found and their references.

CAB Abstracts

CAB Abstracts is an international, bibliographic database that covers veterinary medicine and other life sciences topics, including agriculture, environment, applied economics, food science, and nutrition. CAB Abstract is incorporated in CAB direct together with the other bibliographic database bibliographic database, Global health, a bibliographic database that focuses on research literature in public health and medical health. CAB Abstract up to 2018 contains more than 9 millions publications from more than 120 countries and in 50 languages, even if the majority of the abstracts are in English.[7] Records are selected by subject specialists from more than 8000 serials, books and conference proceedings. This selection process results in some discrepancies that may limit its use for systematic searches. In fact, a study analyzing the use of CAB Abstract to explore the veterinary literature found eleven entries in the CAB Abstracts database that were coded as journal articles, but should have been classified as the correspondence type of publication for the journal *Veterinary Record*, but lack of inclusion of articles in the "Veterinary Medicine Today" section of *Journal of the American Veterinary Medical Association*.[8] Similarly to Pubmed, CAB Abstracts has option of simple and advanced searching. The latter permits to restrict the search of keywords to specific data fields, basically search boxes, that will be connected by similar Boolean operators to PubMed. The data fields include similar fields to other databases such as title or authors, but also original fields specific to CAB (CABI indexing fields), including organism descriptor and geographic location, fields that could be convenient to limit searches to a species or a geographic area. Currently no specific search strategy to retrieve veterinary studies have been demonstrated effective. When search strategies previously developed in human medicine[9] to retrieve clinically relevant research were modified and run on the CAB Abstracts database the results were disappointing, with sensitivity ranging from 12% to 86% and specificity for most searches lower than 40%.[8]

Google Scholar

Google Scholar is a freely accessible web search engine that indexes scholarly literature across a multitude of publishing formats and disciplines. Released in beta in November 2004, Google Scholar includes journal and conference papers, theses and dissertations, academic books, preprints, abstracts, technical reports and other scholarly literature from all broad areas of research. Based on a 2014 study, it is estimated that Google Scholar covers nearly 87%, approximately 100 million documents, of the 114 millions of English scholarly documents available on the web.[10] Google Scholar from its definition has "search robots [that] generally try to index every paper from every website they visit"[11]; unlike the other databases discussed, Google Scholar does not scrutinize journals before inclusion. This aspect is negative from one side because this policy results in the inclusion of predatory journals or other journals that may have limited scientific validity; however, this policy is beneficial because it usually offers a more comprehensive search.[12] the inadequacies of Google Scholar have been early summarized in 3 major weaknesses: a lack of sufficient advanced search features, a lack of transparency of the database content, and uneven coverage of the database.[13] Some of these inadequacies have been corrected or limited in the past year, but some remain. A further weakness is that Google Scholar only shows the first 1000 hits of any search and searches cannot be compared because of the lack of a search history. Finally, repeatability of searches over time in Google Scholar has been found inadequate.[14] Whereas in traditional bibliographic databases, search strategies are designed to retrieve all articles that meet certain criteria based on field codes, in Google Scholar references are selected matching text words, based on algorithms that may change over time, often unexpectedly.[14]

Other search engines and databases

Other free search engines include Microsoft Academic and CiteSeerX. Other subscription-based tools include Elsevier's Scopus and Clarivate Analytics' Web of Science. The main strength of Scopus is the international coverage (22% of journals included are non-English); Web of Science covers a narrower range of materials.[15]

Social Media

The use of social media has increased tremendously over the past decade, with usage rates spanning from 5% American adults in 2005 up to 69% in 2018.[16] In 2011, the results of a survey including 4033 physicians found that 65% of them use social media for professional purposes,[17] and in 2016 72% of the oncology physicians (149/207) replying to a survey reported use of social media.[18] When 10 strategies to improve the visibility and dissemination of research findings were listed by a public health journal, the effective use of social media was listed fourth, together with dissemination through personal blogs and making articles open access.[19]

There are many potential applications of social media for dissemination of health care information. Many major health organizations are currently using hashtag campaigns to spread awareness on specific health topics (eg, #YESMAMM, a 2011 campaign to raise awareness about breast cancer and early detection). These methods are becoming increasingly popular especially on social media sites such as Instagram and Twitter. Of the posts related to health awareness campaigns on Instagram, Facebook, and Twitter, 90% to 99% of the posts were considered by health care professionals to be sharing correct information, with the social media site with the greatest credibility being Twitter.[20]

Other that for purely educational purposes, social media can be used to reach the lay public for scientific reasons. Both Facebook and Instagram have been used to recruit participants for randomized, controlled trials on an intervention for prevention of burn injuries.[21] The cost per enrolled participant was AUS $13.08. Saturdays were the most effective day of the week for advertising results. The most popular time of day for enrolments was between 5 and 11 PM. Participants were representative of the population with regard to age and education levels.[21]

In addition, social media can be analyzed to monitor experiences of patients (or clients, in veterinary medicine) while receiving health care, to improve their experience.[22] When patients are asked about the usefulness of social media in the health care setting, the majority of respondents felt that social media provides benefit to patient experience (80%).[23] In the same survey, patients were asked whether they would feel comfortable with the clinic posting a picture of their infant, and a little more than none-half of respondents (56.3%) responded positively. The vast majority of patients (96.2%) felt comfortable communicating electronically with their clinic. These data are important to the veterinary practitioner, because there are well-known similarities between the view that parents and pet owners may have in regard to their loved ones. The veterinarian should never assume that a pet owner is comfortable with the dissemination of their pet's images, and any type of dissemination should be always supported by written informed consent.

YouTube

YouTube is an American video-sharing site created in February 2005 that is ranked as the second-most popular site in the world, and has hundreds of hours of content uploaded each minute.[24] As of the end of 2018, every YouTube subscriber can share videos up to 15 minutes each in duration, and users with good compliances can share videos up to 12 hours in duration. The maximum size for videos is 128 GB and can have a resolution of up to 7680 × 4320 pixels (8K). In addition to standard videos, YouTube allows to upload and view 180° and 360° virtual reality videos. Once a video is uploaded, the software automatically generates captions using speech recognition technology (but captions can also be added by manually entering them, for greater accuracy).

Having an online video repository is an unevaluable resource for health care professionals. In fact, when medical students, residents, and faculty of 1 institution were asked what was the most frequently used educational video source for surgical preparation, 86% indicated YouTube.[25] When the educational quality of YouTube videos on specific surgical techniques was analyzed, the majority of the videos uploaded were of good or moderate quality (72% [51/71]). There was an association between educational quality and duration of the videos (longer videos had better educational quality), with a cutoff for determination of good quality of 7:42 minutes. Interestingly, the number of likes or dislikes was not predictive of video educational quality, indicating a possible inability of the lay public to discriminate between videos with better educational content.[26] It is encouraging to think that the educational quality of YouTube videos on specific surgical techniques was good overall, but is unpredictable what the quality of YouTube in veterinary medicine could be.

Twitter

Twitter, Inc., is an American online news and social networking service on which users post and interact with tweets—messages limited to 280 characters. Tweets can be commented on, liked, and shared (retweeted) post, liked, and retweet tweets; however, unregistered users can only read them. The widespread use of hashtags (#) on Twitter is revolutionary in the way that permits a live adjournment on everything written on the topic of interest. The possibility to mention other individuals, including brands, in tweets, results in the opportunity for interactions that are otherwise limited in other social media. Twitter has been heavily used and studied in human health care. Because it is often the lay public that is going to initially be exposed to tweets, topics of popular interest may be more effective. When Twitter was used to disseminate evidence to health care providers caring for children, the most effective topics were related to vaccination and pain management, both topics of broad interest.[27] Twitter has been used for several health campaigns, and, for example, has been found more effective than conventional smoking cessation programs for decreasing smoking relapses.[28] Its use in exotic animal medicine has limitless applications, including spreading appropriate husbandry information, use for online journal clubs, or simply connecting veterinarians during major conferences.

Instagram

Instagram is a social networking service launched in 2010 that currently has more than 1 billion monthly active users. It allows users to upload photos and videos that can be organized with tags and location information. The posts can be shared publicly or with preapproved followers. The simplicity of browsing other users' content by tags (hashtags) makes this social network extremely appealing for the dissemination of information in specialized fields.

There is a strong, significant correlation between the association between the number of followers to the hospital's Instagram and the US News 2017 to 2018 Best Hospital Rankings for adult hospitals.[29] Correlation does not imply causation, and it is impossible to establish whether the hospital's reputation may be influenced by its social media presence or that the reputation or rank of a hospital drives social media followers, but this phenomenon highlights the relevance of this social network in health care.

Other applications than simple knowledge dissemination could lead to huge advances in the medical care of exotic species. In human medicine, automated estimation techniques were used to identify individuals at risk for substance use and addiction from their Instagram profiles.[30] The potential to apply analogous mechanisms to exotic animal practice are invaluable. It could be possible to identify animals that are fed an inappropriate diet and correct their husbandry on a large scale.

Facebook

Facebook, Inc, is an online social media and social networking service company launched in 2004, that reached 2.2 billion monthly active users in 2018. Facebook has been successfully used to disseminate medical information, including to disseminate targeted information to ethnic minorities.[31] It is particularly effective in reaching the older female population and is a cost-effective alternative to print-based advertisements.[31] Facebook allows to post photos, videos, written text, or links and other users can like, comment on, or share the content produced. This last feature is characteristic of Facebook and has led to certain content being shared millions of times, resulting in so-called viral posts. Users may join common interest user groups and may follow pages (profiles) made by organization and business companies, among others. Common reasons that human patients described for joining specific Facebook groups or pages included seeking support, education, making friends, and providing support to others.[32]

Groups are an extremely popular way to gather users together and in specific health care fields (eg, congenital abnormalities). Facebook groups had more than the double the membership as Facebook pages.[32] Groups may be openly accessible or private, and there is significant risk that information present on that specific group is provided by a minority of users who may or may not have sufficient expertise or training. In fact, 84% of patients (932/1103) in Facebook groups would like health care professionals to actively participate in their group.[32] Also, 97% of the respondents would like to join a group linked to their primary hospital.[32]

Facebook pages can be a way for institutions, companies, and professionals to disseminate health information to a larger audience. Currently, it seems that the most effective way to disseminate health information on Facebook pages is by using pages focused on specific patient-centered problems rather than pages for an academic journal or for professional societies. In fact, in dermatology, the engagement rate was much higher for the former type of Facebook page, resulting in a yearly engagement rate of 1.5 versus rates of 0.3 and 0.7 for academic journals and professional societies, respectively.[33]

Snapchat

Snapchat is a mobile phone app used worldwide. As of January 2018, it was estimated that 78% of US persons between 18 and 24 years old used Snapchat. The app evolved from being centered on person-to-person content sharing to posting temporary short videos or pictures that are visible by users' followers. Also, a discover section allows companies to show ad-supported short-form content. One of the principal features of Snapchat is that these videos are only available for 24 hours after their publication, making its use in health care substantially different than the other social media platforms. There is little research done on how medical information could be disseminated on Snapchat, or on the benefits that Snapchat may have on health care. Snapchat was selected as the most probable platform (as opposed to Facebook) for items depicting negative behaviors (related with drinking misuse in the survey),[34] and it is currently unclear if this phenomenon could apply to negative behaviors associated with exotic pet ownership.

Professional and Scholar-Oriented Social Networking Web Sites

There are a number of social networking web sites that are being developed for academics or researchers. Academia.edu and ResearchGate are the more used sites. Both of these platforms can be used to share papers, monitor their impact, and follow research (and researchers) in specific fields. ResearchGate, according to a study the academic social network with more active users,[35] has an additional focus on asking and answering questions and find collaborators. Users can upload research output including papers, data, chapters, negative results, patents, research proposals, pre-prints, methods, presentations, and software source code. The uploading of pay-walled articles still needs to follow certain rules. When copyright infringement has been systematically assessed, investigators found that more than one-half of the uploaded papers were posted illegally, because the publisher's version was uploaded.[36] In contrast, LinkedIn is a more general business and employment-oriented web site, that allows members (both workers and employers) to create pro-files and connections to each other. In a survey of Australian physicians, LinkedIn was the most widely used social media platform (51.6%).[37] A specific use of each of these social networking web sites could favor knowledge dissemination.

Limitations of Social Media for Knowledge Dissemination

Although from a theoretical point of view, social media should increase the exposure of scientific publications, in the real world it may be more complicated than that. In a study where 130 articles recently published were randomized to social media expo-sure (blog post, Twitter ,and Facebook) or no exposure at 3 different time points after first online publication, social media exposure did not have a significant effect on tradi-tional impact metrics, such as downloads and citations.[38] It is likely that a solid group of followers are required to see an impact of social media on scientific research dissemination.

SUMMARY

The past decade has substantially changed the way information is retrieved and disseminated. In scientific information retrieval, there remain limitations, such as the presence of a paywall or differences in databases. Database and search interface pro-viders should agree on common standards in terminology and search semantics to make their professional tools as useful as they are intended to be.[39] The possibility to publish preprint article in social networking web site for scholars will decrease the lag time required from the acceptance of an article to its publication, which can be cumbersome in veterinary medicine. From a dissemination standpoint, the boom of social media provides an unprecedented opportunity to implement health promo-tion programs.[40] It is encouraging to think that health care is transitioning to a more open information access, but it is mandatory to educate veterinarians to make them able to critically appraise the information retrieved. Same as other for branches of medicine, veterinary medicine should develop and embark recommendations on the appropriate use of social media.[41] Oversimplification, resulting in a too strong a mes-sage or presenting data with a loss of context are risks of using social media in health care, and should be a concern for the veterinary community. However, by being aware of the limitations and the risks related to the abuse of current technologies, the future of knowledge dissemination is exciting.

REFERENCES

1. US National Library of Medicine. MEDLINE, PubMed, and PMC (PubMed Cen-tral): how are they different?. Available at: https://www.nlm.nih.gov/bsd/difference.html. Accessed November 1, 2018.
2. McKeever L, Nguyen V, Peterson SJ, et al. Demystifying the search button: a comprehensive PubMed search strategy for performing an exhaustive literature review. JPEN J Parenter Enteral Nutr 2015;39(6):622–35.

3. Katchamart W, Faulkner A, Feldman B, et al. PubMed had a higher sensitivity than Ovid-MEDLINE in the search for systematic reviews. J Clin Epidemiol 2011;64(7): 805–7.

4. Damarell RA, Tieman JJ. Searching PubMed for a broad subject area: how effective are palliative care clinicians in finding the evidence in their field? Health Info Libr J 2016;33(1):49–60.

5. US National Library of Medicine. PubMed tutorial: introduction to Boolean logic. Available at: https://www.nlm.nih.gov/bsd/disted/pubmedtutorial/020_380.html. Accessed November 1, 2018.

6. Curti S, Gori D, Di Gregori V, et al. PubMed search filters for the study of putative outdoor air pollution determinants of disease. BMJ Open 2016;6(12):e013092.

7. CABI. Online Information Resources: CAB Abstracts. Available at: https://www. cabi.org/publishing-products/online-information-resources/cab-abstracts/. Accessed November 1, 2018.

8. Murphy SA. Applying methodological search filters to CAB abstracts to identify research for evidence-based veterinary medicine. J Med Libr Assoc 2002; 90(4):406–10.

9. Haynes RB, Wilczynski N, McKibbon KA, et al. Developing optimal search strategies for detecting clinically sound studies in MEDLINE. J Med Inform Assoc 1994; 1(6):447–58.

10. Khabsa M, Giles CL. The number of scholarly documents on the public web. PLoS One 2014;9(5):e93949.

11. Google Scholar. How complete is your coverage?. Available at: https://scholar. google.com/intl/us/scholar/help.html#coverage. Accessed November 1, 2018.

12. Shultz M. Comparing test searches in PubMed and Google Scholar. J Med Libr Assoc 2007;95(4):442–5.

13. Vine R. Google scholar. J Med Libr Assoc 2006;94(1):97.

14. Bramer WM. Variation in number of hits for complex searches in Google Scholar. J Med Libr Assoc 2016;104(2):143–5.

15. Scopus content coverage guide. Available at: https://www.elsevier.com/__data/ assets/pdf_file/0007/69451/0597-Scopus-Content-Coverage-Guide-US-LETTER-v4-HI-singles-no-ticks.pdf. Accessed November 1, 2018.

16. Pew Research Center. Social media fact sheet. Available at: http://www. pewinternet.org/fact-sheet/social-media/. Accessed November 1, 2018.

17. Modahl M, Tompsett L, Moorhead T. Doctors, patients & social media. 2011. Available at: http://www.quantiamd.com/q-qcp/social_media.pdf. Accessed November 1, 2018.

18. Adilman R, Rajmohan Y, Brooks E, et al. Social media use among physicians and trainees: results of a national medical oncology physician survey. J Oncol Pract 2016;12(1):79–80, e52-60.

19. Tripathy JP, Bhatnagar A, Shewade HD, et al. Ten tips to improve the visibility and dissemination of research for policy makers and practitioners. Public Health Action 2017;7(1):10–4.

20. George N, Britto DR, Krishnan V, et al. Assessment of hashtag (#) campaigns aimed at health awareness in social media. J Educ Health Promot 2018;7:114.

21. Burgess JD, Kimble RM, Watt K, et al. The adoption of social media to recruit participants for the Cool Runnings randomized controlled trial in Australia. JMIR Res Protoc 2017;6(10):e200.

22. Rosenkrantz AB, Labib A, Pysarenko K, et al. What do patients tweet about their mammography experience? Acad Radiol 2016;23(11):1367–71.

23. Broughton DE, Schelble A, Cipolla K, et al. Social media in the REI clinic: what do patients want? J Assist Reprod Genet 2018;35(7):1259–63.
24. Alexa. The top 500 sites on the web. Available at: https://www.alexa.com/topsites. Accessed November 1, 2018.
25. Rapp AK, Healy MG, Charlton ME, et al. YouTube is the most frequently used educational video source for surgical preparation. J Surg Educ 2016;73(6):1072–6.
26. Frongia G, Mehrabi A, Fonouni H, et al. YouTube as a potential training resource for laparoscopic fundoplication. J Surg Educ 2016;73(6):1066–71.
27. Dyson MP, Newton AS, Shave K, et al. Social media for the dissemination of Cochrane child health evidence: evaluation study. J Med Internet Res 2017;19(9):e308.
28. Onezi HA, Khalifa M, El-Metwally A, et al. The impact of social media-based support groups on smoking relapse prevention in Saudi Arabia. Comput Methods Programs Biomed 2018;159:135–43.
29. Triemstra JD, Poeppelman RS, Arora VM. Correlations between hospitals' social media presence and reputation score and ranking: cross-sectional analysis. J Med Internet Res 2018;20(11):e289.
30. Hassanpour S, Tomita N, DeLise T, et al. Identifying substance use risk based on deep neural networks and Instagram social media data. Neuropsychopharmacology 2019;44(3):487–94.
31. Dunn PH, Woo BKP. Facebook recruitment of Chinese-speaking participants for hypertension education. J Am Soc Hypertens 2018;12(9):690–2.
32. Jacobs R, Boyd L, Brennan K, et al. The importance of social media for patients and families affected by congenital anomalies: a Facebook cross-sectional analysis and user survey. J Pediatr Surg 2016;51(11):1766–71.
33. Kim W, Vender R. Use of Facebook as a tool for knowledge dissemination in dermatology. J Cutan Med Surg 2014;18(5):341–4.
34. Boyle SC, Earle AM, LaBrie JW, et al. Facebook dethroned: revealing the more likely social media destinations for college students' depictions of underage drinking. Addict Behav 2017;65:63–7.
35. Van Noorden R. Online collaboration: scientists and the social network. Nature 2014;512(7513):126–9.
36. Jamali HR. Copyright compliance and infringement in ResearchGate full-text journal articles. Scientometrics 2017;112(1):241–54.
37. Baird SM, Marsh PA, Lawrentschuk N, et al. Analysis of social media use among Australian and New Zealand otolaryngologists. ANZ J Surg 2018;89(6):733–7.
38. Tonia T, Van Oyen H, Berger A, et al. If I tweet will you cite? The effect of social media exposure of articles on downloads and citations. Int J Public Health 2016;61(4):513–20.
39. Boeker M, Vach W, Motschall E. Semantically equivalent PubMed and Ovid-MEDLINE queries: different retrieval results because of database subset inclusion. J Clin Epidemiol 2012;65(8):915–6.
40. An R, Ji M, Zhang S. Effectiveness of social media-based interventions on weight-related behaviors and body weight status: review and meta-analysis. Am J Health Behav 2017;41(6):670–82.
41. Borgmann H, Cooperberg M, Murphy D, et al. Online professionalism-2018 update of European Association of Urology (@Uroweb) recommendations on the appropriate use of social media. Eur Urol 2018;74(5):644–50.

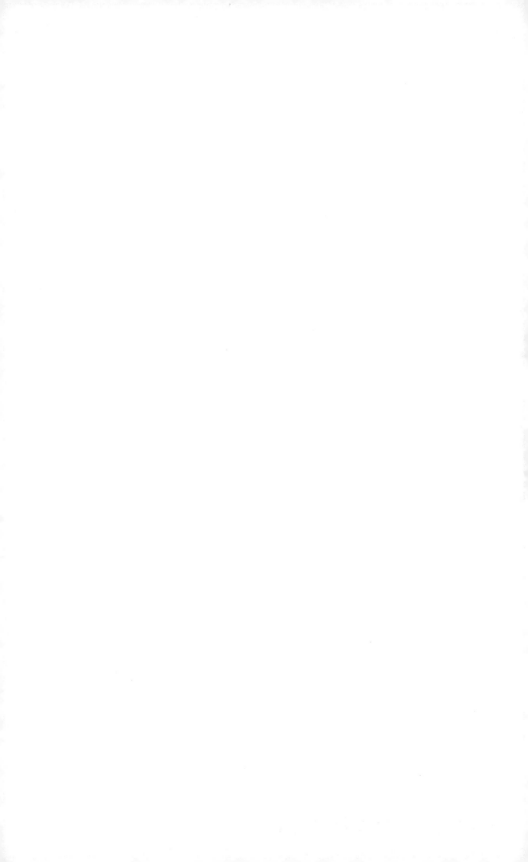

Printed and bound by CPI Group (UK) Ltd, Croydon, CR0 4YY

03/10/2024

01040407-0004